BACK
TO
HEALTH

A
Comprehensive
Medical and Nutritional

Yeast Control
Program

BACK TO HEALTH

A
Comprehensive
Medical and Nutritional

Yeast Control
Program

Dennis W. Remington, M.D.
Barbara W. Higa, R.D.

Illustrated by
LaRene Gaunt

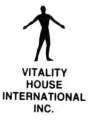

VITALITY
HOUSE
INTERNATIONAL
INC.

Copyright© 1986, 1989 by
Vitality House International, Inc.
1675 North Freedom Boulevard, #11-C
Provo, Utah 84604-2570

Telephone: 801-373-5100
To Order: Call Toll-Free 1-800-748-5100

First Printing, October 1986

Second Printing, October 1987

Third Printing, May 1989

Fourth Printing, June 1991

Fifth Printing, February 1994

This collection of recipes has been gathered and adapted from a variety of sources. All recipes have been adapted to meet the yeast-free criteria.

Library of Congress Catalog Card Number: 86-50490

ISBN 0-912547-03-0

Printed by Publishers Press
Salt Lake City, Utah

Table of Contents

Chapters

Appendices

List of Diagrams

List of Tables

Acknowledgements

We would like to acknowledge C. Orian Truss for his pioneering work and observations in candidiasis. His contributions to relieving the suffering of mankind, by making people aware of Candida, will long be appreciated.

We also thank those chronically ill patients who insisted upon pursuing treatment during our initial exploratory stages with Candida. We learned much from listening and are grateful to them.

We also appreciate the efforts of Margaret Wagner and Dr. Remington's staff who helped prepare and evaluate many of the recipes listed in Appendix 6.

Thanks to Mitch Stowell for creating the title of this book and his many hours of computer time -- both in teaching and in word processing.

Many thanks to Kathy Frandsen for her careful editing of the materials presented herein.

About the Authors

Dennis W. Remington, M.D., is a family physician in private practice with a special interest in preventive medicine and nutrition, exercise, and food and chemical allergies. He has developed several innovative concepts in weight management. He previously served as director of the Eating Disorder Clinic at Brigham Young University's Student Health Center in Provo, Utah. He is a member of the American Society of Bariatric Physicians and the American Academy of Environmental Medicine. He was the founding president of the Society for the Study of Biochemical Intolerance. He is a coauthor of *How to Lower Your Fat Thermostat, The Bitter Truth About Artificial Sweeteners*, and the audio-tape program, *The Neuropsychology of Weight Control.*

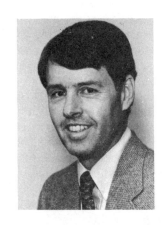

Barbara W. Higa, Registered Dietitian, works in a medical practice with patients suffering from food and chemical allergies, obesity, and yeast problems. A graduate of Brigham Young University, she completed her dietetic internship at the Veterans Administration Hospital in Los Angeles, and taught quantity food production at Brigham Young University. She has instructed physicians from the United States, Canada, and Australia on new allergy treatment and yeast treatment techniques. She is a popular guest lecturer, and specializes in developing delicious recipes for healthy eating. She is the mother of four children. She is a coauthor of *The Bitter Truth About Artificial Sweeteners* and the audio-tape program, *The New Neuropsychology of Weight Control.* She is author of *Desserts to Lower Your Fat Thermostat.*

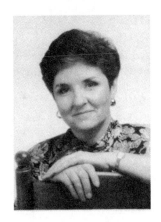

Introduction: Back to Health

If has been estimated that one in every three people, suffer from chronic problems caused by an overgrowth of yeast *(Candida albicans)*. And if you are like most victims of chronic yeast problems, you have been troubled by a variety of symptoms--ranging from mild to totally debilitating--that have had you completely baffled. Chances are, you didn't even know what caused your suffering.

Even if you knew your problems were related to yeast overgrowth, you probably couldn't find any easy-to-understand, practical information about your problem and how you could successfully treat it.

That's where this book comes in. We wrote *Back to Health* for you to use under your doctor's care and supervision--and we wrote it because many other people have the same questions and need the same instructions as our patients over the last few years have needed. Although *Back to Health* is a self-help guide that you can use on your own, we encourage you to seek medical help. If you are troubled by lingering health problems after your prolonged efforts to treat a yeast problem, please consult with your physician.

HOW TO USE BACK TO HEALTH

In the first 11 chapters you will find a brief description of the yeast problem, an outline of the common symptoms it causes, help in diagnosing the problem, instructions for taking medication, dietary guideline, and follow-up advice. If you still have questions after reading these chapters, make sure to carefully read Chapter 12, a trouble-shooting guide that answers the most common questions about yeast infection. You'll notice that the chapters are peppered with case studies, which illustrate the principles we discuss in each chapter. You can skip over them if you wish to save time.

You will find a host of helpful suggestions in the appendices, which contain recipes (Appendix 7) and menu suggestions (see Appendix 6) that will make it easier for you to follow the dietary guidelines. You will also find specific information on the way yeast relates to other problems, such as weight control, allergies, hypoglycemia, and premenstrual syndrome.

There's also a comprehensive doctor's section (see Appendix 8); if you think that you might have a yeast problem, we encourage you to show this section to your physician. He or she may not be completely convinced that yeast is responsible for your problems, but we hope your physician will be convinced that the treatment is safe, and will be willing to prescribe the necessary medication for a trial of therapy.

Remember that any new medical concept is bound to be surrounded by controversy at first; healthy skepticism is good and we invite any physicians who are interested to test these principles out. In the meantime, don't let a little controversy keep you from trying a safe treatment plan that can dramatically improve the quality of your life!

This is the fourth edition of *Back to Health*. We strive to keep it up-to-date and make helpful additions as we find further information. If you use any products that are especially helpful or have any suggestions, please write us in care of the publisher. Read this book, try out the treatment suggested, and follow the guidelines--and we wish you success in getting back to health!

An Important Notice

The book was written to serve as a source of information and to act as a reference to both the professional and the non-professional who are seeking help in dealing with the many debilitating problems associated with an overgrowth of yeast or Candida albicans. The information in this book is meant to complement the advice of your physician, not replace it. You will experience the best results consulting your physician and should carefully follow his or her advice regarding medication usage and other aspects of the treatment of yeast-related illnesses. Accordingly, either you or the professional who examines and treats you must take responsibility for any use made of the information in this volume.

Dennis W. Remington, M.D.
May 1, 1989

Chapter One

YEAST—THE VILLAIN

Yeast. Sounds innocent, doesn't it?

In proper proportions, it might be. After all, there is a type of yeast that lives within all of us. We're unsure of its exact function, but it doesn't seem to be a problem when it's under control.

But let it get out of control, and watch out! It can cause problems literally from the top of your head (headaches) to the tips of your toes (cramps in the bottom of your feet). It can manifest its symptoms inside (pain and malfunction in your organs) and out (eczema and hives). And it doesn't stop with your body—yeast can also work its cruel havoc on your mind and your emotions.

Do you find it difficult to believe that one little organism can cause so much grief? Over twenty years ago, Orian Truss, M.D., a pioneer researcher, began to notice the clearing of a number of seemingly unrelated problems in patients he was treating for other fungal ailments. Through his innovative research, he has proven that yeast can cause a multitude of problems. To understand more about yeast and its impact on your body, it's important that you understand the basic way that microscopic organisms behave.

It's really a matter of competition: each of us has millions of microscopic organisms living on our skin, in our intestinal system, and in other parts of our bodies. Normally, they establish a balanced relationship with each other and with their host—you—by "competing" for their space. In other words, they produce chemical substances that are toxic to other organisms to protect their own interests.

One of the best-known examples of this kind of competition is penicillin. Sir Alexander Fleming, who discovered penicillin, noticed that a fungus he accidentally got on a culture plate killed the surrounding bacteria. His reasoning? The fungus must have been producing a chemical that was lethal to bacteria. He worked to refine the fungus, and the antibiotic penicillin was developed. Penicillin became a potent antibiotic because the fungus manufactured a toxin—penicillin—that could kill surrounding bacteria that were threatening to get all the food!

That kind of competition goes on throughout your body constantly. In your intestinal tract, however, it isn't mere competition—it's perpetual chemical warfare. Many factors influence the outcome, one of the most important being your own immune system. You produce antibodies that, in some cases, completely destroy the microscopic organisms. In other cases, though, the organisms stubbornly resist, and are able to survive despite your immune system.

It doesn't end there. The organisms can in some cases produce chemical substances that interfere with your ability to destroy them—the same kind of competition they wage with surrounding organisms. If your immune system becomes ineffective and you are no longer able to destroy these organisms, they will overrun you.

That's where yeast comes in. There are about 900 species of yeast, and a number of them can inhabit your body. The major yeast in humans is Candida albicans. In some ways it is similar to the yeast used to make bread. An oval-shaped organism that multiplies rapidly by budding, it sends out small hair-like structures called mycelia.

We're not sure why yeast are present in our bodies or what function they serve. The only thing we are sure of is that they help decompose and recycle our bodies when we die. We don't want them to start doing their jobs prematurely, but if yeast multiply too rapidly and start to take over, that's exactly what it can feel like.

It doesn't have to happen. We have already treated more than one thousand patients that we've suspected of having yeast problems. We are convinced that Candida albicans is a major cause of health problems in our society, and we have seen a number of chronic conditions improve dramatically with treatment.

To help you understand the yeast problem, we will outline common symptoms that seem to be caused by yeast, explain what happens with each, and outline a treatment program that we have found to be extremely successful. We will limit ourselves to the most common symptoms that are the most successfully treated. Throughout the chapters that follow, we use the terms "yeast problem" and "candidiasis" (infection by fungi of the Candida family) interchangeably; both refer to the condition of disease-causing overgrowth of Candida albicans.

Remember that these explanations are theories only; it may take years to prove them conclusively through scientific testing. The important part is not to determine whether the theories are correct, but to determine instead whether the outlined treatment will solve the problems you have!

Chapter Two

WHAT YEAST DOES TO YOUR BODY AND MIND

Where there is war, there are casualties—and your body is no exception!

The war being waged inside your body due to yeast overgrowth boasts its own casualties: you develop a variety of troublesome symptoms that can crop up just about anywhere in your body. That's one of the worst parts of candidiasis—symptoms can be so varied and so scattered that they don't even seem related to the same condition. The result? It's easy to miss candidiasis.

The rundown of potential symptoms and health problems resulting from candidiasis reads almost like a catalog of the human body. To understand how such a broad spectrum of symptoms can result from yeast overgrowth, it's important to understand *how* candidiasis produces its symptoms.

How Yeast Causes Symptoms

Candidiasis, or yeast overgrowth, can cause symptoms in any of the following ways:

Local Yeast Infections. Candida organisms can invade various body tissues, resulting in local infections. The most common sites include the mouth (thrush), gastrointestinal tract, vagina, urinary tract, prostate gland, skin, and fingernails or toenails.

Changes in the Immune System. Remember—yeast is waging a war for its very survival inside the body. Under normal conditions, your immune system would destroy the yeast. But in a situation of yeast overgrowth, the yeast produce their own toxins—or poisons—that cripple the immune system and prevent it from doing its job. Your immune system can no longer destroy the yeast, but there's more: your immune system may eventually become so crippled that it can no longer fight off other kinds of infections, such as viral and bacterial infections. This makes you prone to repeated urinary or respiratory infections.

Your immune system may also become altered in such a way that you become sensitive to—commonly called "allergic to"—various chemical odors or foods. Why? Your immune system may be reacting as part of its attempt to fight off yeast. We're not sure exactly how it happens. One theory is that yeast invades and damages the intestinal wall, which normally acts as a filtering system to keep food particles and chemicals from entering your body. With an impaired intestinal lining, large food particles, toxins from microorganisms and other substances may pass through and enter the bloodstream. The body may then treat these particles and chemicals like foreign invaders—and it may produce antibodies in defense.

The result?

Your body responds with typical allergic reactions, such as eczema and hay fever, or it responds with reactions such as headache, dizziness, heart palpitations, anxiety, fatigue, muscle aches, or a number of other symptoms.

That's not all. At first, you may only react to the yeast in your body. As your immune system battles for control, however, you may begin reacting to related yeasts (such as yeast in bread or brewer's yeast) and fungus in foods—such as those in bread and hard cheese—and fungal spores in the air—such as mildew and molds. Any exposure to these causes unpleasant symptoms, and repeated exposure can lead to chronic health problems.

At first, you'll react to only a few foods, chemicals, and odors. Gradually, you may develop a larger number of symptoms, your symptoms may become worse, and eventually you may begin reacting to a wider variety of foods and chemicals such as gasoline fumes, perfumes, or cleaners.

John had been healthy all of his life, but at age forty-five he began to be troubled by intestinal cramping and bloating, deep depression, and extreme nervous tension. He noticed that his stomach would swell immediately after eating such foods as ice cream. His pain became unbearable, so he consulted his family doctor. He was treated with a broad-spectrum antibiotic for an unrelated infection and his symptoms were suddenly aggravated and caused chronic heart fibrillation. John got so sick that he was forced to quit his job as an electronics technician. He went to a series of doctors with the same list of symptoms and was told the following: 1. The only way you can get gas into your digestive tract is to swallow it, so stop swallowing air. Then the doctor ordered $1,500 of laboratory tests, many of which were very uncomfortable. 2. You have a problem with your gall bladder and it needs to be removed. 3. You have nothing physically wrong with you, so you need to see a psychiatrist. The psychiatrist diagnosed depression and prescribed Elavil. 4. You have a spot on your lung. 5. The chiropractor said it was a pinched nerve and prescribed a number of treatments.

All of the above treatments and diagnoses left John feeling confused, angry, and more sick than ever. When he came to our office he was in such an anxious state that he wasn't sleeping, he was hallucinating, and felt he was going to die. We started him on the yeast control program described in this book. During his first week on the program, all of John's symptoms worsened; by the end of the second week, however, he was at least fifty-percent improved, and his heart fibrillations had completely stopped. After only six weeks on the program, he felt he was eighty-percent improved, he was working half days again, and continuing to enjoy gradual improvement of his other symptoms.

Chemicals Produced by Yeast. As long as yeast has something to feed itself with (like sugar), it reproduces rapidly. As yeast reproduces and grows, it releases a number of chemicals in the process. Two that are particularly devastating are called acetaldehyde and ethanol—and both act as poisons on the various tissues of the body. Most people are aware of the problems that ethanol (a type of alcohol) can cause in those that drink too much of it. Most people are also aware that it is the yeast that converts the various sugar sources into ethanol to make alcoholic beverages. The yeast in your body acts in a similar way ingesting the sugars in the food you eat and produces ethanol as a by-product. Acetaldehyde is then produced as the ethanol is broken down and is about six times more toxic to brain tissue than ethanol. Dr. Orian Truss suspects that these chemicals could be responsible for many of the symptoms associated with yeast overgrowth because they cause the following defects:

1. **Cell membrane defects.** Under normal conditions, red blood cells carry oxygen throughout the body; red blood cells must be flexible enough to squeeze down to about one-seventh their normal size in order to travel into the body's tiny capillaries. The chemicals released by yeast cause the red blood cell walls to become more rigid. As a result, they have difficulty squeezing into the tiny capillaries—and the transport of life-giving oxygen to all the tissues and organs of the body is impaired. Deprived of sufficient oxygen, these tissues and organs lose their ability to function.

Red blood cells aren't the only ones affected. Yeast toxins damage white blood cells, too, compromising their ability to fight off infection. Normally, a white blood cell fights infection by wrapping part of itself around a bacteria or other foreign invader, swallowing the invader, and eventually destroying it. A white blood cell that has been made brittle and rigid by yeast toxins simply can't do the job. The result? You can't fight off infection as easily.

There's more. Defective cell membranes may interfere with the ability of sugar to penetrate the various cells, a job normally accomplished with the help of insulin. When cell membranes are damaged, the insulin will have trouble doing its job—and insulin levels may have to be increased. As you'll see later, this may result in low blood sugar and cause you to gain weight!

Thyroid hormones also have trouble penetrating the cell membranes. Since thyroid hormones regulate metabolism, the result is slow metabolism, low body temperature, fatigue, and intolerance to cold. Unfortunately, laboratory tests can't diagnose this kind of a problem, because they read the level of thyroid hormones in the bloodstream—they don't read the ability of the thyroid hormones to function within the cell.

Sodium, potassium, calcium, and other minerals also have trouble penetrating the cell walls. The result can be fluid retention, electrolyte imbalance, and a number of other problems.

Messages that one cell sends to another can also be hindered by yeast toxins. How? Normally, one cell sends a message to another cell by releasing a special chemical; the second cell (in a nerve or muscle) absorbs the chemical and picks up the message. When damaged by yeast toxins, the cells can't send or pick up messages properly—and a number of muscle and nervous system symptoms can result.

2. **Enzyme destruction.** Enzymes are the chemical helpers in your body that help build, help break down, and help produce energy and heat. Yeast toxins can inactivate or destroy some of your enzymes—and can, as a result, slow down all the functions of your body. Enzymes, for example, help break

down sugar stores to keep your blood sugar at ideal levels; when yeast over-growth destroys enzymes, you may develop abnormally high or low blood sugar levels.

3. **Abnormal hormone response.** Hormones regulate your various body functions by traveling through the bloodstream to vital areas of the body. Yeast toxins interfere with that process: the hormones are produced, and they enter the bloodstream, but they have trouble getting to their intended destination. Even though you have plenty of hormones in your bloodstream, they can't do the intended job if they don't achieve adequate levels at the intended site!

Symptoms Caused by Candida Albicans

A wide variety of symptoms can be caused by Candida albicans. Not all of them occur at once in all people; you may have only a few, or only one. The following are common candidiasis symptoms:

Allergic Reactions. Allergic reactions—defined by Webster's as "a condition of unusual sensitivity to a substance or substances which, in like amounts, do not affect others"—are very common with candidiasis. Antibodies may be present, causing the immune system to flare up, but in many cases antibodies are not involved. Allergy symptoms may include asthma, congested nose, and hives, but symptoms may also include problems like headaches, dizziness, diarrhea, weakness, cramps, arthritis, irritability, and depression.

In some cases, the allergy is easy to identify: you react soon after exposure to the substance, you react every time you are exposed to the substance, you react after exposure to even a tiny amount of the substance, and your reactions follow a specific and predictable pattern.

It's not always that easy, though. Sometimes the reaction may be delayed for several hours after exposure to the substance. Or you may not react every time you are exposed. Or the reaction may be cumulative: you may react only after many exposures or after exposure to a massive amount of the substance. Many of the symptoms that result from candidiasis may actually be hidden allergic reactions to various substances—and that's not always easy to determine.

Effective yeast management can improve your tolerance to those substances. In other words, the allergy still exists, but it takes a greater exposure to cause a reaction. If you develop migraine headaches after getting a whiff of cigarette smoke, for example, after a few months of treatment you may be able to sit in a smoke-filled room for thirty minutes before getting a headache. See Appendix 2 on allergies for more information.

Sally was in her mid-twenties. She had suffered since she was a young girl with many respiratory infections, and she had taken many antibiotics for them. In addition to fatigue, nausea, abdominal pains, and diarrhea, Sally had begun to have unpleasant reactions to some of her food. At first, she only had mild stomach upset with wheat, but soon began to react to several types of fruit, and suspected a number of other foods. Her symptoms became increasingly worse. Besides severe abdominal cramps, she began having headaches, muscle aches, and fatigue after eating problem foods. In fact, she began having problems after almost every meal, and began to believe that she was allergic to every food.

With effective yeast treatment, she began to notice that her reactions from eating were becoming less severe. After a number of weeks, she could eat several of her problem foods with no reaction at all. After four months of therapy, all her major symptoms were gone, and she was no longer aware of any adverse reactions from foods.

She discontinued therapy, and seemed fine for a number of months. She began introducing sugars back into her diet over Thanksgiving weekend, and between then and Christmas attended a number of social functions at which she ate a variety of goodies. By Christmas, she was beginning to have fatigue, headaches, muscle aches, and intestinal disturbances again. Shortly after Christmas, she again began noticing mild reactions to various foods. She continued to use sugars, and, in fact, couldn't leave them alone. By early spring, her symptoms were almost as bad as before she started the yeast program, and she returned to the office to resume yeast treatment. Several months of therapy cleared her of her symptoms, and she no longer reacted to foods. When we last saw her, she was feeling very well and was determined to be careful with her diet after this painful lesson.

Gastrointestinal System. When you eat—especially foods high in the sugars that feed yeast—the yeast produces a lot of carbon dioxide. The result? You suffer from gas and bloating. (While good yeast management often clears up gas and bloating, remember that other factors—such as other gas-producing microscopic organisms, swallowed air, milk intolerance, and food allergies— can also cause gas and bloating.)

Direct invasion of the intestinal lining by yeast can cause abdominal pain, gastritis, gastric ulcer, and ulcer-type symptoms; Candida albicans has been found in gastric ulcer craters. Yeast may also indirectly cause ulcers by causing an increase in the amount of stress hormones or prostaglandins the body secretes. Prostaglandins—hormone-like chemicals produced by the body—protect the lining of the gastrointestinal tract by reducing inflammation; when yeast interferes with the production of these prostaglandins, the body's natural protection is lost.

Yeast can also cause increased pressure in the stomach, causing the valve between the stomach and the esophagus to open. The result? Heartburn—a burning pain that results when stomach acids and digestive juices flood the esophagus, corroding or irritating its lining.

Common with yeast overgrowth is diarrhea (often accompanied by cramping pain due to yeast's direct invasion of the intestinal tract), constipation (due to destruction of friendly bacteria in the intestines), or a pattern of alternating diarrhea and constipation. Both diarrhea and constipation may be related to allergic reactions and prostaglandins, both of which are in turn related to yeast overgrowth. Intestinal cramping—often called "spastic colon" or "nervous bowel"—usually responds well to effective yeast management.

Sharon developed a number of problems during her first pregnancy. She was troubled by heartburn, nausea, and constipation. A urinary tract infection toward the end of her pregnancy required several courses of antibiotics to clear. Sharon then developed a vaginal infection, diarrhea, abdominal cramping, gas, and bloating. After the pregnancy and a bout with post-partum depression, she gradually regained her strength and began to feel better. But episodes of abdominal cramps along with alternating constipation and diarrhea continued, and at times became severe. Over the next ten years, she visited a number of doctors for diagnosis; several X-rays and sigmoidoscopies were all normal. She was diagnosed as having a spastic colon.

A high-fiber diet, various types of antispasm medications to control cramping, and tranquilizers to control her anxiety (thought to be the major source of her bowel problems) gave her temporary relief. After developing yet another vaginal yeast infection and worsening of her spastic colon after a course of antibiotics for a urinary tract infection, she heard about yeast problems and came to our office for treatment.

Within three days of starting yeast treatment, she noticed a decrease in the cramping; by the end of the first week, the diarrhea had stopped. By the end of the second week, the gas and bloating were mostly gone, and tight-fitting clothes around her waist no longer caused her discomfort. After two months of treatment, the only symptom left from the previous ten years was the occasional gas after certain foods.

Remember: yeast overgrowth can cause gastrointestinal symptoms, such as heartburn, gas, and diarrhea, but it is not the only potential cause. Other microorganisms (including Amoeba and Giardia), parasites, diet, excessive stress, and other factors can also cause gastrointestinal symptoms. Symptoms that do not respond to yeast treatment should be further investigated.

Respiratory System. Sore throat and sore mouth are commonly caused by direct invasion of yeast; when yeast is present in large numbers, you can see white patches on the throat and inside of the mouth. Yeast also indirectly causes chronic or repeated canker sores.

Yeast can contribute to sinus infections, bronchial infections, and pneumonia. Infections of the nose (characterized by thick green or yellow secretions or crusting), chronic cough, and asthma are also common with candidiasis.

Anna first developed asthma in her pre-teen years after a very bad cough that was cleared only after several courses of antibiotics. The asthma became worse with each respiratory infection, which seemed to happen frequently. The problem was year-round, and allergy testing showed no reaction to the usual pollens, weeds, trees, and other inhalants. Anna's asthma also became worse with pregnancies.

When we saw thirty-two-year-old Anna in our office for the first time, she had been taking several doses of asthma medication daily for close to twenty years. She even needed cortisone at times to keep the asthma under control. She had a number of other symptoms typical of yeast overgrowth, and was started on a trial of yeast treatment.

She was slightly better at the end of one week, at which time she was given the Candida antigen. Within a few hours of starting this antigen, she noticed a clearing of her lungs, and by the second day she was able to reduce the dosage on her medication. One week after starting the antigen, she was no longer taking any medication, and had no asthma symptoms at all. Two months after starting treatment, she had a mild flare-up of asthma along with a mild cold, but neither the infection nor the asthma required any treatment with medication—a first for her. One year later, she became pregnant, which usually triggered asthma, but even that did not cause problems for her.

She also reported a clearing of her chronic stuffy nose, and noted a marked improvement in her energy. In the two years since starting treatment, she has only had two or three minor asthma flare-ups with low-grade infections and heavy dust exposure, none of which required medication.

Cardiovascular System. Palpitations, rapid pulse rate, and pounding of the heart are common with candidiasis—but it's not because yeast directly infects the heart, blood vessels, or lymphatic system. What happens, then? Yeast can interfere with the balance of hormones that regulate the cardiovascular system—especially the stress hormones, which can cause palpitations and rapid pulse. Allergic reactions to the yeast itself or to various foods and chemicals can also result in cardiovascular symptoms.

Imbalances caused by yeast can also cause fluid retention and cold, clammy hands and feet because of reduced blood flow and increased perspiration.

Kathy came into the office for help with her severe depression, anxiety, headaches, and fatigue. These symptoms had come on gradually over the twelve years of her marriage, and seemed to get worse after each of her five pregnancies. In addition, she reported frequent episodes of pounding, rapid heartbeat, and constant cold, clammy hands and feet.

Several weeks of yeast treatment made substantial improvement in most of her symptoms. The episodes of rapid pulse and pounding heart stopped completely. After two months of treatment, her husband noticed that her hands and feet had become warm. That was no small accomplishment; in the fifteen years of their acquaintance, he never remembered a time when her hands and feet had felt warm, even in the summer.

Genitourinary System. One of the most common manifestations of yeast is the vaginal "yeast infection." It is characterized by discharge, itching, swelling, tenderness, and pain; many women suffer from chronic and disabling vaginal yeast infections. While unpleasant vaginal symptoms are caused by direct yeast invasion, they may also be the result of an allergic reaction to the yeast causing itching and burning.

Yeast can also directly infect the lining of the urinary bladder, causing urinary burning, frequent urination, lack of bladder control, and bedwetting. Men can develop itchy rashes on the mucous membranes of the penis and chronic prostate problems as a result of yeast infection.

Imbalanced prostaglandins and hormones, common in candidiasis, can cause menstrual cramps and may cause or aggravate premenstrual syndrome (PMS), characterized by a wide variety of troublesome symptoms during the two weeks prior to menstruation. (See Appendix 5 for a more detailed discussion of yeast's impact on PMS.)

Gail, now in her late thirties, had suffered from severe menstrual cramps since her mid-teen years. She was essentially incapacitated for one day a month by this problem, and quite uncomfortable for another two days. In addition, she noticed about eight to ten days of irritability, swelling, bloating, sugar cravings, and headaches just before the onset of her period. After one month of yeast treatment, the pains were mostly gone, and by the end of three months of treatment, she no longer had any discomfort with her periods. The swelling and bloating before the period were reduced, and the irritability and headaches were not as severe. Additional nutritional supplements over the next six months further improved Gail's premenstrual symptoms, although she still had a few mild problems.

Musculoskeletal System. Muscle weakness, night leg pains, muscle stiffness, and deep muscle pains—especially in the shoulder and neck muscles—are extremely common in candidiasis. Cell membrane defects often prevent nutrients from getting into the muscle tissues and waste products from getting out, which could contribute to muscle weakness and soreness. Good yeast management often helps, especially when combined with calcium, magnesium, and potassium supplements.

Some muscular problems—such as slow reaction time, poor coordination, poor motor skills, falling, and the tendency to drop things—can be indirectly caused by yeast because of impairment in the way nerves and muscles send messages and because of changes in blood sugar levels.

While arthritis is sometimes the result of an allergic reaction to yeast (the antibodies attack not only the yeast, but the joint tissues as well), it is not the only factor. Although some cases of arthritis respond well to yeast management measures, other cases do not.

Eric had many typical yeast symptoms, including tension headaches, pains in his knees (thought to be caused by his overweight condition), and a constant pain in his right shoulder, severe enough at times to be incapacitating. This shoulder pain had been constant for twenty-five years, and he had seen many doctors. A number of X-rays had been taken, and various explanations had been given for its cause. Medications and injections only gave partial and temporary relief.

Within three days of starting yeast treatment, Eric's shoulder pain disappeared completely. It did come back about three weeks later for a few days when he indulged in some sweets, but has not returned in the year that we have followed his progress. The muscle tightness in his neck and shoulders, along with the headaches, also went away, although they have come back a few times when he has been under excessive stress. Even the pains in his knees have mostly disappeared, and he is now able to exercise comfortably.

Skin. Direct yeast invasion commonly causes skin infection, usually in moist areas, such as under the breasts and in the groin. Yeast is a common cause of diaper rash. Hives and eczema can also be an allergic reaction to yeast (as well as a result of allergies to other substances).

Harold had suffered from severe eczema on his trunk, upper legs, arms, and face for most of his thirty-seven years. Even the areas not actively involved with the rash were thick and hard. Cortisone creams had helped a little, but the extensive areas of skin involved made creams rather expensive. He was aware of a few foods that seemed to make the eczema worse, and food allergy treatment caused partial clearing. A yeast management program also helped. Within a few days of starting the Candida antigen, his rash was markedly improved, and by the end of one week, his skin had become soft and supple. He remained entirely rash-free for several months, until he went out of town for Thanksgiving. During the holiday he was exposed to various chemical substances to which he was sensitive, and abandoned his yeast control diet. The rash returned at that time, but cleared again with continued treatment.

Central Nervous System. One of the most common symptoms of yeast overgrowth is headache—candidiasis can cause sinus headaches (resulting from blockage of the sinuses), muscular contraction headaches (resulting from deep muscle pain in the shoulders or neck), and migraine headaches (resulting from spasms in the arteries of the scalp). Migraine headaches can also be the result of allergic response. Still other yeast-related headaches can result from low blood sugar, rapid changes in the blood sugar levels, low body temperature, and the poisons secreted by the yeast.

High levels of stress hormones resulting from yeast overgrowth can cause anxiety, irritability, restlessness, panic attacks, sudden anger, and sleep disturbances. (Imbalances of hormones in the brain, which can also cause these symptoms, may also be the result of poor nutrition, genetics, and impaired thought processes.) When excessive amounts of stress hormones start coursing through the bloodstream, minor stresses that would normally cause no symptoms will cause severe illness.

Yeast can also cause problems with general brain function, causing poor short-term memory, inability to concentrate, fuzzy thinking, and confusion.

Beth's health had deteriorated since her late teens, when she had a number of infections treated by antibiotics. She had four pregnancies during her twenties, all of which seemed to cause further deterioration in her condition. By the time she was in her early thirties, she suffered from a wide range of digestive problems, aches and pains, and fatigue. Her worst problems, however, related to brain function. She had become increasingly forgetful, found it hard to concentrate, and suffered from bouts of depression, anxiety, and sleep disturbance. Her coordination seemed to be bad at times, and she began dropping things and running into doorways. She had trouble focusing her eyes, and suffered from dizziness. A sister with similar problems who had been helped with yeast treatment tried to convince her to come to our office. She finally decided to seek help when she hit a parked car—three times—while trying to get out of a parking space. (We were relieved that someone else had driven her into our parking lot!)

Within days of starting treatment, her intestinal problems began to improve. At the end of two weeks, she felt a little more clear-headed and was not as dizzy. She began to feel like her old self again within two months, and her symptoms kept improving. After four months of treatment, she felt better than she had since she was a teen-ager! Her confidence was back, she was coping well with her family, the depression was gone, and her coordination had returned to normal. Other than a slight fatigue, she felt completely well.

Fatigue. Fatigue is extremely common in candidiasis. There could be a number of reasons: impaired metabolism doesn't enable the body to get enough fuel, and impaired enzymes don't produce energy. Fatigue can also be the result of lack of motivation or lack of interest that accompanies depression.

Weight Gain. Weight gain is an extremely common symptom of candidiasis; many people find that sudden weight gain corresponded to the time when yeast overgrowth first occurred. Many of the problems associated with yeast—such as cravings for sugar, interference with normal hunger, high insulin levels, low metabolism, and factors that interfere with activity (such as fatigue and muscle pain)—all play a role in weight gain. Effective yeast management generally results in weight loss (for those who are overweight) without direct attempts at "dieting." (For more detailed information on the impact of yeast on weight gain, see Appendix 4.)

Helen first started to gain weight with her second pregnancy, and continued to gain following her pregnancy. She also had recurring yeast vaginitis. She was very tired and weak as well, even after the pregnancy. Dieting made the fatigue much worse, and although she initially lost fifteen pounds, she gained twenty-five pounds a few months later. She tried a strict powdered protein diet a year later, and this time she got the flu, which turned into bronchitis. She was more tired than ever, and after the illness (which did not respond very well to either of the antibiotics she used), she began having headaches, indigestion, fluid retention, and joint aches. She became depressed, and could no longer stay with the powdered protein diet. She quickly gained back the twenty pounds that she had lost, along with an additional twelve pounds. An antidepressant helped her depression, but seemed to make the weight go up even higher. Repeated diets only made her depression worse—she could no longer face life without her cola drink, and her weight kept increasing. She finally gave up on her weight, and in spite of eating very little, seemed to stay about ninety pounds overweight.

When she came to our office, Helen was more concerned with her many other problems than her weight; she just wanted to feel well again. She started a yeast control program, and after two weeks had lost nine pounds. When we questioned her, she assured us that she was eating about the same amount of food, but was skipping breakfast. We encouraged to her eat breakfast, and even to add a snack in the middle of the afternoon when she had a period of daily fatigue. In spite of eating more food, she lost an additional seven pounds over the next two weeks. The puffiness around her face was gone, and she described gaining only a few pounds—instead of her usual six to eight pounds— before her last period.

By the end of one month of treatment, Helen's joint pains and muscle stiffness were gone, and she could comfortably walk for thirty minutes. Her energy was greatly improved, her depression had lifted, and she had become interested in again pursuing some of her old hobbies. In spite of eating what she considered to be a huge amount of food (compared to her previous semi-starvation regime), she continued to lose weight. By the end of the second month, she was walking forty-five minutes a day and had lost a total of twenty-two pounds. By the end of one year, Helen was almost eighty pounds lower than her beginning weight. Her weight stabilized there, and she continued to feel well, even though she had stopped the anti-yeast medication some eight months earlier.

(**Note:** More information about the mechanism for causing yeast-related symptoms is found in Appendix 8, designed for physicians and others trained in health related fields.)

Chapter Three
WHAT MAKES YEAST GROW

If yeast is normally present in controlled numbers in your body, what happens to make it multiply out of control? A number of factors make yeast grow too rapidly. Knowing what those factors are helps us in diagnosing a yeast problem and in designing effective treatment.

Poor Nutrition. One of the major contributors to yeast overgrowth is poor nutrition—and one of the major culprits is sugar.

Have you ever made bread? Have you ever observed what happens when you mixed the yeast and sugar in warm water? The yeast bubbled wildly, almost exploding out of the container. Why? Yeast—both baker's yeast and Candida albicans—thrives on sugar! Yeast metabolizes sugar very quickly, producing ethanol (alcohol), acetaldehyde (another form of alcohol), and carbon dioxide gas in the process. (The natural sugars found in fruits and vegetables do not seem to cause as rapid a reaction.)

The problem? The average person in the western world consumes about 125 pounds of refined table sugar (sucrose) every year! That would be bad enough from a yeast standpoint. But there's more: when you eat too high a percentage of highly refined foods, including sugar, you are deprived of vitamins, minerals, and other essential nutrients. It's a vicious cycle: these nutrients are essential to a healthy immune system, which is crucial to keeping yeast under control.

The same thing happens to people who are on calorie restricted diets: when they aren't consuming enough food, they usually aren't getting adequate nutrition. We've noticed that patients who are on strict, calorie-controlled diets are susceptible to many more colds, flu, and other infections. A crippled immune system that can't fight off infection is also in trouble when it comes to controlling yeast overgrowth.

Impaired Immunity. Obviously, impaired immunity can result from poor nutrition, but there are other causes for a weak immune system. Heredity plays a major role: some people seem to inherit an impaired ability to keep various infections—including yeast—under control. Drugs play a part, too. Cortisone (both pills and injections), for example, may interfere with the immune system and encourage the overgrowth of yeast.

Antibiotics. Used to treat bacterial infections, antibiotics can also kill many of the friendly bacteria that normally live in the intestines. The problem? These "friendly" bacteria are great competitors in the continuing chemical war of the intestinal tract, and they secrete chemicals that normally control yeast growth. When the friendly bacteria die, the yeast win the war.

An interesting experiment conducted several years ago shows the effect of antibiotics on yeast growth. A number of healthy people had throat swabs to check for the presence of Candida albicans; about one-third of the people did have Candida. All were then given tetracycline—a common antibiotic frequently used to control acne—for three days. Their throats were recultured. The result? All of them had Candida!

Long-term use of antibiotics (such as daily use for a period of months or years to control acne) seems to be a particular problem. So do high doses of antibiotics or a pattern of switching from one antibiotic to another. Some antibiotics—such as those that specifically kill normal bacteria in the intestines or the "broad-spectrum" antibiotics designed to kill many different kinds of bacteria—seem to be the worst offenders.

In fact, candidiasis may not have been a very common problem before the introduction of the broad-spectrum antibiotics. In the last thirty years, many new antibiotics with the ability to kill a wider spectrum of bacteria have been developed. Unfortunately, doctors often prescribe these antibiotics liberally. Only recently have we become aware of some of the problems that can result.

It's not just the antibiotics we take, either—of growing concern are the antibiotics given to the animals we eventually eat. Animals are given antibiotics to treat and prevent infection, but there's more: some antibiotics stimulate growth in animals. Ranchers and producers who want to fatten their profits may use antibiotics to fatten their animals. If you eat a lot of meat that contains even traces of antibiotics, you may develop a bacteria-yeast imbalance in your intestines.

Pregnancy. The hormonal changes of pregnancy produce favorable conditions for yeast growth. We know that vaginal yeast increases during pregnancy, resulting in vaginal itching, swelling, and discharge. It's probable that intestinal yeast increases, too. Typical candidiasis symptoms—heartburn, constipation, fatigue, food and sugar cravings, weight gain, fluid retention, intolerance to odors, and emotional changes—are also the "typical" symptoms associated with pregnancy.

Women are much more prone to candidiasis than are men, which seems to point a finger at female hormones. In fact, the female hormones used for oral contraceptives seem to favor yeast growth. Yeast growth also flourishes during the premenstrual phase of the cycle, when progesterone is present. The typical premenstrual complaints—such as fluid retention, emotional swings, food cravings, weight gain, and vaginitis—are characteristic of candidiasis.

Chapter Four
DIAGNOSING CANDIDIASIS

With such a wide variety of symptoms that mimic so many other diseases, how do you know that your problem is yeast?

It's not always easy!

One of the most reliable diagnostic tools, that of taking a culture, has proved effective in identifying many diseases caused by bacteria and other microorganisms. But cultures don't usually identify yeast.

Why?

Cultures are great for identifying organisms that aren't usually found in the body. That's a problem, because yeast is normally found in the body in controlled numbers. If yeast is grown on a culture from samples taken from your body, it only means that you have yeast present. It does not tell us about their numbers, or whether they are causing you any problems.

Another generally effective diagnostic tool, testing for antibodies, is also ineffective in determining candidiasis. Why? Antibody testing works on the theory that if you have been exposed to a certain organism, your body will have developed an antibody against that organism. Blood tests can detect antibodies. Through blood tests, then, technicians can generally determine what organisms you have been exposed to.

Why doesn't it work in diagnosing yeast?

Because all of us have yeast in our bodies—and all of us have antibodies against yeast. In fact, at least seventy-nine different yeast antibodies have been identified. Each person doesn't produce or need all seventy-nine, but a certain number of antibodies are required of a healthy immune system to keep yeast under control.

How, then, are researchers diagnosing candidiasis?

Dr. Orian Truss has identified a number of biochemical abnormalities that are often present with candidiasis; these biochemical abnormalities can be detected through a battery of laboratory tests that detect such things as red blood cell filtration rate, amino acid levels, fatty acid levels, and so on. Unfortunately, these abnormalities can also accompany other conditions, and the laboratory tests are not yet specific enough to guarantee candidiasis diagnosis. New immune-function blood tests recently developed also hold some promise.

One of the most promising methods of diagnosis is a careful medical history. A detailed list of symptoms that are known to accompany candidiasis and that usually improve with treatment has been developed into a questionnaire; a scoring system aids in diagnosis. If you have a high score on the yeast questionnaire—especially if your symptoms first occurred after antibiotic use or in association with some other factor known to aggravate yeast overgrowth—you probably have a yeast problem.

You may have a yeast problem even if your score is relatively low—especially if your problems started suddenly after you took a course of antibiotics. You may have noticed that your diarrhea or ulcer symptoms flared up suddenly after you took several courses of antibiotics to clear a sore throat. These less involved cases of candidiasis usually respond quickly to treatment.

SCORING SYSTEM FOR IDENTIFYING YEAST PROBLEMS

INSTRUCTIONS: If you are troubled by any of the listed symptoms, then place an ⊠ in the space following that symptom.

BRAIN SYMPTOMS:
Depression, loss of interest or pleasure ☐
Anxiety, irritability, easily angered, trouble sleeping ☐
Trouble thinking clearly, poor memory, poor concentration ☐
Fatigue, weakness ☐

GASTROINTESTINAL SYMPTOMS:
Intestinal gas, bloating, abdominal fullness ☐
Constipation, diarrhea, or both alternating ☐
Heartburn, acid indigestion, gastritis, intestinal pain or cramping ☐

MUSCULOSKELETAL SYMPTOMS:
Muscle stiffness with normal activity, muscle cramps, deep pains in legs, arms and back ☐

SUGAR METABOLISM:
Cravings for sugar, carbohydrates or alcohol ☐
Feel sick if don't eat regularly ☐

TOTAL _____

SCORING:
If you have answered yes to:
8 or more of the above questions—yeast is almost certainly a problem
6 or more of the above questions—yeast is probably a problem
4 or more of the above questions—yeast is possibly a problem
less than 4 of the above questions—yeast less likely to be a problem

The best diagnostic tool of all, however, is to try the treatment! Start the treatment, and see what happens. If you improve dramatically, you have candidiasis—and you should continue treatment. If you see no improvement after six to eight weeks of treatment, your symptoms are most likely due to something else.

Are you appalled by the thought of undergoing treatment without a firm diagnosis? Consider your alternative: a battery of blood tests, X-rays, and other specialized procedures to track down the source of all your symptoms. Many of our patients have been through thousands of dollars' worth of tests, only to find the test results completely normal. And, as was explained, the most reliable diagnostic tests usually don't pinpoint candidiasis. Effective yeast management is extremely safe and relatively inexpensive—something that can't be said for some traditional diagnostic tests!

Diagnosing Candidiasis in Children

While the yeast questionnaire is a good way to diagnose candidiasis in adults, it doesn't work well for children.

The children's questionnaire and information regarding diagnosing, prevention, and treatment of candidiasis in children is found in Appendix 1.

It's possible—if not probable—that thousands of adults and children suffer from candidiasis without even knowing it. But these men, women, and children can overcome many of the symptoms that trouble them with simple, effective, low-risk treatment procedures designed to help the body regain a normal balance of yeast in the body.

Ready to begin?

Just turn the page!

Chapter Five

YEAST TREATMENT MEASURES: BEGIN WITH MEDICATION

Effective treatment of candidiasis involves seven steps:

1. Take medication to kill yeast.
2. Take Lactobacillus bacteria supplements to restore the balance of organisms in the intestinal tract.
3. Follow yeast control diet.
4. Exercise regularly.
5. Take various nutritional supplements as appropriate.
6. Reduce stress.
7. Strengthen the immune system.

The first step in a yeast treatment program is yeast-killing medication, which is outlined in this chapter; following chapters outline the other six parts of the treatment program.

Remember: yeast is a normal part of your body, and your goal isn't to get rid of it completely! (Even if you wanted to, you probably couldn't eradicate all the yeast in your body.) Instead, your goal is to reduce the amount of yeast enough to get rid of your symptoms and bring you back to health.

Remember, too, that candidiasis is a chronic infection, and chronic infections are sometimes slow and difficult to treat. Improvement is often gradual. While you may notice an immediate and dramatic improvement in some of your symptoms, it may take much longer to notice the improvement in others.

As you begin the treatment program, use the scoring form in Chapter 11. Rate your symptoms before treatment starts, and then at weekly intervals for nine weeks. By doing this, it's easy to identify any improvement. If you are consistent in following the treatment for eight weeks and notice no improvement at all, yeast is probably not your problem, and you should consider other possibilities.

If you do notice improvement, you're on your way, and you should continue treatment!

How long?

Since each case of candidiasis is unique, there is no set answer. As a general guideline, you should continue the treatment program, month after month, as long as you are noticing improvement. When an entire month goes by without any further significant improvement, then you can consider discontinuing treatment. Reduce your active yeast-killing medication to half dosage for one month, and watch for the return of symptoms. If no symptoms return, discontinue the medication completely. Keep using the scoring system every two-weeks to keep track of your progress.

What if symptoms reappear?

Start taking your medication again **at the first sign of troublesome symptoms!** Don't wait until most of your symptoms have reappeared before you start taking your medication. Once you resume treatment, stay on the treatment program for at least two additional months. If your symptoms return after you have stopped taking medication several consecutive times, stay on the full treatment program for at least six months before discontinuing the treatment again.

Do you have to look forward to years of treatment?

Probably not! In some severe cases, treatment may take years, but most cases of candidiasis respond to treatment within a few months. We recommend three months of continuous treatment as a minimum; but if your case is more severe, you will need to continue treatment for a longer period of time.

PRESCRIPTION YEAST-KILLING MEDICATION

Nystatin: Several antifungal medications kill Candida albicans; we prefer the one with the generic name Nystatin (also labeled Nilstat or Mycostatin). Working by direct contact with the yeast cells, Nystatin damages the cell walls and kills the yeast. When taken orally, even in large doses, it is not absorbed into the bloodstream in quantities large enough to cause side effects or to pose a risk. Because Nystatin works in the intestinal tract with its large surface area, you need a substantial dose to be effective.

Nystatin is a prescription item available in both pure powder and pill form; since the powder does not contain food dyes, excipients, or the other additives usually found in pills, we recommend that you use it to begin treatment—especially if you are prone to allergic reactions. Mix it in a glass with a little water; you can eat something immediately afterward to get rid of the unpleasant taste. Another method is to mix the daily amount of nystatin in 8-oz of water, then drink 2-oz of the mixture at four intervals during the day. If you have frequent problems with soreness of the tongue, mouth, or throat or if you have frequent canker sores, swish the Nystatin solution around in your mouth for a minute or two before you swallow it to allow contact with the Candida in your mouth.

While side effects are rare, if you find that the Nystatin solution upsets your stomach, you might try taking it during the middle of your meal.

Nystatin powder can be difficult to find, and must be specially ordered from the manufacturer. Once the lid is opened, the product needs to be dispensed within thirty days, so only those pharmacists near doctors who use Nystatin extensively are likely to stock it. If your doctor is willing to give you a prescription for Nystatin, he or she may know of a pharmacist who stocks it. If not, you can ask your pharmacist to order the Nystatin powder from Lederle Laboratory; your pharmacist will probably be willing to order the Nystatin if you can find several other people who will be purchasing it.

Note: There is a form of powdered Nystatin that is a topical powder intended for use on the skin; it may be the only form of Nystatin listed in your pharmacist's drug book. This form of Nystatin is not intended for internal use. Verify that your pharmacist is giving you the proper powder.

Most pharmacies stock the pills: Nystatin, which is a reddish-brown-coated pill, is less expensive than Nilstat, which is a pink-coated pill. One pill is equivalent to one-eighth of a teaspoon of powder. There are also generic brands available.

The usual starting dose is two pills (or one-fourth of a teaspoon of powder) four times a day. After one week, increase the dose to four pills (or one-half of a teaspoon of powder) four times a day. Some people who are extremely sensitive may experience a worsening of their symptoms as the yeast begin to die off, releasing toxins. If you notice only mild worsening of your symptoms, continue the treatment as outlined. If your symptoms are significantly worse, start with one pill (or one-eighth of a teaspoon of powder) four times a day. Very sensitive people may have to reduce the nystatin dosage to one-sixteenth of a teaspoon or even less to find a tolerated dose. Increase the dosage by one pill (one-eighth of a teaspoon of powder) each week until you reach the suggested treatment dose.

If you are pregnant or nursing, consult your physician before taking Nystatin. Although no problems have been reported from using Nystatin during pregnancy, and although the drug contains no warnings, we suggest that you wait until you are past the thirteen-week point in your pregnancy before taking Nystatin. If your symptoms are severe, or if you get pregnant while on treatment, you may wish to continue taking the Nystatin, but don't exceed one-fourth of a teaspoon (2 pills) four times daily. Since very little Nystatin is absorbed into the bloodstream, very little--if any--gets into the breast milk, so taking it during breast-feeding appears to be safe. Nystatin is tolerated in even high doses by infants.

Nizoral: If Nystatin causes unpleasant symptoms, you might want to try one of the other yeast-killing medications, such as Nizoral. Nizoral, is active against a broader range of yeast organisms. Absorbed into the bloodstream, Nizoral appears to be effective against yeast infections outside the intestinal tract, such as those that affect the skin, or the fingernails or toenails.

While Nizoral has several advantages, it also has disadvantages. Because it has caused liver problems in some people, you should have laboratory tests for liver function before you start treatment and every thirty days that you are using the Nizoral. Any liver problems that develop are reversible, and stopping the medication will prevent serious liver damage. Overall, Nizoral is relatively safe--probably safer than aspirin!

The recommended dose of Nizoral is one pill (200 mg) a day for one week; if you tolerate the Nizoral well, increase the dose to two pills (400 mg) a day, taken at the same time. After a few months, reduce the dose back to one pill a day; if that dosage continues to control symptoms, keep it at that level. Take

Nizoral with meals to aid in absorption. If you are using antacids, anticholinergic medication or acid inhibitors (such as Tagamet or Zantac), take it at least two hours after you take the Nizoral.

Diflucan (Fluconazole) is a systemic antifungal which is absorbed more completely than Nizoral. It works well even in the absence of stomach acids and can be taken at any time. The manufacturers recommend a liver function test after one month on Diflucan. Although this medication appears to have less potential for liver problems, we do perform a routine liver enzyme test.

Recommended dosage for adults is 200 mg the first day as a "loading dose," then 100 mg daily after that. Diflucan comes in 50 mg, 100 mg, and 200 mg pills.

The main drawback with Diflucan is the high cost (about $7.00 per pill).

NONPRESCRIPTION YEAST-KILLING PRODUCTS

If you are unable to tolerate the prescription medications, or if you can't find a physician in your area treating yeast related illnesses, nonprescription products are available. While it is our experience that they are not as effective as the prescription medications, many of the patients we've seen have reported reasonable results with these products:

Caprinex. A high quality, sustained release caprylic acid product, designed to continuously release as it moves through the upper and lower intestines. Sodium caprylate has been extensively studied. At low doses it shows a fungistatic action by inhibiting the separation of buds from the parent cells. At high doses it destroys the integrity of the cell wall, causing the cell to leak and collapse. The recommended dosage is 1 capsule in the morning and 1 capsule in the evening taken with meals.

Capricin. A timed-release preparation containing caprylic acid complex coated with a protective layer, Capricin provides a slow, uniform release of caprylic acid along the entire length of the intestinal tract. Available in capsules, Capricin dosage as recommended by the manufacturer is four capsules three times a day; we recommend that you start with one capsule three times a day, increasing to two capsules three times a day within a few days if you tolerate it well. Gradually increase to four capsules three times a day. Continue the full treatment dose of four capsules three times a day for at least sixteen days, and then gradually reduce the dosage to a maintenance dose of two capsules twice daily.

Capricin, which is relatively safe at recommended dosages, is distribratred by Pro Biologic.

Caprystatin. Similar to Capricin, Caprystatin contains caprylic acid in a delayed-release form. A 100-mg enteric-coated capsule of pure caprylic acid, Caprystatin should be taken on an empty stomach; medication is released in both the upper and lower intestinal tract. Recommended dosage is one capsule two times a day for the first week; two capsules two times a day for the second week; and three capsules two times a day during the third and following weeks. Caprystatin is distributed by Ecological Formulas.

Kaprycidin-A. Caprycidin-A is a 325-mg capsule of mineral caprylate; since Kaprycidin-A is released in the stomach, it's main advantage is for yeast problems in the stomach. While it is buffered to prevent intestinal irritation, it should still be taken on a full stomach. Recommended dosage is one capsule two times a day for the first week; two capsules two times a day during the second week; and three capsules two times a day beginning with the third week and continuing throughout treatment.

Kaprycidin-A is distributed by Ecological Formulas. It is recommended that Caprystatin and Kaprycidin-A be taken simultaneously, possibly reducing total treatment time.

Candistat. A 300-mg capsule of caprylic acid, Candistat works in much the same way as Capricin works. Candistat is distributed by AMNI.

Tanalbit. Tanalbit, available in 500-mg capsules, is based on the deep-intestinal action of zinc-salicylo-tannate. The tannic acids in Tanalbit are natural antifungal substances that destroy fungi, including their spores and mycelia. Tanalbit is distributed by Scientific Consulting Service, Ind.

Cantrol. A combination of Primadophilus, Pau D'Arco, a hypoallergenic antioxidant, linseed oil, and Evening Primrose Oil in portion-controlled packets. Cantrol is a nutritional approach to the control of Candida. Cantrol is distributed by Nature's Way Products, Inc.

Garlic. Used for many years as natural antibiotic, garlic seems to work against fungal infections, including yeast. One major problem with using garlic is its strong odor (which permeates the entire body, not just the breath). Some of our patients have tried garlic, and some reported good results. The deodorized garlic products have the active ingredient (allicin) removed, therefore having no antibiotic effect. A new odor controlled garlic product, **Garlicin,** by Nature's Way Products, Inc. controls the odor while retaining the active ingredient, allicin, and has been found to kill Candida.

Pau D'Arco (Taheebo Tea or Lapacho). Another natural antifungal product is Pau D'Arco, made from the back of a fungus resistant tree. It may be taken in capsule form or by brewing a tea (Taheebo Tea). Some have had success in treating fungal infection symtoms with this product. Follow package directions for brewing and for dosage recommendations.

Mycocidin. A fatty acid concentrate (undecylenic acid) which is derived from castor bean oil. Each capsule contains 50 mg of Mycocidin fatty acid concentrate in a base of extra-virgin olive oil. The usual dosage is 3 to 5 capsules, three times a day. Treatment should continue for at least 4 weeks. Stubborn cases of candidiasis may require months of treatment. Mycocidin is distributed by Thorne Research, Inc.

Recommendations

Choose your anti-yeast medication based on what is available to you, what you tolerate, and what seems to give you the best results. We recommend that you start with prescription medication, and switch to nonprescription only if you can't tolerate the prescription drugs or they do not work in reducing your symptoms. If your problems are severe, you might ask your doctor about combining yeast-killing medications; there seems to be no added risk in taking two medications together. If you are highly allergic and seem to react to various products after a few days, you might ask your doctor about alternating the medications--taking one for a few days, then another one for the next few days, then a third for the next few days before repeating the cycle.

We recommend that you seek the help and advice of a competent physician before beginning any medication, and that you take medication under a physician's supervision. If you take yeast-killing medications for eight weeks with no significant improvement in symptoms, you should discontinue the medication. A list of doctos who are willing to treat patients for candidiasis is kept by:

Price-Pottenger Nutrition Foundation
5871 El Cajon Blvd
San Diego, CA 92115

Send a self-addressed stamped legal-size envelope, with five dollars, and a list of physicians treating yeast problems will be sent to you.

Most members of the A.A.E.M. also treat candidiasis and allergies. They will send you the name of the physicians in your geographical area, information regarding clincial ecology and environmental medicine, and a list of educational publications. Please send $3.00 along with a self-addressed stamped legal-size envelope. Their address is:

American Academy of Environmental Medicine
P.O. Box 16106
Denver, CO 80216

or you may call them at 303-622-9755.

Remember, if you take yeast-killing medications for eight weeks with no significant improvement in symptoms, you should discontinue the medication.

Chapter Six

LACTOBACILLUS SUPPLEMENTS: RESTORING HEALTH TO YOUR INTESTINAL TRACT

Yeast-killing medication does a great job of killing the yeast—but that's only part of the battle plan! You need to recolonize your intestinal tract with normal, healthy bacteria, and the best way seems to be with Lactobacillus bacteria.

Why?

Not only are they present in the intestinal tract in the greatest number under normal conditions, but they have plenty of benefits as well. They produce natural antibiotics that not only kill Candida, but also control a wide range of unhealthy bacteria and possibly some virus infections (including polio!). They help normal function of the intestinal tract, preventing diarrhea and constipation.

Lactobacilli help digest food, especially milk sugar—which means that some people who cannot tolerate milk under normal conditions can tolerate it when taking Lactobacillus supplements. They also produce a number of the B vitamins, essential to health. In one experiment, Lactobacilli were even shown to reduce serum cholesterol levels. Various studies have shown that Lactobacilli may help prevent and treat both canker sores and fever blisters, and some suggest that they may play a role in inhibiting the growth of certain types of cancer cells.

You can't automatically restore a healthy intestinal balance just by taking a few Lactobacilli. It takes time, it takes a regular dose, and it takes a potent form of Lactobacilli (some strains can't survive in the intestinal tract). If you have allergies, you need to choose a Lactobacillus product that is free of milk, soybeans, corn, and other substances that commonly cause allergic reactions.

Read the labels, and choose a potent brand. Since 50 to 98 percent of the Lactobacilli are killed by the acids in your stomach, preferably find a brand that is encapsulated in enteric-coated capsules which don't break down until they reach the intestines—or else you need to boost your dose.

We recommend that you start with one to ten billion organisms a day (start at the lower end if you do not tolerate the supplement well), gradually increasing your dosage. You should continue taking it for one month longer than you take your yeast-killing medication. Monitor your intestinal symptoms carefully: if they return, you should continue taking Lactobacilli for several more months. (Lactobacilli could be safely taken for a lifetime, but your goal is to establish a normal intestinal balance that does not require outside intervention.)

Diet has a profound influence on the balance of microorganisms in the intestine, so follow these guidelines while taking Lactobacillus supplements:

1. Get plenty of carbohydrates. If you can tolerate it, drink one or two glasses of low-fat or skim milk a day—more if you are pregnant, nursing, or a child. Lactobacilli can't survive in the intestines without a good source of carbohydrates.

2. Avoid refined carbohydrates—such as sugar and white flour—because they promote rapid yeast growth, thus interfering with the Lactobacillus population.

3. Avoid large amounts of animal protein; animal protein reduces the Lactobacilli population and increases the level of bacteria that act to putrefy food (and that dump toxins into your bloodstream).

4. Eat a low-fat diet: the bile that is secreted into the intestinal tract to help digest fats is poisonous to Lactobacilli bacteria. As a side benefit, a low-fat diet may help protect you against cancer of the colon, cancer of the breast, and other cancers, as well as heart disease!

Take a good look at those simple dietary guidelines: they are guidelines that promote general good health. Not only will these guidelines help you reestablish intestinal balance, but they will result in much better overall health!

The following Lactobacillus supplement products can be used; check the label and the expiration date to make sure that the product is still potent. All Lactobacillus products (sometimes listed under the general label of acidophilus) should be refrigerated to help protect potency.

Primadophilus (Entrin). A hypoallergenic, high-potency capsule distributed by Nature's Way Products Inc. Entrin is distributed by Murdock Pharmaceuticals. Each capsule contains 2.8 billion Lactobacilli acidophilus organisms per enteric-coated capsule. Enteric means that the capsules do not dissolve in the stomach, but release their active micro-organisms directly in the intestines, where they will be most beneficial. They have been specially formulated to be free of the common allergens such as wheat, corn, soy, yeast, and chemical preservatives. It is safe for all but those who are extremely sensitive to milk. Recommended dosage is one to three capsules daily.

Vital-Dophilus. A high-potency Lactobacillus acidophilus distributed by Klaire, Vital-Dophilus is free of milk, yeast, and soy. Recommended dosage is one-eighth of a teaspoon twice a day, taken with meals.

Cardophilus. Distributed by Allergy Research Group, Cardophilus is a high-potency acidophilus cultured from carrot juice. Each capsule contains a minimum of 600 million organisms, and it is yeast- and dairy-free. A recommended initial dosage is two capsules twice a day, taken with meals.

Other useful products include **Megadophilus** by Natren and **Maxidophilus** by Ethical Nutrients.

Bifidus Bacteria: Infants and young children have a slightly different strain of Lactobacillus in their intestines, called Lactobacillus bifidus. It would be better to use the bifidus strain for babies and very young children. The adult strain of Lactobacillus gradually becomes more numerous and by the age of seven, they dominate. Several brands of bifidus bacteria are available, but may be hard to find. If you can't find the bifidus variety, the adult strain can be substituted.

Bifido Factor. Recommended especially for infants and children under the age of seven, Bifido Factor by Natren should be given once daily between meals. Recommended dosage is one-eighth to one-fourth of a teaspoon, dissolved in 4 oz of water.

Vital-Plex. A high-potency, hypo-allergenic micro-organism combination by Klaire Laboratories containing the strains of Lactobacillus acidophilus KL-1, Lactobacillus bifidus, and Streptococcus faecium. It has 10 billion plus organisms per gram in only ¼ teaspoon. Vital-Plex is completely free of milk, soy, yeast, grain, M.S.G. and other allergens.

DDS Acidophilus. DDS provides two billion viable bacteria per gram and is available in capsule, tablet, and powder forms. It is manufactured by UAS Laboratories and is free of dairy, corn, soy, wheat, and preservatives.

Latero-Flora. (Bacillus Laterosporus - BOD strain) is a unique strain of bacteria capable of improving the balance of friendly bacteria in the intestinal tract. It is manufactured by Bio-Genesis.

Chapter Seven

VITAMIN AND MINERAL SUGGESTIONS

The facts on nutritional supplements are in: if you eat properly, you do not need to take vitamins or minerals. Unfortunately, too many people do not eat properly! Vitamin and mineral deficiencies have been clearly described, and most people who have taken high school health classes are probably familiar with vitamin-deficiency diseases like scurvy, rickets, beri-beri, and pellagra. Some people are completely well nourished, and others have a severe, clear-cut vitamin-deficiency disease. Between those two extremes, many people have slight or moderate symptoms typical of vitamin or mineral deficiency.

Diagnosing the early stages of vitamin and mineral deficiency is difficult for several reasons:

1. One symptom may result from a deficiency of several different vitamins. A sore tongue, for example, can result from a deficiency of three or four different vitamins.

2. It is quite unlikely that you have a deficiency in only one isolated vitamin. Several different nutrients are most likely somewhat low.

3. Other essential nutrients, such as amino acids and fatty acids, can also be low, causing symptoms similar to those of vitamin and mineral deficiencies.

4. Food chemicals may also cause problems, either because of deficiency or through a toxic effect.

5. When deficiencies are combined with yeast overgrowth, other toxins, and food or chemical allergic reactions, a very complicated pattern of symptoms may emerge.

If you suffer from many different symptoms and scored high on the yeast questionnaire, you may have vitamin and other nutrient deficiencies. There are several different reasons why deficiencies occur:

1. Inadequate nutrient intake. In an attempt to control weight, many people have eaten small amounts of food for many years. Others with food allergy have gotten sick so often after eating that they have reduced their total food intake or they may eat an unbalanced diet as they try to avoid problem foods. Refined foods from which certain nutrients have been removed may also lead to deficiencies when eaten in excess. Even though some of the known vitamins and minerals are replaced after the processing, many other nutrients probably remain deficient.

2. Impaired absorption of nutrients from the intestine. Some people have problems with their intestinal tract, resulting in poor breakdown of food. If there are not enough acids in the stomach, or if the pancreas does not produce enough digestive enzymes, then food breakdown is incomplete. Genetic factors can cause deficiencies of certain digestive enzymes. Diarrhea— resulting from infection, allergy, or other reasons—can cause foods to move through the intestines very quickly, not allowing time for complete absorption of the available nutrients.

3. Lack of intestinal bacteria that produce vitamins. Humans have a very interesting relationship with some of the bacteria normally found in the intestines. We provide them with a home and with nutrients, and they in turn produce several of the B vitamins essential to our health and well-being. After use of antibiotics or with yeast overgrowth, there may be inadequate numbers of vitamin-producing bacteria to provide enough vitamins.

4. Essential nutrients may be broken down and lost from your body. Many nutrients are cycled repeatedly through your body. Minerals, for instance, can enter your kidneys where they are either reabsorbed or eliminated. Under some conditions, excessive nutrients can be excreted causing a deficiency.

Although the presence of some vitamins and minerals can be tested simply with laboratory tests, others are more difficult to assess. Much research is being done, and hopefully we will soon be able to do an inexpensive and complete screen of all the known vitamins, minerals, and other essential nutrients. In the meantime, we have to do the best we can with the limited information and tools available to us.

Making sensible recommendations for nutrient supplements is very difficult, even on an individual basis when the doctor can examine and test the patient. To make recommendations for the general population is even more difficult. A Senate Select Committee of nutritional experts meets every five years to study new scientific data and adjust recommended daily amounts (RDAs) of various vitamins and minerals; these RDAs are designed to maintain the good nutrition of practically all healthy people in the nation. In 1985, after much study and a great deal of heated debate, the committee finally made some recommendations, but they were rejected by those who appointed them.

Remember that the vitamin and mineral RDAs are only the amounts that will prevent a nutritional deficiency state in healthy nonstressed individuals; the RDAs do not reflect the ideal or optimal amount of these nutrients, especially for nonhealthy or stressed individuals. If leading authorities cannot agree on the amount of nutrients that will prevent disease, then there certainly can't be agreement on the amount of nutrients required for optimal health. It is even more complicated to make nutritional recommendations for optimal health for people who are deficient to start with, or who have problems absorbing and retaining nutrients.

One thing is certain: any recommendations will be soundly criticized by various authorities—some experts believe the recommendations are too high, others too low. The following suggestions then, are made after much study and discussion. Your own particular needs can best be assessed by a professional who has studied nutrition.

Let us emphasize again that no amount of concentrated nutritional supplements, whether natural or synthetic, will take the place of nutritious, unprocessed food. We simply don't know enough about which various food constituents are needed for optimal health. Remember too, that you must absolutely eat enough food to provide for your needs. If you have been eating only small amounts of food, read Appendix 4 (even if you are thin), which helps you know how to tell when you have eaten enough.

Remember that people with yeast problems are very prone to react adversely to various chemicals—including the dyes, fillers, excipients, and yeast in vitamin pills, as well as the vitamins themselves. It is very common for a patient who has been faithfully taking a particular vitamin pill to stop taking it for a time, and then to discover when introducing it again that the pill makes them sick! For this reason, we suggest the following:

1. Stop all nutritional supplements when you begin your treatment. After three or four weeks, add them back to your diet one at a time. Watch very closely for adverse reactions to the supplements; if there is any question, stop them again for a week, and then reintroduce them. Don't introduce a new food and a new supplement on the same day.

2. If you already have a vitamin supplement that you have taken and that you seem to tolerate, continue with that one. If you are looking for vitamin and mineral supplements, **try to find one that is yeast-free and as allergy-free as possible.** If any vitamin suppliers wish to send us, through the publisher, information and samples about any product they believe might be useful for yeast treatment or supplementation, we will include it in the next printing of this book, if we agree that it is a useful product.

NUTRITIONAL SUPPLEMENT SUGGESTIONS

1. **Multiple vitamin** supplements that contain most of the known vitamins and minerals in reasonably low doses. Take one or two tablets or capsules daily, or follow manufacturer's recommended dosage.

2. **B-complex vitamins.** Although most multiple vitamin supplements do have some B vitamins, we feel that extra B vitamins are helpful. We do not recommend high or megadoses of B vitamins, although they may be fine for some conditions under the supervision of a physician. Find a B-complex that has about four to six times the RDA (no more than ten times the RDA), and avoid the ones that have considerably larger amounts of some B vitamins than others. Most vitamin complexes list the amount of each vitamin by weight (usually in mg. or mcg.) and by the percentage of the RDA that is supplied. To determine balance, you need to look at the percentage of RDA for each vitamin, since the RDA by weight for various vitamins will vary considerably from one vitamin to another.

3. **Vitamin C** is generally well tolerated at 2,000 to 8,000 mg. daily. This dosage could be divided into two to four daily doses.

4. **Calcium and Magnesium** are often found in a combined product. The usual ratio is two or three parts calcium to one part magnesium. In our opinion, patients with yeast problems should have a 3:2 or 4:3 ratio of calcium to

magnesium. You can take calcium at 600 to 1000 mg. daily, and magnesium at around 500 to 600 mg. daily.

5. **Zinc** is recommended at 15 to 60 mg. daily. It is often found in adequate amounts in multiple vitamin formulas. When we are dealing with a compromised immune system, we often will have the patient take as much as 100 mg. per day for one to two months only, and then drop back to the recommended levels. This should be done under a doctor's supervision as high levels of zinc for too long can cause a copper imbalance.

6. **Potassium** can be taken in supplement form or by using No Salt in place of regular salt. If you don't like the taste, you may mix it with equal parts of sea salt. Those with continued muscle pains, leg aches, or fatigue in spite of the other supplements may benefit from higher doses of potassium, but these should be taken only under a doctor's supervision, since impaired kidney function may cause toxic levels of potassium to build up quickly.

FOR THOSE WITH MULTIPLE ALLERGIES

Antioxidant Vitamins

Some forms of allergy may improve considerably with the use of antioxidant nutrients. These products help to get rid of free radicals (electrically unbalanced molecules) that might otherwise attach themselves to various locations and cause problems. The most important of these nutrients include vitamins A, C, D, and E; selenium; and glutathione. Antioxidant vitamins are available such as **Anti-Ox** from Allergy Research Groups, **Anti-Oxidant Formula** from Murdock Pharmaceuticals Inc., or from other sources. The usual dose is one to four capsules daily.

Essential fatty acids are especially important in strengthening the immune system. A discussion follows.

Essential Fatty Acids

Clincial research suggests that Gamma Linolenic Acid (GLA) is useful as nutritional support in patients being treated for hyperlipidemia, diabetes, eczema, allergy, rheumatoid arthritis, hypercholesterolemia, cirrhosis, premenstrual syndrome, cystic fibrosis and schizophrenia. It is absent from cow's milk, though plentiful in human breast milk, almost always absent from the diet, and it is found in most common foods. Excellent sources of Gamma Linolenic Acid include Borage Oil and Evening Primrose Oil.

There is now considerable scientific evidence that fish oils will lower the level of lipids (cholesterol and other harmful fats in the blood stream), and will reduce the risk of developing heart attacks. Fish oils are an excellent source of Omega 3 fatty acids. The best fish are high-fat, cold water northern fish including salmon, sardines, tuna, mackerel, and rainbow trout. If the taste of fish oil is unpalatable, they are available in an encapsulated form which are very easy to take.

Organic Flax Seed Oil is a good source of essential Omega 3 and Omega 6 fatty acids. Vegetarians often will use this source of oil to obtain Omega 3 fatty acids in place of fish oils.

FOR THOSE WITH HIGH BLOOD PRESSURE OR HIGH BLOOD LIPIDS (CHOLESTEROL)

As previously described, essential fatty acids may help to lower the level of lipids in the blood stream. Eliminating cigarette smoking and eating a diet high in fiber and low in fat is also necessary in lowering cholesterol.

Essential fatty acids also appear to lower high blood pressure--along with using calcium, magnesium, and potassium supplements, exercise, and some of the dietary recommendations including no added salt. Fish or marine oils are available in 1000 mg. capsules there are many good sources available. The usual dose is 1000 to 4000 mg. one to two times daily with meals.

DANGERS FROM VITAMINS AND MINERALS

Excessive amounts of the fat-soluble vitamins (A, D, E, and K) can build up in your body and become toxic. Although some patients and physicians have reported using huge dosages of these vitamins with no problems, others have reported problems at doses only a few times higher that the RDA levels. Some minerals, including selenium and iron can also be toxic at too high a dose. Even the B vitamins which were formerly thought to be entirely safe, are now known to be somewhat toxic in large doses. Except under special circumstances, huge doses of supplements will not be any more effective than smaller doses. Be conservative and patient, since results with nutritional supplements may take some time to achieve.

SOME SUITABLE VITAMIN PRODUCTS

We have made no attempt to do a comprehensive search of available nutritional supplements. There are a multitude of supplements available from a multitude of companies. We have found that there isn't one particular supplement that is tolerated by all people. The best way is to stick with reasonable amounts of vitamins and minerals rather than using mega doses, and if you don't seem to feel well with one particular brand, then try another.

Chapter Eight

THE YEAST CONTROL DIET: IT'S WHAT YOU EAT THAT COUNTS!

So far, you've concentrated on trying to reduce the number of Candida albicans in your body. Your strategy has been to kill those yeast and replace them with friendly bacteria, right?

Then the next logical step is to avoid eating foods that feed the yeast!

The rationale behind the yeast control diet is really pretty simple: (1) avoid foods that feed the yeast, and (2) avoid adding further yeast and fungus-containing foods.

We recommend that you begin by following a very strict regimen for four weeks. After that, if you see improvements in symptoms, start experimenting—you may add many of the foods back into your diet, one at a time, while you see how you tolerate them. With this kind of a careful approach, you'll be able to judge exactly what you can eat to remain symptom-free. This kind of careful approach also enables you to identify foods that may be causing allergic reactions.

Four main concepts need to be stressed:

1. **Most food from plant sources has natural fungal inhibitors** that prevent the plants from being destroyed by fungus in the air and soil. When you eat these foods in a whole or unprocessed form, they could inhibit some of the yeast growth in your intestines, but processing the food destroys that capability. Wheat is a great example: the outer layer, which protects the wheat while it is growing (and, therefore, contains the most fungus inhibitor), is the layer that is stripped off when white flour is milled!

Even foods that are high in carbohydrates—which normally feed yeast—can help control yeast if their natural chemical inhibitors are left intact. Refining carbohydrates removes those chemicals. What's left? Refined carbohydrates that act as a quick food source for yeast! You should avoid the refined and processed carbohydrates—which include sucrose (table sugar), fructose, corn syrup, honey, molasses, maple syrup, maple sugar, date sugar, and white flour.

2. Other yeast management programs suggest a diet restricted in all carbohydrates; but we believe that **carbohydrates should be eaten as long as they are complex carbohydrates** (such as those found in whole grains and vegetables). You need to establish a healthy balance of bacteria in your intestinal tract — and those bacteria need carbohydrates for fuel!

So how do you give healthy bacteria fuel without giving yeast fuel? Simple: yeast thrive on simple carbohydrates — such as sugar, refined flour, and fruit juice--but have a tough time breaking down complex carbohydrates, which the friendly bacteria thrive on. A good rule of thumb is to steer clear of simple carbohydrates, and eat plenty of wholesome complex carbohydrates.

A high complex-carbohydrate, low-fat diet with few animal proteins seems to provide an optimal balance of nutrients for good health. The American Cancer Society, the American Heart Association, and the American Diabetes Foundation are all stressing a diet high in complex carbohydrates and low in fat.

3. **Avoid foods that contain yeast and fungi.** Some people react allergically to yeast; others have an allergic reaction to the metabolic by-products (toxins) produced by the yeast. We've found that most people do much better when they eliminate foods that contain yeast. In addition to possible allergic reactions, toxins produced by these fungi may add to those produced by the yeast in your intestines and illness can occur.

4. **Eat enough food!** We can't stress that enough. We've seen many people who have developed candidiasis either during or after a restrictive, low-calorie diet. Plenty of medical evidence tells us that inadequate food intake over an extended time will cause many problems--including fatigue, weakness, depression, irritability, sleep disturbance, headaches, muscle aches and pains, numbness and tingling, altered sensation (feeling pain when touched), frequent urination, and water retention. Not eating enough food can eventually lead to medical problems, including high blood pressure, diabetes, and obesity.

One last note: don't concentrate on the negative! Don't get overwhelmed with what you cannot eat. Instead, emphasize the positive changes you're making! And use the delicious recipes in Appendix 8 and the menu suggestions in Appendix 7--you'll find out that a good yeast-control diet can be satisfying, delicious, and fun!

PHASE I: FIRST FOUR WEEKS

For the first four weeks, strictly follow these dietary guidelines:
You may eat

1. All meats, fish, poultry, and eggs. For weight control, eat lean beef not more than two to three times per week; emphasize skinless chicken, turkey, rabbit, water-pack tuna, fresh fish, and veal. Eat no more than two to three eggs per weeks, and substitute egg whites for egg yolks in your cooking.

2. All vegetables (a complete list is found in Appendix 6), including scrub bed potatoes, yams, and sweet potatoes. Tomatoes and avocadoes can be eaten.

3. All legumes such as lentils, peas, soy beans, dried beans - pinto, navy, northern, kidney, etc.

4. All whole grains, including barley, corn, millet, oats, brown rice, and wheat. Use whole wheat pasta products (such as noodles, macaroni, spaghetti, and lasagna), or vegetable pasta such as spinach noodles, etc. Brown rice can be used as a pasta substitute or cooked cauliflower is good under spaghetti sauce. Popcorn is a good snack.

5. Whole-grain muffins, biscuits, pancakes, waffles, rice cakes, whole wheat tortillas, and corn tortillas (most tortillas do not contain yeast, a few brands do, check the ingredients). You may use baking soda and baking powder in your recipes. You may also add one to two tablespoons of honey to your muffin recipes in place of the specified amount of sweetener. Honey is suggested as it makes a more moist and slightly sweeter product. You can substitute one to two table-spoons of fructose, rice syrup, or sugar if you would prefer. A very small amount of sweetener is acceptable when mixed with a whole grain (complex carbohydrate) flour as the body processes it like a complex carbohydrate rather than a straight sugar. Also, by using a small amount of sweetener, it makes the transition from eating a lot of sugar to practically none, a little easier.

6. Hot or cold cereals, such as:

Wheatena	Shredded Wheat
Oat bran	Spoon-Size Shredded Wheat
Cream of Rice	Shredded Wheat and Bran
Zoom	Puffed Wheat
Oatmeal	Puffed Rice
Wheat Hearts	Roman Meal
Grits	Cracked Wheat

Health food stores have an additional variety of no-sugar-added cereals available. Fruit juice sweetened cereals are acceptable.

7. Unprocessed nuts and seeds (not salted and not roasted). You should avoid roasted nuts because the oils used in the roasting process become unhealthy when they are heated to the high temperatures required by roasting. Peanuts and peanut products (peanut butter) should be avoided, since peanuts — grown underground — are a moldy nut. In place of peanut butter, you may try other nut butters, such as almond butter or cashew butter (these can be found in health food stores). For weight control, use nuts, seeds, and nut butters sparingly (all are high in fat content).

8. Butter and cold-pressed oils, such as walnut, linseed, olive, sunflower, and safflower. Olives are allowed. It is healthier to use butter and oil sparingly and avoid all fried foods, especially for those who are overweight.

9. Milk, plain yogurt (use as a sour cream substitute), buttermilk, cream cheese, ricotta cheese, and cottage cheese. Avoid sweetened yogurt or yogurt that contains fruit. For weight control, drink 1 percent or skim milk, use low-fat cottage cheese, and do not eat cream cheese.

10. Use catsup, mustard, mayonnaise, miso, and soy sauce very sparingly; extremely sensitive people may need to eliminate all five completely from their diet.

Foods to Eliminate:

1. Avoid all sugars and sugar-containing foods, including table sugar, fructose, corn syrup, honey, molasses, maple syrup, maple sugar, and date sugar.

2. Avoid white flour and refined grain products of any type, including white pasta products (white-flour spaghetti, macaroni, and so on).

3. Avoid yeast breads and pastries; avoid anything that contains yeast, including bread, brewer's yeast, baker's yeast, multiple vitamins and B-complex vitamins manufactured from yeast sources, and crackers and pretzels that contain yeast.

4. Avoid all cheese except cottage cheese, ricotta cheese, and cream cheese.

5. Avoid alcoholic beverages.

6. Avoid all fruit juices and fruits (fresh, canned, and dried). Fresh lemon juice or lime juice can be used in water, or as a substitute for vinegar in salad dressings. **Note:** In children, we eliminate fruit juice only, they may eat fresh or unsweetened canned fruit.

7. Avoid all coffees, all teas, and all herbal teas.

8. Avoid leftovers that have been in the refrigerator too long. Freeze extras unless they will be eaten during the next 2 to 3 days.

9. Avoid obvious fungus, such as mushrooms.

10. Avoid peanuts and peanut products.

11. Avoid processed meats, such as bacon, sausage, ham, hot dogs, luncheon meats, corned beef, and pastrami.

12. Avoid all products soaked in vinegar, such as pickles, relish, and sauerkraut. Lemon juice may be substituted for vinegar in recipes.

13. Avoid all artificially sweetened drinks and food products.

After one to two weeks on this strict diet, you may try adding to your **muffin recipes** various unsweetened fruits — such as mashed bananas, unsweetened crushed pineapple, unsweetened applesauce, diced and peeled apples, and so on. Why? Many people don't have problems with cooked fruits. Again, your own body is your guide: watch your symptoms. If you don't feel as good as you did before adding the cooked fruits to your muffins, eliminate them again.

Stay on Phase I for four weeks. If you are extremely sensitive to foods and chemicals, you may need to remain on the Phase I diet for an indefinite period of time. Again, let your symptoms be your guide.

PHASE II: GRADUALLY ADDING FOODS

After four weeks on Phase I, gradually add back whole grain yeast breads and fresh fruits. The order in which you add foods is up to you. Add only one new item back into the diet at a time. If you seem to tolerate the new food, continue to eat it several times a day for two days. If you still feel okay on the third day, you can continue to use that food, and start another new food. For example, if you start bread on Wednesday, start it in the morning, eat several slices that day, then the next day, and on Friday morning. If you still feel okay, start a new item (for example, apples) by mid morning or noon. Eat several apples Friday, Saturday, and one on Sunday morning. If you still feel okay after that, begin another new item (for example, oranges). You may continue to eat bread and apples on a regular basis, and each food that you establish as well tolerated.

Next add back any of the following cheese: romano, provalone, parmesan, asciago, mozzarella, or Swiss, and see how you tolerate them. Continue to avoid obviously moldy cheeses, such as bleu cheese or roquefort. When you are feeling well, add other cheeses. If you are concerned about your weight, continue to use cheese very sparingly (it is very high in fat).

Finally, add back any of the other restricted foods, but continue to avoid sugars, fruit juices, and alcoholic beverages.

Often, we will find that each individual food by itself may not cause any problem as it is added back, but if you eat a lot of these previously avoided foods during a day, then you might get some symptoms back. For example, if you had toast and a banana for breakfast and a sandwich and a fruit salad for lunch, then had dinner rolls and a cheese main dish for dinner, you might not feel as well as when you ate these items one at a time.

Finally, try adding back any of the other restricted foods, but continue to avoid sugars, fruit juices, and alcoholic beverages.

As you gradually and carefully add back foods, watch for food allergy or intolerance. Once you have followed Phase I strictly for four weeks, you will probably feel much better—and it will be obvious if you eat something that causes a reaction. If a food causes severe symptoms, especially if it happens more than once, eliminate it from your diet permanently.

If your reaction is mild, try the rotation system: eat that food (and related foods) no more than once every four days. This kind of rotation will either reduce your reaction or eliminate it completely. Obviously, rotation will not help eliminate a fixed food allergy, (an allergic reaction that occurs every time you eat a certain food). See Appendix 2 for more information regarding allergies.

A very small number of our patients felt better when they restricted their carbohydrate intake. If no significant improvements in symptoms are made after one to two months, you may wish to try this approach.

Three Final Notes

As you add back food and establish your permanent diet, you should keep three final notes in mind:

1. **Avoid table sugar.** A large percentage of people tolerate sugar very poorly. Even though we're not sure why, one factor seems to be the rapid ingestion of sugar by yeast and its quick conversion to toxic by-products. When you use refined sugar instead of whole foods for your calories, you deprive yourself of important nutrients—and you have to put up with unpleasant symptoms and strong sugar cravings in the meantime!

The nutrients found in whole, unrefined foods seem to play a major role in keeping the body healthy; in preventing heart disease, cancer, and other degenerative diseases; in balancing neurotransmitters, allowing the brain to function; and in strengthening the immune system. Even though white flour is not as refined as white sugar is, and even though most people tolerate it better, whole-grain products are much better from a nutritional point of view.

2. **Avoid alcoholic beverages.** Alcoholic beverages contain yeast. But there is another problem: when alcohol is metabolized, it is broken down into acetaldehyde—the same chemical that causes so many problems when yeast is

metabolized by your body. Because you are already overloaded by yeast by-products, even a small amount of alcohol can cause a toxic reaction.

3. **The kind of oil you use is important!** At the beginning of the century, oils were extracted by a large roller that pressed the oil out of the seeds. People soon learned, however, that the oils went rancid quickly, giving them a short shelf life. To solve the problem and prolong shelf life, the food industry developed the process of hydrogenation, which allowed unlimited shelf life without refrigeration.

As with many solutions, this one carried a disadvantage: hydrogenation caused the natural "cis" form of the fatty acids to change into a "trans" for, which is harmful to the body.

Cold-pressed oils--found in most health food stores under the Hain label--are the answer. The cold pressed oils, which include soybean, olive, safflower, linseed, and walnut oil, promote the formation of healthy prostaglandins, hormone-like substances that are necessary to your immune system. Fish oils are also very healthy, especially northern cold-water fish oils. Bad prostaglandins result from animal fats, hydrogenated fats, and hydrogenated oils (such as margarine, vegetable shortening, and commercial oils). Bad prostaglandins also result when oil is overheated in cooking or deep frying.

Cold-pressed oils have another advantage: they contain two fatty acids, omega-6 and/or omega-3, that are essential to health but deficient in most American diets.

As you work with your diet, listen to what your body is trying to tell you! The foods you eat may have been causing problems you never imagined. Part of your job entails careful observation to determine which problems are caused by yeast and which might be caused by allergic reactions to the food you eat!

Approach your diet with a positive attitude! The information in Appendix 6 and Appendix 7 will help in cooking and meal planning as you start on the road back to health.

Chapter Nine

EXERCISE AND STRESS REDUCTION

Exercise is quickly taking center stage as being vital to overall good health: it increases your energy level, vigor, and strength. It reduces body fat and builds up muscle tissue. It improves metabolism. And it helps control weight.

There's more! Exercise promotes the development of fat-burning enzymes. It improves sugar metabolism. It reduces stress, anxiety, and depression while it improves sleep and elevates your moods.

But all these rave reviews are just the beginning!

Why?

Because exercise also helps control yeast overgrowth! How? It helps strengthen the immune system—and a strong immune system is essential for keeping yeast under control.

A consistent, effective exercise program is essential to a good yeast management program. As you start your exercise program, follow these guidelines:

Begin your exercise program very gradually. Start out by exercising for a short period of time at a modest pace; overdoing will cause joint damage, pain, and other unpleasant symptoms. You can start by trying for fifteen minutes of walking at a time, but, depending on your physical condition, you might need to start with less than that. Choose a time and pace that seems suited for you.

Exercise at a comfortable pace. Exercise should make you feel good. If you feel worse afterward, then slow down! A good guide is to exercise slowly enough that you can carry on a conversation while you are exercising—if you are too breathless to talk, then you're overdoing it. Even after you have been exercising for many months, you need to do it at a comfortable pace.

Eat plenty of wholesome, nutritious food. If you want your body to perform properly, you need to feed it adequately! You won't have the energy to exercise—nor will you find it enjoyable—if you are starving yourself. If you want to become healthy, eat enough of the right foods. If weight control is important to you, don't try to lose weight through severe restriction—we know that doesn't work! Instead, learn how to promote good health while losing weight by following the guidelines in Appendix 4. Many additional ideas may be found in *How to Lower Your Fat Thermostat*, by Dr. Dennis Remington, Dr. Garth Fisher, and Dr. Edward Parent, published by Vitality House International.

Emphasize exercise that uses large muscle groups in a rhythmic fashion. These exercises, done at a moderate pace for a prolonged period of time, are called aerobic exercises. You'll notice the greatest improvement in your overall health from aerobic exercises, such as walking, running, jogging, swimming, aerobic dancing, using a treadmill, jogging on a mini-trampoline, using an exercise bicycle, or using a rowing machine. Exercises that enhance flexibility or build only certain muscle groups may help increase strength, but aerobic exercises are of greatest value.

Emphasize the types of exercise that you can do anywhere. If you enjoy swimming or aerobic dancing, do them—but don't limit yourself to exercises that require special equipment, special locations, or certain instructors! Many people stop exercising because their dance class breaks up for Christmas vacation, because the pool has been drained so it can be painted, or because they go on a business trip away from their exercise cycle. If you are fit and enjoy it, walking or running are probably the best exercises. Plan for a bad-weather option you can use in case of storms; a mini-trampoline or exercise cycle works well for this purpose, but use these only as alternatives to a good walking or jogging program.

Exercise at least three times a week. If you can, exercise every day! Increasing or maintaining your fitness level requires a minimum of three periods of exercise a week. Significant improvements and weight loss are best accomplished with daily exercise.

Exercise at least thirty minutes at a time. Many of the helpful biological changes begin only after prolonged exercise. If you are trying to lose weight, you need to build up to forty to sixty minutes at a time. (Remember to start gradually—you can't pound the pavement for a full hour your first time out!)

DON'T STOP WITH YOUR BODY

You've found out how to exercise your body—but don't stop there! Your mind and your moods need a workout, too, and may influence your ability to successfully treat yeast overgrowth.

One of the greatest detriments to health is stress—the bodily changes produced whenever a person is exposed to nervous tension, physical injury, infection, cold, heat, X-rays, or anything else, according to Dr. Hans Selye. If you're under too much stress, your body loses its ability to cope—you can even exhaust your body's ability to manufacture stress hormones.

Eliminating the overgrowth of yeast in your body is a great beginning, but it's just that—a beginning. You need to do whatever you can to enhance your body's ability to cope with all kinds of stresses. Follow these guidelines:

Eliminate as many harmful physical influences as you can— including prolonged exposure to excessive heat or cold, preservatives and additives in food, environmental pollution, automobile exhaust, industrial wastes, and smog. Spend as much time as you can in clean air. Did you realize that some new houses—especially those that are tightly insulated—pose more of a hazard than outside air? Toxic fumes are emitted from the sub-flooring, underlay, carpet, adhesives, caulking compounds, foam insulations, and even from furnace and water heater exhaust. It helps to keep your windows open—or at least cracked open—whenever weather conditions permit.

Emotional and psychological stress can come from working too many hours, trying to accomplish too much, or worrying about money. Slow down. Cut out some of your activities. Reduce the amount of money you spend on consumer items (like new cars) and investments that might cause financial pressure. Above all, try to stop worrying—analyze your situation carefully, make the best decision, and try to solve your problems in the best possible way.

Take a good look at your relationships, too: marital problems, rebellious children, or critical parents can bring on guilt, anger, fear, and frustration. Consider seeking professional help, or reading some of the excellent self-help books on the market that are geared toward helping you improve your interpersonal relationships.

Finally, utilize your inner resources—your spirit, or your psyche, mobilizing your spiritual powers. You've probably read about the power of positive thinking: it's real, and it works! In his book, *Anatomy of an Illness,* author Norman Cousins describes how he overcame a serious illness through laughter and humor. Read it, and consider some of the other self-help books on the market that can help you mobilize your inner resources and get back to health!

Chapter Ten

STRENGTHEN YOUR IMMUNE SYSTEM AND WIN THE WAR!

If you have a yeast problem, chances are that your immune system is weak. If your immune system is weak, you're going to eventually lose the war that is being waged inside your body.

If you're a winner instead of a loser, round out your yeast management program by strengthening the troops--your immune system!

How?

Remember smallpox vaccinations? How about polio? They worked on a principle of injecting dead smallpox bacteria or polio viruses into your body--and your body reacted by building up an immunity. The same thing can happen with yeast!

Dr. Orian Truss advocates the use of Candida immunization as an important part of treatment. We have little hard scientific evidence to support the use of Candida extract in treating chronic candidiasis, but it has been used successfully for years in the control of chronic vaginal yeast infection--dermatologists have found that it stops much of the itching, burning, and tissue damage.

If Candida extract does work like other immunizations work, you would be less likely to develop a recurrence of candidiasis after your active treatment is stopped!

There's another potential advantage to treatment with Candida extract: it may reduce allergic responses. Here's how it would work--if you are allergic to Candida or to the toxins it secretes in your body, you can be treated with small doses of Candida antigen to reduce your sensitivity. Careful control of the immunization process can result in a dilution of the Candida extract that actually relieves symptoms while it strengthens your immunity! This process, called "neutralizing," is explained in more detail in Appendix 2.

Anna, a thirty-year-old who had been troubled by constant asthma since her childhood, had required medication several times a day to control it. She also had typical candidiasis symptoms. Within a few days of starting Candida extract antigen, which she simply put under her tongue, her asthma stopped entirely; she needed no more medication. Over the next year, she had only one or two mild asthmatic episodes along with respiratory infections, but otherwise remained clear.

Betty, a forty-five-year-old with many chronic candidiasis symptoms, had suffered from severe daily headaches for years. When she placed her first neutralizing dose of Candida antigen under her tongue, her headache disappeared completely within sixty seconds. She was able to keep herself free of headaches for the next week--five or six hours after using the antigen, she would feel a headache coming on, and she would use the antigen again.

But that's not all! Betty noticed that her chronic depression was improved, and her energy was coming back.

Gradually, Betty stopped getting better. The antigen didn't seem to be working--in fact, she felt worse when she used the antigen. When we rechecked her, we found that her tolerance had changed, so we gave her a new concentration of Candida extract. By continuing to make occasional adjustments, we were able to help Betty control her symptoms.

Since many of the unpleasant symptoms associated with candidiasis seem to be caused by allergy, you should try the immunization process if you can find a doctor who is willing to administer it; it seems to be effective both in injection form (given once or twice a week) or in sublingual form (given in drops under the tongue). Appendix 2 gives specific instructions for a doctor who wants to start the technique.

Finally, there is scientific evidence that you can improve the immune system's ability to fight infection with vitamins, minerals, and food supplements as appropriate; nutritional supplements that seem especially important in controlling candidiasis include the B vitamins (preferably, a yeast-free supplement), antioxidant formulas, additional Vitamin E, Vitamin C, Zinc, and Beta carotene, and essential fatty acids such as Omega 3 (Fish Oils) and Borage Oil or Evening Primrose Oil.

Chapter Eleven

TREATMENT CONCLUSION

Remember that candidiasis is a chronic disease, and it will not clear up overnight. It takes time and effort to make improvements. Be patient, and you should be well rewarded for your efforts. To help track your progress and keep you enthused about your results, you should use the symptom scoring system at the end of this chapter. Score yourself before treatment begins and each week of treatment thereafter. It is easy to forget how badly you felt a number of weeks before, and sometimes it helps to be reminded of your progress, especially if you should become discouraged.

Make sure that you continue treatment long enough to get your health problems under control. If you stop too soon, the symptoms often return, and it is sometimes hard to get started again on the treatment program. Don't stop treatment suddenly; taper off your medication gradually, and stop medication entirely only when you feel just as well with reduced dosages. Watch closely for the return of any symptoms after reducing or stopping the medication, and don't hesitate to get back on treatment if symptoms should return.

Keep in mind that candidiasis is not cured, merely controlled. A healthy diet with adequate calories and nutrients is necessary to maintain an effective immune system. Make the necessary lifestyle changes so that healthy eating becomes natural, easy, and enjoyable. Don't allow yourself to feel deprived or punished when others around you are indulging in inappropriate foods. The dietary changes we recommend are not only useful for continued yeast control, but also are ideal for prevention of other chronic disease states such as cancer, hypertension, heart disease, and diabetes.

Make changes as needed in your life to get stresses under control. Don't hesitate to seek help from a psychologist or other counselling professional to help reduce stress. Handle any problems that keep your stress levels high.

Make sure that you seek help from an experienced doctor if you have any trouble getting your symptoms under control. There are a lot of new developments in this area, and our chances of helping you are increasing as new information is continually emerging.

SYMPTOMS QUESTIONNAIRE

As you begin the yeast program, mark your symptoms in the first column only. Mark the other columns on a weekly basis to follow your progress. Keep track of each symptom in the following manner:

No trouble (leave blank)	[ ]
Mildly troublesome	[1]
Moderately troublesome	[2]
Severely troublesome	[3]

Date

Neurological

Trouble getting to sleep	[	][	][	]	[	][	][	]	[	][	][	]
Trouble staying asleep	[	][	][	]	[	][	][	]	[	][	][	]
Difficulty waking up	[	][	][	]	[	][	][	]	[	][	][	]
Trouble staying awake	[	][	][	]	[	][	][	]	[	][	][	]
Tired most of the time	[	][	][	]	[	][	][	]	[	][	][	]
Weakness	[	][	][	]	[	][	][	]	[	][	][	]
Lack of endurance	[	][	][	]	[	][	][	]	[	][	][	]
Depression	[	][	][	]	[	][	][	]	[	][	][	]
Loss of pleasure/interest	[	][	][	]	[	][	][	]	[	][	][	]
Crying spells	[	][	][	]	[	][	][	]	[	][	][	]
Agitation	[	][	][	]	[	][	][	]	[	][	][	]
Excess worry	[	][	][	]	[	][	][	]	[	][	][	]
Phobias or fearful	[	][	][	]	[	][	][	]	[	][	][	]
Panic attacks	[	][	][	]	[	][	][	]	[	][	][	]
Anxious or nervous	[	][	][	]	[	][	][	]	[	][	][	]
Suspicious	[	][	][	]	[	][	][	]	[	][	][	]
Irritability/anger	[	][	][	]	[	][	][	]	[	][	][	]
Delusions	[	][	][	]	[	][	][	]	[	][	][	]
Hallucinations	[	][	][	]	[	][	][	]	[	][	][	]
Tremor	[	][	][	]	[	][	][	]	[	][	][	]
Seizures	[	][	][	]	[	][	][	]	[	][	][	]
Shaky feeling	[	][	][	]	[	][	][	]	[	][	][	]
Hyperactive	[	][	][	]	[	][	][	]	[	][	][	]
Balance problems	[	][	][	]	[	][	][	]	[	][	][	]
Feel faint	[	][	][	]	[	][	][	]	[	][	][	]
Blackouts	[	][	][	]	[	][	][	]	[	][	][	]
Dizziness-light headed	[	][	][	]	[	][	][	]	[	][	][	]
Spinning	[	][	][	]	[	][	][	]	[	][	][	]
With position change	[	][	][	]	[	][	][	]	[	][	][	]
Difficulty concentrating	[	][	][	]	[	][	][	]	[	][	][	]
Trouble thinking clearly	[	][	][	]	[	][	][	]	[	][	][	]
Indecisive	[	][	][	]	[	][	][	]	[	][	][	]
Confusion	[	][	][	]	[	][	][	]	[	][	][	]
Memory disturbance	[	][	][	]	[	][	][	]	[	][	][	]
Learning disability	[	][	][	]	[	][	][	]	[	][	][	]
Difficulty with speech	[	][	][	]	[	][	][	]	[	][	][	]
Difficulty with writing	[	][	][	]	[	][	][	]	[	][	][	]
Taste diminished or gone	[	][	][	]	[	][	][	]	[	][	][	]
Decreased sense of smell	[	][	][	]	[	][	][	]	[	][	][	]
Vision-Blurred	[	][	][	]	[	][	][	]	[	][	][	]
Trouble focusing	[	][	][	]	[	][	][	]	[	][	][	]
Double vision	[	][	][	]	[	][	][	]	[	][	][	]

Loss of hearing	[ ][ ][ ]	[ ][ ][ ]	[ ][ ][ ]
Ears ringing	[ ][ ][ ]	[ ][ ][ ]	[ ][ ][ ]
Poor temperature regulation)			
(Frequently too hot or cold)	[ ][ ][ ]	[ ][ ][ ]	[ ][ ][ ]
Headaches-Migraine type	[ ][ ][ ]	[ ][ ][ ]	[ ][ ][ ]
Stress type	[ ][ ][ ]	[ ][ ][ ]	[ ][ ][ ]
Sinus type	[ ][ ][ ]	[ ][ ][ ]	[ ][ ][ ]
Numbness	[ ][ ][ ]	[ ][ ][ ]	[ ][ ][ ]
TOTAL	___ ___ ___	___ ___ ___	___ ___ ___

Urinary System

Frequent urination	[ ][ ][ ]	[ ][ ][ ]	[ ][ ][ ]
Burning on urination	[ ][ ][ ]	[ ][ ][ ]	[ ][ ][ ]
Hesitation to start urination	[ ][ ][ ]	[ ][ ][ ]	[ ][ ][ ]
Obstruction to urine flow	[ ][ ][ ]	[ ][ ][ ]	[ ][ ][ ]
Loss of urine with straining,			
coughing, or activity	[ ][ ][ ]	[ ][ ][ ]	[ ][ ][ ]
Urinary tract infections	[ ][ ][ ]	[ ][ ][ ]	[ ][ ][ ]
Bed wetting	[ ][ ][ ]	[ ][ ][ ]	[ ][ ][ ]
TOTAL	___ ___ ___	___ ___ ___	___ ___ ___

Gastrointestinal

Mouth ulcers—cankers	[ ][ ][ ]	[ ][ ][ ]	[ ][ ][ ]
Mouth/tongue raw or sore	[ ][ ][ ]	[ ][ ][ ]	[ ][ ][ ]
Heartburn	[ ][ ][ ]	[ ][ ][ ]	[ ][ ][ ]
Indigestion	[ ][ ][ ]	[ ][ ][ ]	[ ][ ][ ]
Excess acidity	[ ][ ][ ]	[ ][ ][ ]	[ ][ ][ ]
Gastritis or acid stomach	[ ][ ][ ]	[ ][ ][ ]	[ ][ ][ ]
Gastric ulcers	[ ][ ][ ]	[ ][ ][ ]	[ ][ ][ ]
Nausea	[ ][ ][ ]	[ ][ ][ ]	[ ][ ][ ]
Abdominal pain	[ ][ ][ ]	[ ][ ][ ]	[ ][ ][ ]
Sore all over	[ ][ ][ ]	[ ][ ][ ]	[ ][ ][ ]
Cramping pain	[ ][ ][ ]	[ ][ ][ ]	[ ][ ][ ]
Upper abdominal area	[ ][ ][ ]	[ ][ ][ ]	[ ][ ][ ]
Lower abdominal area	[ ][ ][ ]	[ ][ ][ ]	[ ][ ][ ]
Gas pains	[ ][ ][ ]	[ ][ ][ ]	[ ][ ][ ]
Intestinal gas	[ ][ ][ ]	[ ][ ][ ]	[ ][ ][ ]
Abdominal bloating	[ ][ ][ ]	[ ][ ][ ]	[ ][ ][ ]
Constipation	[ ][ ][ ]	[ ][ ][ ]	[ ][ ][ ]
Diarrhea	[ ][ ][ ]	[ ][ ][ ]	[ ][ ][ ]
Alternating constipation			
and diarrhea	[ ][ ][ ]	[ ][ ][ ]	[ ][ ][ ]
Rectal itch	[ ][ ][ ]	[ ][ ][ ]	[ ][ ][ ]

Food cravings   [ ][ ][ ]   [ ][ ][ ]   [ ][ ][ ]
Fluctuating appetite   [ ][ ][ ]   [ ][ ][ ]   [ ][ ][ ]
  Loss of appetite   [ ][ ][ ]   [ ][ ][ ]   [ ][ ][ ]
  Sudden hunger   [ ][ ][ ]   [ ][ ][ ]   [ ][ ][ ]
           TOTAL   __ __ __   __ __ __   __ __ __

Cardiovascular System

Chest pain on exertion   [ ][ ][ ]   [ ][ ][ ]   [ ][ ][ ]
Leg pain on exertion   [ ][ ][ ]   [ ][ ][ ]   [ ][ ][ ]
Swelling of feet/legs/hands   [ ][ ][ ]   [ ][ ][ ]   [ ][ ][ ]
Cold hands and feet   [ ][ ][ ]   [ ][ ][ ]   [ ][ ][ ]
Jumping/flopping of heart   [ ][ ][ ]   [ ][ ][ ]   [ ][ ][ ]
Rapid pulse/pounding heart
  for no apparent reason   [ ][ ][ ]   [ ][ ][ ]   [ ][ ][ ]
           TOTAL   __ __ __   __ __ __   __ __ __

Musculoskeletal

Aching generalized   [ ][ ][ ]   [ ][ ][ ]   [ ][ ][ ]
Muscle soreness   [ ][ ][ ]   [ ][ ][ ]   [ ][ ][ ]
Muscle cramps   [ ][ ][ ]   [ ][ ][ ]   [ ][ ][ ]
Muscle weakness   [ ][ ][ ]   [ ][ ][ ]   [ ][ ][ ]
Muscle jerks   [ ][ ][ ]   [ ][ ][ ]   [ ][ ][ ]
Muscle stiffness   [ ][ ][ ]   [ ][ ][ ]   [ ][ ][ ]
Arthritis, joint pain   [ ][ ][ ]   [ ][ ][ ]   [ ][ ][ ]
Back pain   [ ][ ][ ]   [ ][ ][ ]   [ ][ ][ ]
Stiffness of neck
  and shoulders   [ ][ ][ ]   [ ][ ][ ]   [ ][ ][ ]
           TOTAL   __ __ __   __ __ __   __ __ __

Skin

Skin rash   [ ][ ][ ]   [ ][ ][ ]   [ ][ ][ ]
Eczema or dermatitis   [ ][ ][ ]   [ ][ ][ ]   [ ][ ][ ]
Itching or irritated skin   [ ][ ][ ]   [ ][ ][ ]   [ ][ ][ ]
Dry skin   [ ][ ][ ]   [ ][ ][ ]   [ ][ ][ ]
Rough skin   [ ][ ][ ]   [ ][ ][ ]   [ ][ ][ ]
Easy bruising   [ ][ ][ ]   [ ][ ][ ]   [ ][ ][ ]
Flushing/redness of skin   [ ][ ][ ]   [ ][ ][ ]   [ ][ ][ ]
Hives   [ ][ ][ ]   [ ][ ][ ]   [ ][ ][ ]
Acne starting or persisting
  into adulthood   [ ][ ][ ]   [ ][ ][ ]   [ ][ ][ ]
Dandruff   [ ][ ][ ]   [ ][ ][ ]   [ ][ ][ ]
Excessive perspiration   [ ][ ][ ]   [ ][ ][ ]   [ ][ ][ ]
Sweaty hands and feet   [ ][ ][ ]   [ ][ ][ ]   [ ][ ][ ]
           TOTAL   __ __ __   __ __ __   __ __ __

Respiratory

Nose congested											
Only during certain seasons	[ ][ ][ ][ ]			[ ][ ][ ]			[ ][ ][ ]				
Only in some situations	[ ][ ][ ][ ]			[ ][ ][ ]			[ ][ ][ ]				
Constant	[ ][ ][ ][ ]			[ ][ ][ ]			[ ][ ][ ]				
Constant, but worse at times	[ ][ ][ ][ ]			[ ][ ][ ]			[ ][ ][ ]				
Nose runny	[ ][ ][ ][ ]			[ ][ ][ ]			[ ][ ][ ]				
Nose itching	[ ][ ][ ][ ]			[ ][ ][ ]			[ ][ ][ ]				
Sneezing	[ ][ ][ ][ ]			[ ][ ][ ]			[ ][ ][ ]				
Nose bleeds	[ ][ ][ ][ ]			[ ][ ][ ]			[ ][ ][ ]				
Eye itching	[ ][ ][ ][ ]			[ ][ ][ ]			[ ][ ][ ]				
Eye soreness	[ ][ ][ ][ ]			[ ][ ][ ]			[ ][ ][ ]				
Eye watering	[ ][ ][ ][ ]			[ ][ ][ ]			[ ][ ][ ]				
Eye redness	[ ][ ][ ][ ]			[ ][ ][ ]			[ ][ ][ ]				
Crusting/rash on eyelids	[ ][ ][ ][ ]			[ ][ ][ ]			[ ][ ][ ]				
Swelling of eyelids	[ ][ ][ ][ ]			[ ][ ][ ]			[ ][ ][ ]				
Dark circles under eyes	[ ][ ][ ][ ]			[ ][ ][ ]			[ ][ ][ ]				
Ears sore	[ ][ ][ ][ ]			[ ][ ][ ]			[ ][ ][ ]				
Ears — deep itching	[ ][ ][ ][ ]			[ ][ ][ ]			[ ][ ][ ]				
Ear pressure	[ ][ ][ ][ ]			[ ][ ][ ]			[ ][ ][ ]				
Ear fluid	[ ][ ][ ][ ]			[ ][ ][ ]			[ ][ ][ ]				
Sinus pressure or dullness	[ ][ ][ ][ ]			[ ][ ][ ]			[ ][ ][ ]				
Sore throat	[ ][ ][ ][ ]			[ ][ ][ ]			[ ][ ][ ]				
Swelling throat	[ ][ ][ ][ ]			[ ][ ][ ]			[ ][ ][ ]				
Tightness of throat	[ ][ ][ ][ ]			[ ][ ][ ]			[ ][ ][ ]				
Itching mouth or throat	[ ][ ][ ][ ]			[ ][ ][ ]			[ ][ ][ ]				
Drainage from nose or sinuses in throat	[ ][ ][ ][ ]			[ ][ ][ ]			[ ][ ][ ]				
Hoarseness	[ ][ ][ ][ ]			[ ][ ][ ]			[ ][ ][ ]				
Swollen neck lymph nodes	[ ][ ][ ][ ]			[ ][ ][ ]			[ ][ ][ ]				
Shortness of breath	[ ][ ][ ][ ]			[ ][ ][ ]			[ ][ ][ ]				
Trouble moving air in/out	[ ][ ][ ][ ]			[ ][ ][ ]			[ ][ ][ ]				
Asthma or wheezing	[ ][ ][ ][ ]			[ ][ ][ ]			[ ][ ][ ]				
Air not satisfying	[ ][ ][ ][ ]			[ ][ ][ ]			[ ][ ][ ]				
Smothering feeling	[ ][ ][ ][ ]			[ ][ ][ ]			[ ][ ][ ]				
Tight chest	[ ][ ][ ][ ]			[ ][ ][ ]			[ ][ ][ ]				
Chest pain with breathing	[ ][ ][ ][ ]			[ ][ ][ ]			[ ][ ][ ]				
With coughing	[ ][ ][ ][ ]			[ ][ ][ ]			[ ][ ][ ]				
Cough	[ ][ ][ ][ ]			[ ][ ][ ]			[ ][ ][ ]				
Throat infections	[ ][ ][ ][ ]			[ ][ ][ ]			[ ][ ][ ]				
Ear infections	[ ][ ][ ][ ]			[ ][ ][ ]			[ ][ ][ ]				
Sinus infections	[ ][ ][ ][ ]			[ ][ ][ ]			[ ][ ][ ]				
Bronchitis	[ ][ ][ ][ ]			[ ][ ][ ]			[ ][ ][ ]				
Pneumonia	[ ][ ][ ][ ]			[ ][ ][ ]			[ ][ ][ ]				
TOTAL	___ ___ ___			___ ___ ___			___ ___ ___				

Females

Vaginal soreness/burning	[ ][ ][ ]	[ ][ ][ ]	[ ][ ][ ]
Vaginal itch	[ ][ ][ ]	[ ][ ][ ]	[ ][ ][ ]
Vaginal discharge/infections	[ ][ ][ ]	[ ][ ][ ]	[ ][ ][ ]
Loss of sexual interest	[ ][ ][ ]	[ ][ ][ ]	[ ][ ][ ]
Hair growth, face	[ ][ ][ ]	[ ][ ][ ]	[ ][ ][ ]
Irregular menstrual periods	[ ][ ][ ]	[ ][ ][ ]	[ ][ ][ ]
Menstrual cramps	[ ][ ][ ]	[ ][ ][ ]	[ ][ ][ ]

Development of/or
  worsening of symptoms
  during the time prior
  to menstruation:

Headache	[ ][ ][ ]	[ ][ ][ ]	[ ][ ][ ]
Fluid retention	[ ][ ][ ]	[ ][ ][ ]	[ ][ ][ ]
Weight gain	[ ][ ][ ]	[ ][ ][ ]	[ ][ ][ ]
Increased appetite	[ ][ ][ ]	[ ][ ][ ]	[ ][ ][ ]
Irritability	[ ][ ][ ]	[ ][ ][ ]	[ ][ ][ ]
Angry outbursts	[ ][ ][ ]	[ ][ ][ ]	[ ][ ][ ]
Depression	[ ][ ][ ]	[ ][ ][ ]	[ ][ ][ ]
Fatigue	[ ][ ][ ]	[ ][ ][ ]	[ ][ ][ ]
Confusion	[ ][ ][ ]	[ ][ ][ ]	[ ][ ][ ]
Personality change	[ ][ ][ ]	[ ][ ][ ]	[ ][ ][ ]
Change in sex drive	[ ][ ][ ]	[ ][ ][ ]	[ ][ ][ ]
Clumsiness	[ ][ ][ ]	[ ][ ][ ]	[ ][ ][ ]
TOTAL	— — —	— — —	— — —

Neurological Total	— — —	— — —	— — —
Gastrointestinal Total	— — —	— — —	— — —
Cardiovascular Total	— — —	— — —	— — —
Musculoskeletal Total	— — —	— — —	— — —
Respiratory Total	— — —	— — —	— — —
Urinary System Total	— — —	— — —	— — —
Skin Total	— — —	— — —	— — —
Females Total	— — —	— — —	— — —
GRAND TOTAL	— — —	— — —	— — —

Chapter Twelve

TROUBLE-SHOOTING GUIDE: ANSWERS TO COMMON QUESTIONS ABOUT THE YEAST-CONTROL PROGRAM

Once you start your yeast-control program, you'll probably run into some common problems or questions. We've anticipated those questions by including them here—and we've added suggestions on how you can solve many common problems!

After a few days on the yeast control program, I feel worse than ever. What's wrong?

There are several reasons why some people may feel worse during the first few weeks of treatment:

- "Die-Off" reactions commonly occur early in treatment. When the yeast are killed, toxic substances are released that either poison your enzyme systems or cause an allergic reaction.
- Adverse reactions to any of the medication can occur.
- You might be addicted to a food you've been eating—and when you eliminated it from your diet, you can suffer actual withdrawal symptoms. Common foods that cause addiction are sugar, chocolate, caffeine, alcohol, bread, and cheese.
- You might react adversely to foods that you add to the diet in place of foods you stop eating. Some of these foods may be tolerated in small amounts, but if you use more of them as you change your diet, you may begin to react.
- If you are under a lot of stress or worrying about personal problems, you may produce too many stress hormones; these excessive stress hormones can cause many unpleasant symptoms.
- You might have another type of infection, such as the flu or a sinus infection, that is causing symptoms.

If your problems are relatively minor, continue the program as outlined and see what happens. If your symptoms are moderately uncomfortable, reduce your dosage of Nystatin (or other yeast-killing agent) by one-half and see what happens. If your problems are quite severe and unpleasant, completely stop taking all new medication.

If your problem was caused by die-off, your symptoms should usually last only four or five days, and no longer than seven to ten days. If your symptoms disappear completely in spite of continued medication, especially if you start to get over many of the problems for which you began yeast treatment, die-off was almost certainly your problem.

If you reduce or stop the medication and the unpleasant symptoms go away, your problem is probably either die-off or medication reaction. It is usually easy to tell the difference between these two problems. Add your yeast-killing medication back at a small dosage, or continue at the reduced dosage. You may have to experiment to find a tolerable dose—some people can tolerate only as much powder as they can fit on the flat end of a toothpick! Once you find a dosage that causes only mild symptoms, continue it.

With a die-off problem, symptoms usually last only a few days, and then you should start to improve. If symptoms stay the same or get worse, you are probably reacting to the medication. Another clue to medication reaction is that the problems are usually worse within a few minutes to a few hours after taking it; then you'll start to feel better until the next dosage is given. If your main symptoms are digestive (nausea, abdominal pain, indigestion), try taking the medication in the middle of a meal or right after eating. If your problems are more severe, or involve other body systems, you might need to switch to another medication.

If the symptoms are severe but seem to be caused by die-off, continue faithfully with the Phase I diet for a week or so, and then start the medication again at a lower dose. This will usually enable you to continue treatment. After the die-off symptoms have disappeared or become less severe, gradually increase the dosage of medication again until you are taking the full therapeutic dose suggested in Chapter 5.

If you stop the medication for a few days and still don't feel any better, you probably have one of the other above-listed problems. If, along with other symptoms, you have a strong craving for something sweet or for a particular food, try eating or drinking it. If a food addiction is the source of your symptoms, you'll start feeling better within a few minutes—sometimes within a few seconds! If all of your symptoms disappear when you eat or drink the suspect food, food addiction was probably your only problem.

If problems persist, try completely eliminating some of the foods you have been using as a replacement on the yeast-control diet. If you feel better a day or two after stopping a food, try eating it again as a test—if you start to feel sick again, that's your problem. Eliminate that food until later. If you need help with a food addiction or suspected allergy, see Appendix 2.

Although any infection may lead to generalized symptoms like fever, tiredness, aching, dizziness, and decreased appetite, there are usually some localized signs that can help you determine whether you have an infection. An elevated temperature is strong evidence of infection. A urinary infection generally causes urinary frequency, burning, or pain over the bladder or kidney area. A sinus infection generally causes sinus pressure, headache, and nasal congestion. An infected throat usually causes sore throat or lymph gland soreness in the neck. If you think you have an infection, you might want to consult a physician who can confirm it. If you do have an infection, express your reluctance to take an antibiotic unless absolutely necessary. Most infections, even bacterial infections, will clear in a week or so. You can continue your yeast-control treatment during an infection.

If none of the above suggestions seem to solve the problems, and they persist even when you stop yeast treatment, you may be suffering from excess stress. Resume your yeast treatment, and make sure that you include plenty of exercise. Effective exercise may reduce stress hormones enough that you will start to feel better within a few weeks.

My gas and bloating are not any better; in fact, my gas is worse.

Although yeast seem to be a major cause of intestinal gas, and treatment will usually greatly improve this symptom, it doesn't always eliminate gas. A number of different intestinal organisms can also cause intestinal gas as a by-product of metabolism. Sometimes killing yeast allows these other gas-producers to grow, and you get more gas.

You probably know that beans cause gas, but do you know why? Humans lack the digestive enzyme needed to break down a particular carbohydrate found in beans. Other foods can cause gas, too. Many people have inadequate amounts of the digestive enzyme (lactase) necessary to break down milk sugar (lactose). If that's your problem and you drink too much milk, you'll suffer gas, bloating, abdominal cramps, and diarrhea. Excessive amounts of whole wheat products can also cause gas. If you're used to eating white flour and suddenly switch to whole wheat, you'll probably suffer from gas and bloating at first. You'll probably gradually adjust to eating more whole wheat, but you might need to increase it a little at a time to allow your system to adapt.

Gas and bloating commonly result from food intolerance. Although we don't exactly know why, certain problem foods can cause almost immediate gas and bloating—too immediate, in fact, to blame on gas-producing microorganisms. Any sudden development of gas could be caused by new foods you've added to your diet.

Some excess gas may be caused by swallowed air. People often swallow air when they chew gum or when they suffer increased anxiety for any reason.

If you are having increased gas and bloating, watch closely for any pattern. If it gets worse right after a meal, write down what you ate at that time, and then test each food item independently. If you have started chewing more gum, stop, and see if it helps. You may wish to stop all wheat and milk products for a trial period; if that stops the gas entirely, add them back one at a time to find out which one is the culprit. Keep in mind that both could be a problem.

If you can't find the cause and correct the excess gas, you might want to try treating the symptoms. Taking digestive enzymes (ask your pharmacist for names) might help; take them immediately before meals to help quickly break down foods that might otherwise cause gas. Simethicone (found in many antacids, but also by itself in Mylicon and other products) helps to reduce the discomfort from gas. Exercise is also helpful in getting rid of excess gas.

Since starting yeast treatment, I'm not very hungry anymore. Is it still necessary to eat regularly?

Eating very little or eating a diet low in carbohydrates can artificially suppress hunger. If you are eating too little, or not eating enough vegetables and whole-grain products, you need to concentrate on eating a healthier, more adequate diet.

Our concern is with chronic dieters who normally eat only once or twice a day, and even then, give in only to the strongest of eating drives. With yeast management, which brings a reduction in cravings and hunger, these people find they can reduce their food intake even further, and eat even less often. Because of old ideas about energy balance, they often think that they will lose weight effectively by doing this. To get well and to keep weight off, it is necessary to eat plenty of good, nutritious food on a regular basis.

If you have been trying to lose weight by reducing the amount you eat, read Appendix 4, and then start eating! Establish regular meal times, and then eat at those times, even if you are not hungry at first. You will eventually get used to eating on schedule, and should develop normal hunger drives.

Since starting yeast treatment, I am hungry all the time, and just can't get satisfied. What is the problem, and what should I do about it?

When many of the usual foods are eliminated, some people have trouble deciding what to eat, and they just don't get enough food to satisfy their hunger. Like a reduced-calorie diet, this will cause a great increase in hunger. The menu suggestions and recipes in Appendix 6 and Appendix 7 should help you to eat enough good-tasting foods to satisfy your needs.

Food addiction, and subsequent withdrawal, can lead to cravings, hunger, or a strong desire for those particular foods. If your hunger is for a specific type of food (like sweets), you could be going through an addictive, withdrawal reaction. Appendix 2 gives suggestions on how to deal with an addictive problem.

Is it okay to use artificial sweeteners in place of sugar?

Our experience has convinced us that artificial sweeteners cause a number of problems. In the first place, they don't deliver the weight loss that they promise in the diet-drink commercials. In fact, there is now good experimental evidence to suggest that they make people fatter. In addition, they seem to enhance the desire for sweet foods. When using artificial sweeteners on a regular basis, most people will want soft drinks, pastry, cookies, or other sweet things to satisfy them when they get hungry.

It is very important that you stay away from all highly sweetened foods so the healthy foods (which should become the mainstay of your diet for a lifetime) begin to taste good to you. Within ten days to two weeks of avoiding sweetened foods, you'll find that healthy foods taste much better—and sweeter—than they did before!

The response of our bodies and brains to the food we eat seems to be important in controlling hunger and keeping brain chemistry in balance. The use of sugars or artificial sweeteners seems to interfere with this process. When you use sweeteners regularly, healthy foods are just not sweet enough to shut off your eating drive and give you a full, satisfied feeling after eating. Using sweetened foods regularly also impairs production of the neurochemicals that normally make you feel contented and happy after eating.

The newest artificial sweetener, Nutrasweet (aspartame), is a combination of two amino acids, aspartic acid and phenylalanine. Phenylalanine is converted into various neurotransmitters, and taking extra phenylalanine in the form of aspartame may interfere directly with the balance of brain chemicals. It has now been shown experimentally that aspartame does change the balance of neurohormones in various areas of the brain.

Many people use artificial sweeteners instead of eating when they are hungry. In our opinion, using diet drinks or other non-nutrient substances to cut back on eating makes no sense considering what we now know about weight control. Our experience shows that artificial sweeteners have no useful function at all, and only create problems. The sooner you get them completely out of your diet, the better off you will be.

I had rapid improvement at first on the yeast control program, but after a few months, my improvement is very slow. What am I doing wrong?

Sometimes people are completely better in a few months, but most people enjoy rapid improvement at first and then slower improvement. Many people are 50 to 75 percent improved after three months, but require another year or more to improve the rest of the way. Some people aren't 100 percent better even after an entire year. The yeast problem often emerges gradually over the course of many years, and may take a long time for complete reversal of problems. Nutritional supplements may help, but even they take several months to normalize body functions.

As more research is done, we will know more about specific deficiency states or other problems associated with yeast overgrowth. When this happens, we will have better treatment for specific problems, and thus be able to get quicker results.

I have taken Nystatin for six weeks, and faithfully followed the diet with no improvement at all. What do I do next?

If you have no improvement with Nystatin, a Nystatin-resistant strain of yeast may be causing the problem. Try a Caprylic acid product (Caprinex or Capricin), or see if your doctor will give you a trial of Nizoral for two to four weeks. If you improve while using these other products, then continue treatment with them. If there is still no improvement, we have to conclude that yeast is not the cause of your problems.

Other microorganisms may overgrow in the intestines and cause similar problems. If you have many intestinal problems, especially diarrhea, it is certainly possible that you have a Giardia or Amoeba infestation. We often do a stool culture in this situation, but a culture doesn't always identify a bug. We sometimes try Flagyl in this situation, and have seen some very favorable responses. Chronic virus infections now appear to be fairly common, and may cause symptoms very similar to those caused by yeast. Much research is being done on methods to identify and treat these chronic viral states.

Allergies or adverse reactions to various foods and chemical substances can cause a wide range of problems. Although yeast overgrowth is very often at the root of an immune-allergy problem, it is not the only reason for people to begin allergic reactions. See Appendix 2 for further information.

I made a lot of improvement and felt good after one month of treatment, but then some of the symptoms came back and I don't feel as well. What is the problem?

Many people discover allergic reactions to foods that they try to add back into the Phase II diet. These are usually fairly rapid responses, and easy to identify. In some cases, a delayed reaction to an added food may cause problems. In other cases, a food may cause no reaction when you add it the first time, and you may assume it's safe—but when you start using it as a regular part of your diet, a cumulative allergic reaction may occur. Go back to the Phase I diet. If you begin to feel better, one or more of the foods that you added back to the diet were probably the problem. This time, add only one new food every three days, watching for delayed reactions. Then use each new food item only once every four days (in other words, rotate your foods). See Appendix 2 for further information.

It is also possible that yeast-containing products have toxins that will cause problems, and even though you don't respond immediately after eating a slice of bread, you may not feel as well when you are eating yeast products. By experimenting, you should be able to tell whether yeast products are a problem for you. Even if you think yeast breads and other yeast products are safe, it is a good idea to use them in small amounts, and find ways other than yeast bread to eat your whole-grain products.

If you are a female with ovaries intact, it is possible that feeling bad again may be due to cyclical hormonal changes. Most women are somewhat familiar with premenstrual syndrome, or PMS (see Appendix 5 for information about PMS). Chart your symptoms on a calendar; if you consistently have a pattern of good days alternating with bad days that is related to your cycle, you could have PMS. Sometimes feeling bad again after initial improvement is a result of arriving at the bad time of the menstrual cycle. If the worsened state continues for more than three weeks, then PMS is probably not the culprit.

Allergy to chemicals or inhalant plant materials could also make you feel worse. When the pollens begin to flourish, many people don't feel as well. Some people have an interesting allergy pattern in which they can tolerate certain foods most of the year, but during the pollen season, they react. The reaction might occur to a combination of elements in the food and the pollen, or something common to the two might be cumulative enough to cause a reaction.

Any new exposure to chemical substances may cause problems for you. You might react to a new carpet, a pesticide you or your neighbor have sprayed on the lawn or trees, fumes from turning your furnace on for the first time in the fall, pollution build-up from an inversion or other change in climatic conditions, a new perfume that you have started wearing, a new bath soap, fabric softener, laundry detergent, air freshener, or many other things.

As you become more familiar with these types of problems, you will probably be able to identify and correct your difficulties. Professional help from a doctor interested in these problems may also be beneficial.

I got a rash after starting on Nystatin. What do I do?

The rash is probably an allergic reaction to either Nystatin, the Lactobacillus product, or something in the diet. Stop the Nystatin and the Lactobacillus. The rash should go away within a few days. If it hasn't started clearing up within one week after you stop taking the medications, it is likely that something in the diet is causing trouble. It is also possible that an unrelated problem is causing the rash, and just started at that time by coincidence. You should see your doctor if it has not cleared adequately by the end of one week. If itching accompanies the rash, take 25 to 50 mg of Benadryl three times a day.

If the rash goes away in a few days after stopping the medications, it is probable that one of them was the cause. Add back the Lactobacillus product cautiously (one small dose daily), since it seldom causes severe reactions. If the rash does return, stop Lactobacillus immediately. If no rash occurs, the Nystatin probably caused the problem. Because of the potential for a second reaction being more severe, it is not a good idea to try Nystatin again. Stay with the diet, and when the rash is completely gone, try some other yeast-killing product.

My child has vomiting and diarrhea, and I am supposed to give him clear liquids. What do I do?

Most clear fluids are either mainly sugar or fruit juice. For someone with a healthy immune system, these products may cause no problem. But to be safe, use something without refined sugar. Apple juice seems better than refined sugar, and can be used diluted with water for a baby. Beef broth is also an acceptable clear fluid. The most important consideration is to prevent dehydration, and if you can't get enough fluid into the child through apple juice and beef broth, by all means add soft drinks or jello water.

Since diarrhea is notorious for disrupting the normal balance of intestinal microorganisms, it is a good idea to use Lactobacillus for two weeks after any episode of diarrhea.

When can I begin taking the Nystatin pills instead of the powder?

By the time you are taking the powder at the full dosage (one-half of a teaspoon four times a day), and are free of die-off symptoms, you can switch to the pills. This usually occurs at about the second week of treatment, about the time that the first container of powder is running out (we usually prescribe 20 grams of Nystatin). Since the pills are not broken down until they get into the stomach, they may not help as much as the powder in clearing symptoms of sore mouth, heartburn, and indigestion. Some people use both: powder at home once or twice daily, and the pills when they are at work or away from home. If you have no upper intestinal problems, you may wish to stay with the pills exclusively. Watch for any unusual reactions or unpleasant symptoms. If you have problems, go back to using the powder. If you tolerate the pills, keep using them. Remember that the usual dose is four pills four times daily, for a total of sixteen pills per day. Each pill is equivalent to one-eighth of a teaspoon of powder.

How long do I stay on the Nystatin?

You should stay on Nystatin for at least three months. If you feel completely well by that time, you can reduce the dose and then stop. As long as you are having problems, but continue to experience improvement, you should continue to take Nystatin. Some people who have been ill for a long time, or who have severe symptoms, may need to keep taking it for many months or even years. When you decide to stop taking Nystatin, try cutting the dose in half for one month, watching closely for the return of any symptoms that had cleared with treatment. If you feel just as well with the lower dose, then stop Nystatin completely, again watching closely for any problems. If you begin to experience the return of symptoms, go back on Nystatin again for a month or so before trying to stop it. Don't wait until all your symptoms return before getting back on treatment.

I feel better and have more energy when I eat things that contain sugar. How am I going to survive the fatigue when I'm off sugar?

The fatigue you feel when you stop eating sugar may result partly from simply not getting enough total calories to provide all of your energy needs. Make sure that you are eating plenty of good, nutritious food.

The usual problem, however, is addiction. Many people are addicted to sugar, chocolate, and caffeine. When they stop eating foods with those ingredients, they suffer withdrawal symptoms—one of which is extreme fatigue. Most people will get over these symptoms in a few weeks if they faithfully avoid the problem foods. If your problems get progressively worse after one week, you may need to deal with the addiction more directly. Read the section of Appendix 2 that deals with addiction, and follow those suggestions.

I'm pregnant. Can I go on the yeast control program?

Nystatin appears to be very safe during pregnancy; the Physician's Desk Reference contains no warning about its use during pregnancy. In the small dosages originally prescribed, it does not seem to be absorbed into the bloodstream. In the larger doses that we recommend, small amounts do seem to be detectable in the bloodstream. For this reason, we generally reduce the dosage during pregnancy to one-fourth of a teaspoon, or two pills four times a day. If your problems are not severe, we suggest that you wait until after the first trimester of the pregnancy (the first thirteen weeks) before starting treatment, just to be extra safe. If your symptoms are relatively unpleasant, we recommend treatment, since the risks of continuing intestinal problems with possible malabsorption of food, or emotional problems with extra strains on a marriage relationship, greatly outweigh any potential risk from the medication. Some of the over-the-counter products also seem to be very safe during pregnancy. Nizoral should definitely not be used, unless under extreme circumstances determined by your physician.

If I need to go on an antibiotic, should I take one, or will it cause a worsening of the yeast problem?

Many infections are caused by viruses; even if bacterial, many are mild enough that your own immune system can clear them without antibiotics. An antibiotic should be used to treat a clear-cut bacterial infection that is potentially dangerous. Tell your doctor that you are reluctant to use an antibiotic unless absolutely necessary. He should be willing to work with you, possibly take a culture, or wait for a few more days to see how the infection develops. If he feels strongly that you should take treatment, and you agree, then start the antibiotic.

Some antibiotics are worse than others for causing yeast problems. Plain penicillin or Erythromycin appear to cause less problems than some of the more broad-spectrum antibiotics; they are good choices if appropriate. Taking the Nystatin and Lactobacillus regularly during treatment and for a few weeks after should reduce the risks of worsening the yeast situation from an antibiotic.

Even if you have not recently taken Nystatin, it is a good idea to take it during antibiotic treatment and for one or two weeks following the treatment.

Should I take the Lactobacillus along with an antibiotic, or will it interfere?

The Lactobacillus will not interfere with antibiotic treatment. Some of these Lactobacillus organisms will be killed by the antibiotic, but those that are not destroyed may still have some value. Continue Lactobacillus during the antibiotic treatment and for at least two weeks after you finish the antibiotic.

If I don't follow the diet carefully, is there any sense in taking the medication?

The results are much better with very close adherence to the diet. You should still get some improvement with the medication, even if you don't follow the diet strictly. One of the most significant improvements with yeast treatment is a great reducion in hunger and sugar cravings. The diet gets easier to follow as time goes on. Do the best you can with the diet, and don't be too hard on yourself if you have an occasional problem.

Appendix One
CANDIDIASIS IN CHILDREN

Candidiasis can present unique problems in children, resulting in symptoms and behavioral changes that are not usually seen in adults with candidiasis. Following are guidelines for diagnosing children, a list of potential symptoms, suggestions for prevention, and tips for treatment.

DIAGNOSING CANDIDIASIS IN CHILDREN

Although adults can usually be diagnosed with the help of a questionnaire that assesses symptoms and medical history, that technique does not work well for children. If a child has one of the following predisposing factors and at least two of the following symptoms, candidiasis is highly probable.

PREDISPOSING FACTORS:
1. **Thrush** (white patches in the mouth) or diaper rash as a baby. Although these Candida-produced problems will usually clear up completely, they may indicate the tendency towards chronic problems later.
2. **Poor Nutrition,** regardless of the reason. A child may not eat enough because of poor appetite, or may miss essential nutrients because of a diet that is too high in refined or processed foods. Medical problems could also prevent a child from absorbing the nutrients he does ingest, leading to problems with the immune system.
3. **Antibiotic use** can predispose children to candidiasis. Although frequent antibiotic use is most often the culprit, even occasional antibiotic use can cause candidiasis.

CANDIDIASIS SYMPTOMS IN CHILDREN

1. **Gastrointestinal disturbances,** including abdominal pains, stomach-aches, frequent diarrhea, frequent constipation, alternating diarrhea and constipation, cramps, gas, and bloating.
2. **Behavior and learning problems,** including hyperactivity, learning disability, attention deficit disorders, poor memory, and aggressive or otherwise inappropriate behavior.
3. **Mood problems,** including rapid swings in mood, depression, irritability, anger, frustration, and unreasonable fears.
4. **Muscle problems,** including muscle aches, cramps, muscle fatigue, and incoordinated muscle activity.
5. **Sugar cravings** or strong drive for sugar-containing foods.
6. **Allergic reactions,** including asthma, eczema, hives, runny or stuffy nose, or known reactions to various foods, chemicals, or other substances. Allergy problems that begin after antibiotic use are particularly indicative of candidiasis.

If a child has any of the predisposing tendencies accompanied by two or more of the above-listed symptoms, it would be reasonable to start candidiasis treatment. The risks of the treatment are minimal, and the potential benefits are great.

Occasionally, yeast can cause dramatic problems in children. One extremely bright four-year-old was given repeated antibiotics for a stubborn ear infection. He stopped communicating, lost control of his bowels and bladder, and lived in his own little dream world, hallucinating much of the time. After batteries of tests from a score of doctors, he was diagnosed as psychotic with autistic tendencies. Only his mother's determination to care for him herself kept him from being institutionalized. After almost three years, he was started on an effective yeast management program; within a few months, he was communicating effectively, starting to identify the various letters of the alphabet, and progressing rapidly.

Still another child, at one year of age, was progressing normally: he was beginning to feed himself, was almost walking, and was doing all the other things that a "normal" one-year-old does. After several powerful antibiotics for a resistant infection, he stopped feeding himself and stopped trying to walk. He didn't walk until he was two, and when he was seen in the office at three and a half, he still was not talking—nor was he trying to communicate in any other way. He was extremely active, but he had very poor coordination and balance, and he staggered around, falling frequently. He had almost constant diarrhea. With candidiasis treatment, balance and coordination quickly improved and his chronic diarrhea cleared. Candidiasis was obviously a major factor in his illness.

PREVENTING CANDIDIASIS IN CHILDREN

After taking histories from hundreds of patients with typical candidiasis symptoms, we have noticed that many of them began having problems as children. Now that we understand more about candidiasis in general, we can take certain measures to prevent chronic candidiasis.

Breast-feeding infants when at all possible may do a great deal to prevent candidiasis, as well as other infections. Breast milk contains special Lactobacillus organisms, which are not present in cow's milk or commercial infant formulas. It also has special chemicals which promote the growth of healthy bifidus bacteria. In addition, most infant formulas have added refined carbohydrates (often from corn) that may help feed the Candida organisms. A number of our patients have confirmed that various infections began after breast-feeding was stopped and a cow's milk or other formula was started.

Thrush, a Candida growth in the mouth of infants, should be treated adequately. Unfortunately, most treatment is inadequate. Traditionally, treatment involves Mycostatin oral suspension; the manufacturers' recommendations are to use it for at least forty-eight hours after all signs of thrush have disappeared. The recommended dosage is 200,000 units four times daily, and the stock bottle contains enough medicine for about one week's treatment.

There are several problems with the traditional approach to treatment. First, the Mycostatin suspension is about 50 percent sucrose (table sugar), and may contribute to further Candida growth. Second, both the dosage and the duration of treatment are probably inadequate to reduce the concentration of Candida in the intestinal tract. Third, nothing is done to restore the normal balance of Lactobacillus bacteria. We believe that more aggressive treatment is needed in cases of thrush. (Treatment follows.)

Antibiotics should be used sparingly, and only when a definite bacterial infection is present. Whenever possible, avoid the use of broad-spectrum antibiotics. Penicillin, either V or G, and Erythromycin are adequate for the treatment of most infections and are not as likely to kill healthy intestinal bacteria. Nitrofurantoin is usually very effective for urinary tract infections, and is less likely to contribute to candidiasis than the other antibiotics usually used to treat urinary tract infections.

Whenever an antibiotic is used, Lactobacillus should be used at the same time and for at least two additional weeks. If a child already has candidiasis or develops some candidiasis symptoms during antibiotic treatment, nystatin should be started and continued for at least two weeks after the antibiotic is finished.

Refined carbohydrates and artificial sweeteners should be used very little in a child's diet. Besides contributing to candidiasis, excessively sweet foods often interfere with a child's enjoyment of healthy, nutritious foods. It is hard to get children to eat vegetables when they are allowed highly sweetened food—the vegetables taste bland, or even bitter, by comparison. In addition to eating the right kinds of food, it is also important for children and young adults to eat enough of those foods. Many of our patients developed problems after eating poorly during adolescence. Young women who miss meals or severely restrict food intake to control weight should be taught the basic principles of weight loss (see Appendix 4). Besides contributing to candidiasis, chronic dieting usually makes people fatter and contributes to a wide range of other physical and emotional health problems.

TREATING CANDIDIASIS IN CHILDREN

Thrush in babies should be treated with nystatin oral powder if it is available. A reasonable dose is one-eighth of a teaspoon four times daily, which provides 500,000 units with each treatment (about two and a half times the amount provided by the suspension). Treatment should continue for at least two weeks after all traces of the mouth lesions are gone, and even longer if the baby is fussy, irritable, or has colic. Lactobacillus should also be used for this same period of time at a dosage of one-half to one billion organisms daily to restore a normal balance of intestinal microorganisms. If available, **Lactobacillus bifidus** should be used for children under five years of age. The regular adult strains of Lactobacillus may be acceptable, but the bifidus is a more naturally occurring strain in young children.

The dosage of nystatin in children may be varied considerably depending on the response, because it is very safe even in high doses. A reasonable dose is one-eighth of a teaspoon up to the age of about four, one-fourth of a teaspoon for those aged four to twelve, and one-half of a teaspoon for those twelve and older, with all doses taken four times a day. For children who can't tolerate pills, or who have continued problems with thrush, mouth symptoms, heartburn, upper intestinal problems, or allergy to food dyes, the powder should be continued. Many children are more likely to continue treatment or be more cooperative during treatment if they are given the pill instead of the powder. Ideally, the powder should be used first to establish that it is well tolerated, but if it is not readily available, the pills can be started without any problems in most cases.

Follow a diet that will discourage Candida growth. Whenever possible, feed infants breast milk; if breast-feeding is not possible, use a commercial infant formula until the age of one year. If intestinal problems continue despite candidiasis treatment, the infant may have an intolerance to one of the ingredients in the formula; your physician can recommend a substitute.

Because many researchers feel that too-early introduction of solid foods contributes to food allergies, you should wait to introduce solids if you can—a satisfied breast-fed baby could wait one year, and a formula-fed baby who is doing well could wait eight or nine months. If the baby has candidiasis symptoms, however, you should begin introducing solid foods at the age of six months. Add one food at a time, watching for adverse reactions, such as diarrhea or skin rash, that indicate allergic reaction. If the baby tolerates the food well for three days, introduce another new food. Start with vegetables first, since their more complex sugars help to inhibit Candida. Add fruits only after the baby has learned to enjoy a number of vegetables and cereals. Since fruits are sweet, adding them first will often prevent a baby from liking vegetables and cereals which are more bland.

Cereal products can also be added at the same time vegetables are started, using the same policy of adding only one item at a time. Rice and barley are usually well tolerated, but wheat and corn should not be tried until later in a baby who has shown any allergic tendencies or who has a family history of food allergies.

When adding meats, start with lamb, chicken, and veal. Do not give the baby eggs or any foods containing eggs until he is at least one-year-old.

Introduce fruit by giving the baby, one at a time, applesauce, bananas, and pears. Avoid citrus fruits of any kind until the baby is at least one-year-old, since citrus fruits commonly cause allergy problems.

To diminish the chances of developing food allergies, it is best to rotate a baby's food. It's easy to do: when you use a particular fruit, vegetable, cereal, or meat on one day, don't use that same food again until the fourth day. You don't need to be 100 percent strict with rotating, but it can provide a good general guideline. You might consider modifying the entire family's diet so that the child does not feel deprived or singled out—and the entire family will enjoy health benefits from the dietary guidelines suggested in candidiasis treatment, too.

The young child who is home all day is relatively easy to feed properly. When a child begins school and is confronted with school lunch, it is somewhat more difficult. If you can get a copy of the menu in advance, you can often help the child choose appropriate food. You may need to send a lunch on those days when there are no suitable choices, or you may decide that it is more satisfactory to send a lunch all the time. You might try some of the yeast-free breads listed in Appendix 6 in your child's lunch.

The main problem with children of all ages seems to be getting them committed to follow the program. It does little good to eat well at home if they eat lots of sugar at lunch, after school at the convenience store, and with their friends in the evening. After seeing improvement in their condition, most children are prepared to at least try. Some do better if they are given some type of incentive or reward system for good compliance to the diet.

Most children seem to feel better about following the program routinely if they are allowed an occasional exception. It is tough for some kids to think that they can never again have sugar. An exception at Christmas, Halloween, Easter, for birthdays, or for other special occasions does not usually cause lasting problems. If a good meal is eaten first, it greatly reduces the impact of inappropriate foods. On an empty stomach, a sudden load of sugar can sometimes make a child very ill, especially if he hasn't eaten sugar for some time.

Children who do not appear to have allergies can continue to eat whole fruit, even during the first phase of the yeast control diet; fruit provides a reasonable alternative for children who are used to lots of sweets or in situations where there are not many alternative foods available. Again, it is important to watch for adverse reactions, since fruit is a common culprit in allergies.

You do not have to be perfect in feeding your child in order to see many improvements. By making some reasonable lifestyle changes, most children will do very well. The duration of treatment may be shortened with a child in many cases. They seem to be more resilient than adults, and often recover faster from illness. Continue treatment for at least two months; if all the symptoms are gone at the end of two months, reduce the dosage of nystatin (or the alternative yeast-killing medication you are using). If symptoms don't return, you can stop the medication completely. If symptoms still don't return, you can taper off and then stop the Lactobacillus. Continue to restrict sugar. If symptoms return after an illness or after a period of dietary indiscretion, resume candidiasis treatment until all symptoms have disappeared.

Appendix Two

CONTROL OF FOOD AND CHEMICAL ALLERGIES

Our interest in food and chemical allergy occurred almost by accident as we worked with thousands of people who wanted to lose weight. When we eliminated some of the foods they had relied heavily upon, we noticed remarkable improvement in a wide range of chronic problems—including headaches, arthritis, muscle pains, intestinal problems, skin rashes, heart palpitations, cough, asthma, and nasal congestion. Many symptoms cleared up within a few days. Even emotional symptoms—like anxiety, panic attacks, depression, and sleep disturbance—improved dramatically or disappeared entirely. Oddly, when these patients went off the diet we had placed them on, their symptoms often returned, sometimes within a matter of minutes.

At thirty-three, Kathy had suffered for years from chronic daily headaches, severe heartburn, sore throat and ears, abdominal pain, muscle soreness, infertility, and fatigue. A series of physicians had dismissed her seemingly unrelated symptoms as imaginary. Midway through her first week on the yeast control program, Kathy's headaches vanished. By the end of the week, her heartburn and muscle soreness had disappeared. After six weeks on the program, she continued to enjoy improvement. The careful diet transition helped her pinpoint several suspected food allergies.

Part of the explanation for this phenomenon undoubtedly rests with the fact that many traditional weight control diets are also good yeast management diets—and that many of the symptoms these patients suffered could have resulted from Candida toxins. But that's not all: many of these patients were allergic to the foods they had been eating—without even knowing it.

When you eat foods that you are allergic to, you can suffer a wide range of clinical symptoms that don't necessarily seem like "allergic reactions." When you eliminate the foods from your diet, your symptoms will disappear. Following is an explanation of traditional allergy treatment techniques, a listing of typical allergic reaction symptoms, suggestions for controlling your allergies, and an explanation of new techniques for treatment.

THE DEVELOPMENT OF ALLERGY TECHNIQUES

The word "allergy" was coined in 1906, even though hay fever victims had been treated orally with pollen extracts since the late 1800s. The term allergy means a "state of altered reactivity," or as defined in Webster's Dictionary, "abnormal reactions of the body to substances normally harmless." In 1911, a technique of allergy testing was developed in which allergenic materials were injected into the skin and a local skin reaction indicated an allergic reaction.

The substances causing the reaction were later identified as IgE—a special kind of antibody. It was thought that this antibody reacted to specific proteins within the injected material.

Traditional allergy treatment consists of periodically injecting these substances under the skin, in increasingly concentrated dilutions, over a period of years, gradually building a patient's immunity to the allergen. (Incidentally, this technique works reasonably well for allergies to pollens, mold spores, and house dust, but does not work well against food and chemical allergies.)

Pioneers in allergy treatment research found that by starting the injection at doses that caused no reaction, they had the best success. But they found something else out, too: by administering these specific doses, they were able to actually relieve symptoms. The result was a technique called **neutralizing,**[1,2,3,4,5,6,7,8,9,10] which produces almost immediate relief of symptoms.

Researchers pinpointed a wide range of nonprotein substances that cause adverse reactions, and that could therefore be used in allergy treatment. Among them are ethanol (ethyl alcohol) derived from petrochemical sources, formaldehyde,[11] phenol, glycerol, chlorinated water,[12] and a number of drugs.[13,14,15,16] Food additives—including food dyes, monosodium glutamate, sulfiting agents, and nitriting agents—were also shown to cause reactions. Extracts from pine needles and grass are also used in treatment.[17]

It has been discovered that antigens can be given by several techniques in addition to injecting them. Drops given under the tongue (sublingual) are in wide usage[18,19,20,21,22] now, and several studies have demonstrated their effectiveness.[23,24,25,26,27] This allows a patient to give their own treatments at home, and is not painful like the shots. Some allergists are now using antigens in the nose as well.

A breakthrough in allergy research occurred when Brigham Young University researcher Robert W. Gardner discovered that phenolic compounds or aromatic hydrocarbons—which give plants and foods their odor, color, taste, and play a role in growth and disease resistance—were often the source of the allergy, and that phenolic compounds were therefore valuable in the treatment of many kinds of allergies.[28,29,30] This may become of increasing importance in the treatment of those with candidiasis, since the characteristic allergic response in these people is to chemical odors, which are aromatic hydrocarbons. The entire area of allergy research and treatment is still steeped in controversy, however, with traditional allergists battling researchers who look for new treatment techniques. Specific areas of controversy and disagreement include the following:

1. Traditional allergists accept only a narrow range of symptoms as being related to allergy, including runny, congested nose, watery, burning eyes, asthma, cough, eczema, and hives. Many researchers accept a wide range of physical, psychological, and emotional reactions. In our experience, adverse reactions to various substances have been shown to cause migraines and other

headaches, arthritis, fatigue, irritability, depression, and many other symptoms.

2. Traditional allergists claim that a true allergy will result in a skin reaction caused by IgE antibodies. All other kinds of reactions not caused by IgE antibodies are not accepted as allergic.

3. Many traditional allergists reject the phenomenon of neutralization, which is the basis for many of the new treatment techniques.

4. Traditional allergists seem to reject the idea that foods commonly cause allergies. A textbook on immunology published as recently as 1983 devotes only one paragraph out of its 520 pages to food allergy![31] While some traditional allergists claim that food allergies occur in only a few in every thousand people, other researchers estimate that more than sixty percent of us have some kind of food allergy.

Despite the controversy surrounding allergies, several professional associations have been organized to help physicians learn new allergy treatment techniques. One of the largest, with more than 3,000 members, is the American Academy of Otolaryngic Allergy; others include the American Academy of Environmental Medicine and the Pan-American Allergy Society. New techniques are being taught at various conferences and workshops, and have been described in a number of textbooks.[32,33,34,35,36] A number of studies (some double blind) have demonstrated the effectiveness of these new treatment techniques.[37,38,39,40,41,42]

IDENTIFYING FOOD AND CHEMICAL ALLERGIES

Sometimes it's easy to identify an allergy: you react with specific symptoms right after exposure, you react in the same way every time, and the only time you suffer those symptoms is in association with a certain food, plant, or chemical.

Unfortunately, all allergies don't offer such simple diagnosis. You may not react for many hours after exposure—sometimes not until a day or two later. You might react to a specific food or chemical part of the time, but not all of the time. Or you might be feeling terrible most of the time, so it's difficult to distinguish allergy reactions from other symptoms. Even worse, the allergic symptoms might not correspond with the exposure—a food you eat might cause intestinal upset, for example, but it could also give you a stuffy nose or a headache.

Despite these difficulties, you can often identify your own food and chemical allergies if you understand the nature of these allergies and know what to look for. The most common reactions to food and chemical allergies include the following, which are not listed in order of frequency:

Nasal congestion, sneezing, runny nose, sinus pressure

Itching, red, sore eyes

Cough, tightness in the chest, chest pain, asthma, trouble breathing

Swollen tongue, swollen throat

Heartburn, indigestion, abdominal cramps, diarrhea
Fatigue, muscle weakness, headache, anxiety, panic attacks, trouble sleep-
ing, depression, trouble thinking clearly, trouble concentrating, trouble
remembering things, dizziness
Heart palpitations, rapid pulse, cold hands and feet
Hives, eczema, skin itching

FOOD ALLERGY PATTERNS

Food allergies may cause an **immediate reaction** or a **delayed reaction**
may occur hours or days later. There are several different patterns of allergic
reactions:

1. **Fixed reactions** are those that occur every time you eat a certain food.
Even if you haven't eaten that food for years, you'll have a reaction the next time
you do eat it. (This is typically the only kind of food allergy reaction accepted by
traditional allergists, incidentally.)

2. **Cumulative reactions** occur only after you've eaten a certain amount of
food, or only after you have eaten the same food several times in a period of a few
days. You are able to tolerate a certain amount of the food without suffering a
reaction, but above that certain amount you develop symptoms. A classic example is the child who can eat chocolate without any problems but who develops a
skin rash or diarrhea on Easter morning after eating handfuls of chocolate eggs.

3. **Variable reactions** may be the worst of all: they occur without any logical
pattern. You may be allergic to a specific food only during hay fever season, or
only during the premenstrual phase of your menstrual cycle. You might react
only to the cooking odors, but be able to eat the food in a restaurant if someone
else prepares it.

4. **Addictive reactions** occur when you are addicted to a certain food and
then you avoid it for a period of several hours. You're likely to develop unpleasant symptoms—literally withdrawal symptoms—that can include cravings for the food, irritability, anxiety, depression, weakness, shakiness, fatigue,
headache, and generalized aching. As soon as you eat the specific food, you feel
fine again, usually within a matter of minutes—sometimes within a matter of
seconds! If you avoid the food entirely, you can usually overcome the withdrawal
symptoms within a few days to a week; stubborn cases may require a few weeks
to a few months.

You may get the impression that the addictive food is really helping you out
and is your friend. Don't be deceived! In most cases, these foods also cause
reactions, and are thus classified as allergy-addiction. They may cause
headaches, dizziness, fatigue, arthritis, aching, depression, sleep disturbance,
irritability, and many other problems.

Most of our patients who have given up an addictive food have noticed the
clearing of troublesome symptoms that plagued them for many years. In most
cases, they had no idea that ingesting their favorite foods on a daily basis was
causing these problems.

A food allergy-addiction is a true no-win situation. You feel rotten if you eat the food, but feel worse if you don't. The only sensible solution is to give up the problem food entirely. You may suffer some unpleasant withdrawal symptoms for a few days or even a few weeks, but it should be well worth your effort since you should feel so much better afterwards.

Any food can become addictive; the most common offenders include refined sugar, chocolate, coffee, and cola drinks. Remember that it might not be the *food* itself that you are addicted to, but an ingredient in the food instead. If you are addicted to caffeine, for example, you could get relief by ingesting chocolate, coffee, and cola drinks—but if you are addicted to sugar, coffee would not relieve your withdrawal symptoms like cola drinks and chocolate would. If you are allergic to refined sugar, you won't get relief by eating foods that contain naturally occurring sugars, such as fruits and vegetables.

IDENTIFYING FOOD ALLERGIES

Effective identification of food allergies requires that you understand the symptoms that are related to your allergy and that you figure out what kind of allergy pattern is involved. There is a simple way to test whether you are suffering from an allergy to a particular food: eliminate it completely from your diet for four to five days, and see if your symptoms clear up. Try one of these methods of self-testing:

1. Eliminate only one suspect food at a time from your diet. After eliminating the suspect food completely for four or five days, eat it again and watch for reactions. If you eliminate a certain food from your diet and then experience a strong craving for it within a day or two, accompanied by unpleasant symptoms, you probably have an allergy/addiction reaction to that food. Don't wait for four or five days: try the food again immediately, and watch your reaction. If the cravings and the unpleasant symptoms disappear almost immediately, you are probably addicted to the food. Watch how you react over the next several hours, too, since an addictive food that can relieve withdrawal symptoms can also produce similar allergic reactions.

2. Eat a very limited diet for four or five days, restricting yourself to foods that seldom cause allergic reactions. At the end of five days, begin reintroducing other foods as described above, watching for reactions. This technique is described in more detail in *The Type 1/Type 2 Allergy Relief Program* by Dr. Alan Levin.

3. If you can't get your food allergy problems sorted out, you may wish to try a fast *under the supervision of your physician.*[43] Go on a complete fast for four to five days, eating nothing and drinking only spring water; this regimen allows all the food residues to be eliminated from your body. At the end of the fast, add one food at a time back into your diet. At first, eat only a few bites of the food, and watch for reactions during the next twenty-four hours. If you have a reaction, you probably have a fixed allergy to that food. If you have no reaction, test for a cumulative or variable allergy by eating a larger amount of the food—until you

are completely full—and watching for symptoms. If you still don't react, eat the food again for your next meal. If you do not have any reactions, the food is probably safe to include in your permanent diet. Continue testing foods one at a time until you have tested all the common foods in your diet. A prolonged fast like this is an extreme measure, and is only recommended as a last resort measure.

TREATMENT OF FOOD ALLERGIES

Fixed allergies are best treated by complete avoidance of the problem food. You might want to try the food again after three or four months of aggressive Candida treatment—sometimes the effective yeast management, nutritional support, and antioxidant vitamins and minerals will enable you to tolerate the food in small amounts at infrequent intervals. What you thought to be a fixed allergy might have really been a cumulative allergy, and you may be able to enjoy the food on occasion.

Food allergy/addictions are also best treated by complete avoidance. Aggressive Candida management, good nutrition, antioxidant nutrients and exercise make the withdrawal period easier to tolerate. Continue to avoid the food completely for at least six to nine months; you may find after the abstinence period that you can eat it occasionally without adverse reactions. Keep in mind that it is very easy to become addicted again, and never use a formerly addictive food on a regular basis.

Cumulative allergies are best treated with a rotational diet: you can eat each problem food once every fourth day, but not more often. (A number of doctors suggest that rotating all the food you eat can help prevent the development of food allergies.)

NEW ALLERGY THEORIES

The physicians who are now addressing food and chemical allergies are finding new contributing causes and treatments as they do extensive research. Treatment with various vitamins, minerals, and other antioxidant substances has been shown to reduce some allergic reactions.

The Free Radical Theory: Adverse reactions may result from the action of free radicals, electrically unbalanced molecules which attach themselves to various receptor sites or other locations to cause problems.[44] Normally, a system of antioxidants or free radical quenchers inactivates these toxic substances. Various vitamins (A,C,D, and E) and selenium, as well as enzymes, act as antioxidants. Dr. Stephen Levine describes clearing his own chemical allergies by using these antioxidant supplements. He has also described a revealing experiement in which fasted rats were injected with a toxic substance. This substance was fatal at only 1/25 the dose required to kill normally fed rats.[45] Antioxidants were shown to be protective from these toxic effects. Again, we wish to emphasize the extreme importance of eating plenty of wholesome, unrefined foods in order to provide adequate levels of these protective substances. Those with allergies could also benefit from adding antioxidant supplements. (See Chapter 7.)

Prostaglandins and Similar Hormones: There have been a number of special hormones recently discovered which are controlling hormones. They are all formed from various fatty acids, and seem to balance each other. When some of these hormones are produced in excessive amounts, adverse responses like asthma, arthritis, and menstrual cramps may occur. Drugs found to effectively treat these conditions are now recognized as prostaglandin-blockers.

There are "good" prostaglandins which can counteract the effects of the "bad" prostaglandins. The balance between the "good" and the "bad" depends upon the type of fatty acids in the diet. By changing the diet to eliminate unhealthy fats and increase healthy fatty acids, various symptoms have been shown to improve. Fatty acid supplements may help as well. (See Chapter 7 for suggestions.)

Other diseases may also contribute to allergy, according to some researchers. We know that candidiasis can aggravate allergies, and that effective treatment can reduce allergic reaction. Chronic Epstein-Barr Virus Syndrome, a chronic infection with the virus responsible for Infectious Mononucleosis, is associated with allergies in 65 to 85 percent of those who have the condition. Other virus infections may also adversely affect the immune system causing allergies.

Desensitization and other immune therapy is improving. With a number of new techniques emerging, the next few years should see the development of landmark approaches in the treatment of food and chemical allergies.

GETTING HELP FOR FOOD AND CHEMICAL ALLERGIES

Unfortunately, if you suffer from allergies, you might be caught in the middle of the warring factions: it might be difficult for you to find a physician willing and able to treat you. Many traditional allergists and physicians won't believe that your symptoms stem from allergies to foods and chemicals—you might be told that you are merely depressed or under stress, or that your symptoms are a figment of your imagination. You might even get referred to a psychiatrist. And that's not your only problem: many insurance companies refuse to pay for treatment using the new techniques. If your allergies have interfered with your ability to work, you may not be able to afford the treatment that may really help.

If you suffer from food and chemical allergies, the yeast management diet described in this book has been found to help tremendously for many people. Those with food and chemical allergies often stop reacting after effective yeast treatment. Others may get partial relief from allergic reactions. Additional self-help information is included in the following books: *An Alternative Approach to Allergy,* by Theron G. Randolph, M.D.; *Brain Allergy,* by William Philpot, M.D. (Keats Publishing, Inc.); *The Type 1/Type 2 Allergy Relief Program,* by Alan Levin, M.D. (Jeremy P. Tarcher, Inc., publishers, distributed by Houghton Mifflin Company); and *Food Allergy: New Perspectives,* edited by John Gerrard, D.M. (Charles C. Thomas, Publisher).

If you have severe allergy problems, or if your minor allergies don't clear adequately with yeast control measures, you may wish to find a physician or allergist in your area who can help. When you call the doctor's office for information, ask if the doctor treats food allergies and what methods of treatment are used. To find the name of a doctor nearest you who uses new treatment techniques, you may wish to contact the American Academy of Environmental Medicine, P.O. Box 16106, Denver, Colorado 80216, (303) 622-9755. Send $3.00 and a self-addressed stamped legal-size envelope; they will mail you the physician names in your area along with additional reading material.

1. Rinkel HJ. Inhalant allergy, Part I: The whealing response of the skin to serial dilution testing. Ann Allergy 1949; 7:625.
2. Williams RI. Technique of serial dilution antigen titration. Arch Otolaryngol 1969;89:109.
3. _____. Skin titration: testing and treatment. Otolaryngologic Clinics of No Am 1972; 4:3.
4. Lee C. Relieving acute symptoms of allergy: Definitive testing. Presented at the sixth advanced seminar in clinical ecology. Soc Clin Ecology. Albuquerque, New Mexico, 1971.
5. Hansel FK. Clinical Allergy. St. Louis, MO: Mosby, 1953.
6. Rinkel HJ. The management of clinical allergy. Arch Otolaryngol 1962; 76:489.
7. Rinkel HJ, Lee C, et al. The diagnosis of food allergy. Arch Otolaryngol 1964; 79:71.
8. Lee CH, Rinkel HJ. A new test for the detection of food allergies and pollen and mold incompatibilities. Trans Soc Ophthalmol Otolaryngol Allergy 1962; 3:1.
9. Lee CH, Williams RI, Binkley EL. Provocative inhalant testing and treatment. Arch Otolaryngol 1969;90:81.
10. _____. Provocative testing and treatment for foods. Arch Otolaryngol 1969; 90:81.
11. Lockey SD, Sr. Reactions to hidden agents in foods, beverages and drugs. Ann Allergy 1971; 29:461.
12. Hosen H. Hydrocarbons and other gases, as related to the field of allergy and clinical ecology, p. 262.
13. Mellon MH. Drug allergy. Manual of Allergy and Immunology 1981; pp. 231.
14. Foster DW. Diabetes Mellitus. Harrison's Principles of Internal Medicine, Ninth Ed 1980; pp. 1754.
15. Kirby WM. Chemotherapy of infections. Harrison's Principles of Internal Medicine, Ninth Ed 1980; pp. 573-75.
16. Wendel GD. Penicillin allergy and desensitization in serious infections during pregnancy. N Eng J Med 1985; 312:19.
17. Binkley EL. Botanical Extracts. Clinical Ecology. Thomas 1976; pp. 422.
18. Pfeiffer GO. Sublingual allergy therapy. Trans Allergy Soc Ophthalmol Otolaryngol 1963; 4:82.
19. Pfeiffer GO, Dickey LD. Sublingual therapy in allergy (Instructional course number eight). Trans Am Soc Ophthal Otolaryngol Allergy 1964; 5:37.
20. Pfeiffer GO. Sublingual procedures. Trans Soc Opthalmol Otolaryngol Allergy 1970; 11:104.
21. Morris DL. Sublingual therapy for food allergy. Ann Allergy 1969; 27:289.
22. Mandell M. Symposium on alcohol. Food allergy, food addiction, obesity, alcoholism, and chemical susceptibility. The clinical significance of reactions to ethyl alcohols derived from foods and petroleum. Presented at the Seventh Inter-American Conference on Toxicology and Occupational Medicine, Miami, FL, August 1970.
23. Rapp D. Weeping eyes in wheat allergy. Trans Soc Opthalmol Otolaryngol Allergy 1982; 18/1:159-60.
24. Mandell M, Conte A. The role of allergy in arthritis, rheumatism, and polysymptomatic cerebral, visceral, and somatic disorders: a double-blind study. J Internat Acad Preventive Med 1982; pp. 5-16.
25. O'Shea J, Porter S. Double-blind study of children with hyperkinetic syndrome treated with multi-allergen extract sublingually. J Learn Disabilities 1981; 14:189-91.
26. King D. Can allergic exposure provoke psychological symptoms? A double-blind test. Biological Psychiatry 1982; 16:3-7.

27. Rapp D. Double-blind confirmation and treatment with milk sensitivity. Med J Australia 1978; 1:571-72.
28. Gardner RW. Aromatic and heterocyclic compounds as principal inciters of allergic responses. Presented at Society for Clinical Ecology Fourteenth Advanced Seminar, Callaway Gardens, Georgia, November 4, 1980.
29. Gardner RW. The role of plant and animal phenyls in food allergy. Presented at 37th Annual Congress of the American College of Allergists, Washington, D.C., April 4-8, 1981.
30. Gardner RW. Basic chemistry of allergens. Presented at the Scientific Session at the Dedication of the Princeton Brain Bio Center, Princeton, NJ, June 13, 1981.
31. Barrett JT. Textbook of Immunology. St. Louis, MO: C.V. Mosby Co, 1983.
32. Philpot W, Kalita DK. Brain Allergy. New Canaan, CT: Keats, 1980.
33. Clinical Ecology. Thomas, 1976.
34. Gerrard (Ed). Food Allergy - New Perspectives. Thomas, 1980.
35. Levine AS. Type I Type II Allergy Relief Program. Los Angeles, CA: Jeremy P. Tarcher, Inc., 1983.
36. Randolph TG, Moss RW. An Alternative Approach to Allergy. New York, NY: Harper and Row, 1980.
37. Boris M, Schiff M, et al. Bronchoprovocation blocked by neutralization therapy. J Allergy & Clin Immun 1983; 71:92.
38. Rea WJ, Podell, RN, et al. Intracutaneous neutralization of food sensitivity: a double-blind evaluation. Arch Otolaryngol 1983.
39. McGovern JJ, Rapp DJ, et al. Double-blind studies support reliability of provocative-neutralization test. Arch Otolaryngol 1983.
40. Miller JB. A double blind study of food extract injection therapy: a preliminary report. Ann Allergy 1977; 38:185-91.
41. Miller JB. Influenza: rapid relief without drugs. Clin Med September 1974; 81:16-19.
42. King D. The reliability and validity of intradermal and sublingual provocative testing: A critical analysis of the controlled research. Appendix A: A presentation to insurance companies. Submitted by: SSCE, AAOA, PAAS, 1984.
43. Mandell M, Scanlon LW. Dr. Mandell's 5-Day Allergy Relief System. New York, NY: Pocket Books, 1979.
44. McCord JM. Oxygen-derived free radicals in postischemic tissue injury. N Eng J Med 1985, 312/3:159-63.
45. Levine SA. Free radicals are the toxic species. Allergy Research Review Spring 1984; 3/1.

Appendix Three

HYPOGLYCEMIA

Hypoglycemia, or "low blood sugar," has become the subject of considerable controversy: some doctors think that it is extremely common, while other physicians believe it is quite rare and that most cases are misdiagnosed.

For true hypoglycemia to exist, three conditions need to be present: the blood sugar must be significantly below the normal range; the symptoms in question must occur only when the blood sugar is low; and the symptoms must be quickly eliminated by eating foods that are readily converted into blood sugar. Most hypoglycemia is **reactive hypoglycemia,** which occurs after eating sugar.

To understand hypoglycemia, you need to understand the basics of normal sugar metabolism. Here's what happens:

The major fuel that your body uses for energy is glucose, or blood sugar; you get it from many of the foods you eat. Most glucose comes from carbohydrates, but some proteins and fats can also be converted into glucose. Refined sugar (table sugar or sucrose) is only two sugar units long, and is quickly broken down by the enzymes in your saliva and absorbed into your bloodstream. Unprocessed foods contain carbohydrates in the form of starches, which have many sugar molecules (several thousand in some cases) connected like the links of a chain.

As you chew your food and the enzymes in your saliva and stomach break the food down, dietary fiber is separated from the rest of the food. Simple sugar molecules are then broken off, one molecule at a time, and absorbed into the bloodstream.

Simple sugars are taken to the liver, where they are converted into glucose. Some of the sugar may be stored in the liver as glycogen for later use, while the rest remains in the bloodstream and is circulated throughout the body for fuel.

Fruit sugar is also a simple sugar called fructose. Some people classify it as complex since it is mixed with fiber and other nutrients in the fruit. Fructose doesn't seem to cause as many problems as refined sugars since it doesn't appear to stimulate as much insulin production.

In order for sugar to be used by the cells, the hormone insulin must be present. Produced by the pancreas, insulin attaches itself to the cell membranes and helps transport the glucose into the cells. If there isn't enough insulin, or if the insulin isn't doing its job properly, the glucose doesn't go into the cells; instead, it stays in the bloodstream, creating a condition of high blood sugar. If too much insulin is produced by the pancreas, too much of the glucose goes into the cells and too little remains in the bloodstream. The result is hypoglycemia, or low blood sugar.

How does the body know how much insulin to produce? A variety of signals trigger the insulin production that then helps normalize the level of glucose in the bloodstream. Foods that contain carbohydrates usually taste sweet, and the sweet taste triggers the release of insulin into the bloodstream from the pancreas even before any of the sugar is actually absorbed. This initial release of insulin is called the **cephalic phase.**[1,2] During the cephalic phase, the liver is primed so that it will be able to store much of the glucose that arrives in the bloodstream.[3]

Once the sugar from ingested food enters the bloodstream, the rising level of glucose in the blood triggers the majority of the insulin that is released. When there is an effective cephalic phase of insulin production, much of the sugar is taken into the liver, and the rise of blood sugar is gradual; relatively little insulin is needed to process it. But when the cephalic phase is inadequate, or for other possible reasons, the liver isn't ready to store sugar. It quickly enters the bloodstream, resulting in abnormally high blood sugar. More insulin is produced in an attempt to process all the sugar in the blood, and as a result the fall in blood sugar is rapid.

Several mechanisms in your body prevent the blood sugar level from falling too low. Your digestive process provides a pretty consistent supply of sugar from the food you eat; once that is gone, the liver releases stored glycogen. As a last resort, your body will convert various proteins—especially muscle tissue—into glucose to maintain the blood sugar level. Various enzymes, hormones, minerals, and vitamins are essential for the maintenance of blood sugar levels.[4,5]

It's easier to understand what happens when you can see the process plotted on a graph. Look at Graph 1: under normal conditions, the blood sugar rises and falls gradually, and the level of insulin in the bloodstream rises slightly just before the blood sugar starts to rise (signalling the cephalic phase of insulin production). Now look at the hypoglycemic pattern: there is no cephalic phase of insulin production before the blood sugar starts to rise. The level of insulin rises dramatically, and the level of sugar in the blood rises rapidly at first but then falls dramatically, falling below normal levels.

SYMPTOMS OF HYPOGLYCEMIA

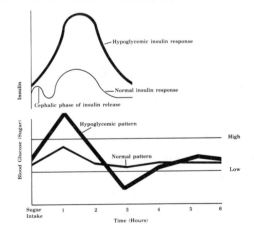

When the level of blood sugar falls too low, your brain and other body cells lack sufficient fuel, and the following symptoms can occur:
Depression
Sleepiness
Trouble thinking clearly
Trouble remembering
Weakness
Fatigue
Poor endurance
Hunger and sugar cravings
When blood sugar gets too low or falls rapidly, your body pumps out various hormones in an attempt to stabilize blood sugar; glucagon, adrenalin, norepinephrine, cortisol, and growth hormone may be produced, and can cause the following undesirable side effects:
Anxiety
Nervousness
Restlessness
Anger
Irritability
Fears
Phobias
Panic attacks
Heart palpitations
Excessive perspiration
Shakiness
Trembling
Dizziness
Mary first developed symptoms of hypoglycemia (low blood sugar) during grade school. She had trouble concentrating and could hardly stay awake during the last hour of school, and then felt very weak as she walked home. A snack made her feel much better, and something with sugar seemed to pick her up faster than anything else. She felt sick if she didn't eat her meals on time, and by the time she was in high school, she had developed the habit of drinking two or three bottles of soda pop per day to boost her energy. Even then, she was fatigued most of the time, and she could hardly function during some classes. She was taken to the doctor, and a glucose tolerance test confirmed that she had hypoglycemia. Several more glucose tolerance tests over the next fifteen years confirmed the original finding, although one test was only borderline.

By staying away from sugars, eating a high-protein diet, and eating six small meals per day, Mary prevented the worst of her hypoglycemic symptoms. But if she was late for a snack by even thirty minutes, she began to feel weak, shaky, and irritable; she often began to perspire, and her heart pounded. She had strong sugar cravings before her periods, and whenever she gave in to them, she suffered headaches, depression, weakness, and dizziness for almost two days.

Mary had many other problems typical of candidiasis, and we started her on a yeast treatment program. By the end of three months, she no longer needed her between-meal snacks. After six months of treatment, she noticed that her strong sugar cravings were gone, but she had indulged in cake and ice cream at a birthday party, with no ill effects afterwards. Her energy and strength were much better, and she no longer had the emotional swings. She felt much the same from one time of the day to the next. If a meal was delayed a few hours, she felt very hungry and still became a little weak, but had none of the other symptoms of hypoglycemia.

FACTORS CONTRIBUTING TO HYPOGLYCEMIA

While we are not certain as to exactly what causes hypoglycemia, we do know that a number of factors may help contribute.

As a result of vitamin or mineral deficiency, obesity, or inactivity, the cells of the body may become resistent to insulin. What happens then? The body produces more insulin to get the job done. At first, while the extra insulin is being produced, the blood sugar level is too high; once all the extra insulin gets into the bloodstream, however, it falls too low.

Prolonged fasting, skipping meals, and adhering to deprivation diets that don't supply enough food can interfere with the cephalic phase of insulin production. When the cephalic phase doesn't work properly, the liver isn't primed to store the excess blood sugar, and too much glucose ends up in the blood. The result? The body pumps out more insulin in an attempt to lower the blood sugar—and when it does its job, the blood sugar level goes too low.

If you consistently eat foods that are sweet, you may condition your body to release insulin only in response to very sweet foods—other foods, such as meat, vegetables, grains, milk, and so on, will no longer trigger the cephalic phase of insulin production because the body doesn't interpret them as being "sweet." If you consistently use foods sweetened with artificial sweeteners, the same thing can happen: the artificially sweet food triggers the release of insulin, but the sugars (glucose) never arrive. After a while, the body recognizes the deceit—and even when you eat genuinely sweet food, your body doesn't produce insulin during the cephalic phase.[6,7]

Eating foods rich in refined sugar can also contribute to hypoglycemia: they are broken down and absorbed more quickly, causing a rapid rise in blood sugar. Extra insulin is pumped out to stabilize the situation, and the excessive insulin causes blood sugar to drop below normal levels. There's an accompanying complication, too—diets high in refined sugar often lack adequate nutrients, so the body cells may begin to resist insulin, as explained earlier.

Hypoglycemia can also result when the pancreas and adrenal glands fail to produce enough hormones to counteract the insulin. Some authorities believe that constant stress, for example, may result in "adrenal exhaustion," crippling the adrenal glands and compromising hormone production. Other potential causes of hypoglycemia include food allergies and Candida toxins, both of which seem to interfere with many of the enzymes critical to sugar metabolism.

Candidiasis seems to be a major cause of hypoglycemia symptoms. Perhaps most of the people we see with suspected candidiasis have typical hypoglycemic symptoms. Yeast toxins somehow interfere with the uptake of sugar by the cells, and also seem to interfere with the breakdown of glycogen and protein to stabilize blood sugar.

DIAGNOSING HYPOGLYCEMIA

The traditional diagnostic test for hypoglycemia is a five- to six-hour glucose tolerance test. After an overnight fast, a blood sample is taken and tested for blood sugar level. You are then given a glucose solution to drink, and your blood is tested half an hour later, an hour later, and then every hour for the remainder of the test. Hypoglycemia is diagnosed if your blood sugar level drops to excessively low levels, if you experience unpleasant symptoms at the same time your blood sugar level drops, and if the unpleasant symptoms vanish when your blood sugar returns to normal.

Unfortunately, it's not all that clear-cut. We used to routinely do a glucose tolerance test on all new weight control patients and anyone with hypoglycemic symptoms, and have administered thousands of them. Many people with perfectly normal tests experienced severe symptoms. Others with no symptoms at all frequently had a hypoglycemic pattern. Much more appears to account for symptoms than the level of sugar in the blood. We now rely more on the clinical picture and do fewer glucose tolerance tests. Various factors may account for the difference between the results of the glucose tolerance test and the clinical picture. Your body may pump out excessive hormones, which succeed in elevating your blood sugar level but that cause a variety of horrid symptoms. As a result, your test would show normal blood sugar levels, even though you suffer numerous symptoms.

There are some individual differences in ideal blood sugar levels. One person may start experiencing symptoms at a blood sugar level that is considered to be normal. Others may function normally with no symptoms at a blood sugar level considered to be in the hypoglycemic range.

There are a number of other problems with the glucose tolerance test, but most of them can be compensated for by careful testing procedures. The following guidelines can increase the test's accuracy as a diagnostic tool for hypoglycemia:

1. Make sure the test lasts for at least five, and preferably six, hours. The original glucose tolerance test was developed to diagnose diabetes, and lasts only three hours—which is not enough time to diagnose a drop in blood sugar levels.

2. Don't use a glucose solution that has been artificially flavored and colored with additives to which you are allergic. Many solutions are made from corn syrup, which is a problem for those sensitive to corn. An allergic reaction often raises or lowers the blood sugar, thus interfering with the test.

Unfortunately, your body processes the glucose solution differently than it processes candy, soft drinks, and other sweets that you normally eat—so the reading on the test may not be entirely accurate. It would probably be better if the physician administering the test gave you the sugar sources that you normally eat, but then other physicians would probably not accept the test results.

3. Precede the test with three days of "carbohydrate loading"—eating foods rich in carbohydrates. Your liver will fill with stored glycogen, preventing the wild swings in blood sugar levels that can otherwise occur during the test. (This is a particular problem for dieters, who tend to eat few carbohydrates and whose test results will be inaccurate.)

4. Even though blood testing is done hourly during the test, alert your physician immediately if you start to experience unpleasant symptoms between test times. Sometimes the drop in blood sugar levels is brief, and hormones stabilize it before it can be detected by hourly blood testing. Testing at ten- or fifteen-minute intervals during problem times when you are experiencing symptoms may pick up a low blood sugar reading which might otherwise be missed.

5. Make sure that the physician interpreting the test takes into account the blood sugar level readings *and* your description of symptoms during the test. Your condition during the test is essential in interpreting it. Even if your blood sugar levels are normal, and you do not have hypoglycemia, you could have some other problem that needs to be addressed if you get sick during the test.

6. Remember that other conditions can produce symptoms similar to those of hypoglycemia. Food addiction, food allergies, and Candida toxins, among other things, can cause hypoglycemic-like symptoms.

TREATMENT OF HYPOGLYCEMIA

The traditional treatment for hypoglycemia has been a low-carbohydrate diet of frequent, small meals, usually six a day. Interestingly, exactly the same diet has been effective in controlling candidiasis—which could indicate that controlling yeast overgrowth is an important part of correcting hypoglycemia.

We have a number of concerns about the traditional approach to treatment of hypoglycemia:

1. **Traditional treatment does nothing to correct the basic metabolic problems that cause the hypoglycemia.** The low-carbohydrate diet controls symptoms, but does nothing to correct the cause.

2. **Low-carbohydrate diets are not healthy for prolonged periods of time.**

3. **The low-carbohydrate diet is clearly less effective than a high-complex-carbohydrate diet in controlling insulin problems.** Extensive research has shown that a high-complex-carbohydrate, low-fat diet is the best in helping normalize insulin production;[8,9,10,11,12,13] diabetics who follow it are often able to stop using insulin entirely. Since hypoglycemia is basically an insulin problem, it may respond to the same kind of dietary guidelines as for diabetes.

4. **Eating small meals may make hypoglycemia worse.** Consistently eating less than you need to make you feel full can stimulate your body's natural starvation defenses—and you feel hungry, crave sweets, and become tired, irritable, and depressed. In addition, eating small meals can inhibit cephalic insulin production, making hypoglycemia worse.[14] Finally, nutritional deficiencies common with eating small meals can aggravate the conditions that cause hypoglycemia.

Sound treatment principles include the following guidelines:

1. **Use effective candidiasis treatment measures when evidence of candidiasis exists.** This has been a most effective treatment for the hundreds of hypoglycemic patients we have treated. Many people who still had troublesome symptoms in spite of careful adherence to a traditional hypoglycemic diet, have been completely cleared of symptoms with effective yeast treatment.

2. **Exercise.** Effective, regular, consistent exercise results in several metabolic improvements that help correct the cause of hypoglycemia.

3. **Strictly avoid refined carbohydrates and artificial sweeteners; eat a diet low in fat, moderate in protein, and high in complex carbohydrates.** The Candida control diet, as outlined in this book, is ideal; if you are also concerned about weight control, limit the amount of fat to levels lower than suggested in this book. Suggestions for appropriate fat content can be found in *How to Lower Your Fat Thermostat* (Vitality House International).

4. **Eat until you feel full at least twice a day.** You can eat more often than that—six times or more, if needed to control symptoms—but at least two of your meals should make you feel full. If you are eating the right kinds of foods and exercising, you should not gain weight.

5. **Use nutritional supplements.** Make sure that you eat healthy, well-balanced meals, but you might also need a nutritional supplement at first. Follow the general guidelines in the text. Dr. Carlton Fredericks[15] also suggests taking methionine (an amino acid) and 100 to 200 mcg per day of chromium.[16] Since chromium usually comes from yeast sources, monitor carefully for any adverse reactions.

Remember that hypoglycemia is a chronic disease that cannot be cured, but a life-long treatment plan that includes good nutrition and consistent exercise can keep it under good control in most cases.

1. van Borstel RW. Metabolic and physiologic effects of sweeteners. Clin Nutr Nov/Dec 1985; 4:215-20.

2. Berthoud HR, Bereiter DA, et al. Cephalic phase, reflex insulin secretion. Diabetologia 1981; 20:393-401.

3. Rohner-Jeanrenaud F, Bobbioni E, et al. Central nervous system regulation of insulin secretion. Szabo AJ ed. CNS regulation of carbohydrate metabolism. New York: Academic Press, Inc 1983; p. 193-220.

4. Bolli GB, Dimitriadis GD. Abnormal glucose counterregulation after subcutaneous insulin in insulin-dependent diabetes mellitus. N Eng J Med 1984, 310:1706-11.

5. Bolli GB, Gottesman IS, et al. Glucose counterregulation and waning of insulin in the somogyi phenomenon (posthypoglycemic hyperglycemia). N Eng J Med 1984; 311:1214-19.

6. Nicolaides S. Sensory-neuroendocrine reflexes and their anticipatory and optimizing role on metabolism. Kare M, Maller O, eds. The chemical senses and nutrition. New York: The Nutrition Foundation 1977; 123-43.

7. Deutsch R. Conditioned hypoglycemia: a mechanism for saccharin-induced sensitivity to insulin in the rat. J Comp Physiol Psychol 1974; 86:350-58.

8. Anderson JW, Sieling B, Chen W-JL. Professional Guide to HCF Diets. Lexington, KY. HCF Diabetes Research Foundation, 1981.

9. Anderson JW. The role of dietary carbohydrate and fiber in the control of diabetes. Adv Intern Med 1981; 26:67.

10. Burkitt DP, Trowell HC. Refined Carbohydrate Foods and Disease. New York: Academic Press, 1975.

11. Miranda PM, Horwitz DL. High-fiber diets in the treatment of diabetes mellitus. Ann Intern Med, 1978; 88:482.

12. Kiehm TG, Anderson JW, Ward K. Beneficial effects of a high carbohydrate high fiber diet on hyperglycemic diabetic men. Am J Clin Nutr 1976; 29:895.

13. Anderson JW, Ward K. High carbohydrate, high fiber diets for insulin-treated men with diabetes mellitus. Am J Clin Nutr 1979; 32:2312.

14. Strubbe JA, van Wachem P. Insulin secretion by the transplanted neonatal pancreas during food intake in fasted and fed rats. Diabetologia 1981; 20:228-36.

15. Fredericks C. New Low Blood Sugar and You. New York: Pedigree Books, Putnam Pub Group, 1985.

16. Offenbacher E, Pi-Sunyer FX. Beneficial effect of chromium rich yeast on glucose tolerance and blood lipids in elderly subjects. Diabetes 1980; 29:919-25.

Appendix Four

THE INFLUENCE OF CANDIDIASIS ON WEIGHT PROBLEMS

One of the benefits of treatment for candidiasis in overweight people is weight loss—even without a conscious effort at "dieting." Extensive research has helped us understand the relationship between the two—and basic knowledge of the problems associated with excess body fat help explain that relationship. (**Note:** Throughout this appendix, we refer to overweight as "obesity," even though obesity is technically defined as 20 percent above ideal weight.)

It has long been believed that obesity resulted simply from eating more food energy (calories) than you needed, with the excessive calories being stored as fat. Reduced food intake (dieting) was thought to be the answer—and we believed that if people would just use some self-control, they could achieve their ideal weight and maintain it.

These old, simplistic concepts don't hold up to scientific scrutiny. It is now well established that on the average, fat people eat no more than thin people.[1,2,3,4,5,6] Many thin people eat huge amounts of food but stay thin, and many fat people remain fat while eating small amounts of food. Some people remain the same weight in spite of huge variations in their food intake during various periods of their lives. It appears, then, that obesity is really a problem with the way we store fat instead of the amount that we eat.

It seems that the amount of fat storage is closely regulated by centers in the brain—in much the same way body temperature, acid-base balance, and electrolytes in the blood are closely regulated by brain centers. We like to refer to these centers as the **fat thermostat.** The fat thermostat attempts to control the body weight by directing you to eat the right amount of food to keep a stable weight. When your body is in need of food, you start to get hungry, and get progressively more hungry until you eat. After your needs are met, you will feel full or satisfied for a number of hours until your body is again in need of fuel, and the resulting hunger encourages you to eat again.

The fat thermostat also seems to fine-tune the weight by controlling a number of bodily processes that either waste energy or conserve it. When you eat more food than you need, the extra calories are merely wasted by heat-producing cycles. You can put on excess weight by eating more than your body can waste, but most people can eat relatively large amounts and still be able to waste the excess calories.

If you don't get enough food, either because you are starving or dieting, energy conservation systems are triggered in an attempt to maintain your body weight even with a considerably lowered food intake. Your body may not burn as much energy to produce heat, your metabolic rate will fall, and you may feel cold and even have a lowered body temperature. You become tired, feel less like moving, and thus are usually less active while dieting, which conserves energy. You may even develop increased levels of fat-storage enzymes, which will quickly cause any weight lost from dieting to be regained as soon as you return to near-normal eating. Even if you eat less than you did before dieting, you can gain the weight back rapidly.

If these theories are correct, and much scientific evidence suggests that they are, then there are only three ways to gain excessive weight:

1. The level at which the fat thermostat "decides" to control your weight (setpoint) can go up to a higher level. Your weight then stabilizes at a higher level.

2. Something may go wrong with the basic metabolic processes through which your body produces and stores fat, burns fat, and wastes energy, causing excessive fat gain.

3. If you consistently eat more than your energy-wasting systems can eliminate, you might gain weight. Anything that interferes with your normal hunger drive can do it—so can eating in response to non-hunger needs, such as eating excessively for reward, entertainment, loneliness, boredom, and so on. This may be a relative factor, and may only cause weight gain when metabolic problems are present. Keep in mind that thin people eat just as often for psychological reasons as fat people.

It is useful to understand the function of the fat thermostat and the factors that influence the level at which it controls your weight. The fat thermostat is a survival mechanism, and its existence has enhanced our ancestors' ability to survive famines. When confronted with famine conditions, not only does the fat thermostat direct conservation mechanisms to increase the chances of surviving the current famine, but it adjusts upward, causing you to gain more weight while food is available so you can better confront the next famine. Each prolonged period of food deprivation may then cause you to gain a few more pounds.

Unfortunately, the fat thermostat can't distinguish between true starvation and a reducing diet. In our clinical experience, most reducing diets have resulted in a five- to ten-pound weight gain in the long term! Some people have been able to diet themselves into grossly obese proportions, and they are right: the harder they try, the fatter they get!

Your fat thermostat seems to keep your fat stores at a level suitable for providing protection from starvation, but also seems to be "concerned" with your mobility. In primitive societies, the ability to move fast in order to hunt effectively, escape from enemies, and migrate long distances to places where food was available also enhanced survival. These two factors (fat storage and mobility) are not compatible: the more fat you store, the less mobile you are. The fat thermostat seems to "choose" a weight level that will give you reasonable fat storage while maintaining reasonable mobility. If you are very active, especially if you are involved in endurance activities, your fat thermostat will somehow adjust itself to a lower level, as if aware that you are better equipped for continued activity if you have less fat to pack around.

If you become less active, the fat thermostat seems to be aware of reduced activity, senses less need for mobility, and "chooses" to favor the other survival mode, that of storing more fat. The setpoint of the fat thermostat, then, is determined to a great extent by your activity level.

Stress may also have an effect on the fat thermostat. It seems that we have only a few basic responses to stress, and one of them is put on more protective fat. For some types of stress (famine, for example), this is a highly appropriate protective mechanism. In other cases, this stress response is rather inappropriate, and may cause a highly undesirable weight gain. In a sense, this is like the well-known **fight** or **flight response** that is very effective in the face of danger that necessitates either fighting your way out of the situation, or running away. In many stress situations when you don't need to fight or run, the fight or flight response occurs anyway—even though you don't need it, and even though it can harm you over prolonged periods of time.

The type of food you eat also seems to determine your fat thermostat setting. A high-fat diet will produce and maintain a much greater amount of body fat than will exactly the same number of calories from low-fat foods.[7] It may be that when we eat animals that have prepared themselves for winter by putting on more body fat, our own control centers are aware that winter is close, and that more body fat would provide better protection against the impending prolonged period when food will not be as available. This protective mechanism also seems to be triggered when you eat domestic animals—which are fat throughout the year—or when other forms of fat make up too many of your total food calories.

A diet high in refined sugar also seems to cause more fat to be gained and maintained than a diet containing exactly the same number of calories, but no refined sugar.[8] Although the mechanism for this is unclear, it seems to have some direct effect on the level of the fat thermostat.

Candidiasis can influence body weight in a number of ways:

1. Candidiasis may help increase the setting of the fat thermostat. Excessive levels of stress hormones, which appear to be present in many people with candidiasis, may have a direct effect on the fat thermostat. Because of various metabolic problems discussed below, there is often an inadequate amount of fuel available for cellular metabolism, resulting in excessive hunger. The same process that causes you to consciously be aware of hunger may be interpreted by your fat thermostat as starvation, resulting in a defensive move upward to a setting that will maintain more protective fat stores.

Those who experience a weight gain for any reason usually try very hard to take it off. They often start missing meals, cutting down on total food intake, or go on various crash diet programs. All of these eating styles may be interpreted as starvation, resulting in an increase in the level of the fat thermostat, causing weight gain.[9] Thus the efforts to get the weight off may be a major factor for making the weight problem worse.

With each of her three pregnancies, Diane gained about fifteen additional pounds which she had trouble losing. Dieting caused a temporary loss, with a rapid return to her previous weight. With the last few diet attempts, she seemed to gain even more weight than before she started the diet. She was about sixty pounds overweight when first seen at our office. She had many other problems typical of yeast overgrowth, and was started on a trial of yeast therapy.

Within the first week of treatment, she lost eight pounds, even though she was eating as much food as she usually did. She described feeling less puffy and swollen, and her craving for sweets diminished. She found it more comfortable to exercise, and no longer had the soreness and stiffness afterwards. She could walk faster and exercise longer without fatigue. She described an increased energy level, and felt much more motivated to exercise. By the end of the second week, she lost thirteen pounds, and by the end of four weeks, she lost twenty-two pounds. After the initial weeks of rapid water loss, her weight loss slowed down to about one to one and one-half pounds per week. By six months, her weight loss was almost fifty pounds, and she reported never feeling deprived and never suffering from hunger. The depression, irritability, anxiety, sleep disturbance, and digestive problems were mostly gone, and she was feeling very good about herself.

2. Yeast toxins seem to interfere with the movement of glucose (sugar) into the various cells of your body, where it is burned for fuel. After you digest your food and it is absorbed into the bloodstream, your blood sugar may rise too high because it remains in the blood instead of penetrating the cells. This acts as a trigger for the release of excessive amounts of insulin, which by itself can make you fat. When given to experimental animals, insulin causes increased hunger and more eating. Even when no more food is given to these experimental animals than is given to control animals, excessive insulin will still cause excessive fat gain. It seems to do this by converting blood sugar into fat, and then storing that fat in the fat cells. Excess insulin also tends to inhibit or slow down breakdown of fat from the fat stores into a fuel that can be used for energy. Insulin, then, can make you fat and keep you fat.

3. Yeast toxins seem to interfere with sugar metabolism in several ways. Besides interfering with sugar absorption by the cells, several other steps in sugar metabolism are blocked. Normally, the sugar forms glucose—the major source of fuel for most body cells. This glucose can come directly from breakdown of various foods in your intestines, especially from sugars and carbohydrates. Proteins in the diet are broken down to amino acids, and amino acids can be converted into glucose by a process called gluconeogenesis (the making of new glucose). After the food from a meal has been completely digested and no further energy is available from that source, sugar stored in the form of glycogen (in the muscles and liver) can then be converted into glucose and used for fuel. About 2,000 calories of energy are available in this form as a reserve between meals or when food is not readily available. Various protein tissues in the body, including muscle tissues, can also be readily broken down to glucose when energy is needed.

These beautifully designed metabolic systems normally keep the blood sugar relatively constant, and provide a steady source of energy at all times. Yeast toxins may, however, interfere with the various enzyme systems which are responsible for mediating all these processes. If you can't effectively utilize your sugar stores, or break down your amino acids for fuel, then you must rely mainly on food presently in the intestines. Between meals, there may be low blood sugar and excessive amounts of hunger, encouraging the ingestion of more food than your body can effectively waste, resulting in weight gain. As you experience this hunger, it will probably be for carbohydrates, and especially for refined sugars, since the sugars are the most readily available source of available fuel.

4. Yeast toxins may also impair fat metabolism. As mentioned earlier, the higher insulin levels are responsible for producing excess amounts of fats, that are stored in the fat cells. Insulin also interferes with the breakdown of fat stores. Fat is normally broken down into components called fatty acids and glycerol, which are further metabolized to produce energy.

Under normal circumstances, fatty acids are burned almost exclusively through muscle tissue. Special enzymes called beta-oxidation enzymes found in muscle cells are necessary in order to burn fatty acids. Very active people, especially endurance athletes, have large numbers of beta-oxidation enzymes, allowing them to burn large amounts of fat for fuel, while inactive people tend to have very few of these enzymes. Most overweight people are just not active enough to have good levels of fat-burning enzymes, and this is made even worse with candidiasis. There may also be an impairment of the enzyme systems responsible for deriving energy from fatty acid metabolism, thus further limiting the amounts of fats that can be used for fuel.

In a sense, these problems that interfere with fat metabolism could be compared to having huge piles of firewood stacked all around your house, a firm contract with someone who keeps bringing more, and only a very small stove in which to burn it.

5. Excessive levels of hunger, especially a craving for sugar and carbohydrates, is very common in candidiasis. The hunger may be a product of a number of problems. For those who frequently cut down on food intake, it is a natural consequence of starvation. Thin people will also get very hungry and preoccupied with food when they are deprived for a time.

Yeast toxins may, however, interfere with the various enzyme systems that are responsible for providing fuel for your various cells. If you can't effectively utilize your sugar stores, or break down your proteins or fat, then you rely almost entirely on food presently in the intestines for your fuel needs. After the energy from the previous meal is gone, you may experience excessive hunger. Many people will satisfy this hunger with the kind of food that brings the most rapid satisfaction: readily digested, processed, or refined foods. Since these substances are broken down more rapidly than unrefined foods, you may again get hungry before you should—leading to more frequent eating or snacking.

Excessive hunger might strike even while you still have food in your intestines. Because of impaired ability to get the sugar that is there into the cells, a feeling of hunger may result. The rise in blood sugar, excess production of insulin, and resulting fall in blood sugar to low levels may intensify this hunger problem. In this situation, there is not enough sugar present in the blood, often leading to even more eating.

Food addiction may play a big role in excess hunger (see Appendix 2). When you have not recently eaten a food to which you are addicted, you will feel a strong, specific hunger drive for that food. Many people try to satisfy that specific hunger by substituting another food, which only adds further unnecessary food to the system but doesn't really stop the hunger. If you eat the addictive food regularly, it may add enough extra calories to your overall food intake to cause weight gain.

All of these causes of excess hunger seem to lead to the ingestion of excessive amounts of food, and to the ingestion of problem foods. The high-energy foods, that are so often relied on to satisfy hunger, are often high in fat and refined sugar, leading to an increase in the setting of the fat thermostat. The refined foods may further accelerate yeast growth and toxin production. The amount of food ingested because of these problems may be more than can be effectively wasted, leaving the body no choice but to store the extra calories as fat. Keep in mind than many thin people have these same problems, but are able to waste the excess.

6. An impairment in the various energy-wasting systems may lead to excessive weight gain. Thin people waste their energy through a basic increase in the metabolic rate, by burning it through the brown fat to produce heat, and through the sodium-potassium pump. This "pump" mechanism normally transports or pumps potassium into the various cells and pumps sodium out. When energy needs to be wasted, it appears that this cycle can be increased in a way that will accomplish this. Other energy-wasting or so-called "futile" cycles are probably also present in some people.

It is thought that many overweight people have impaired energy-wasting systems, and that this may allow the body weight to get well above that "chosen" by the fat thermostat. Besides the problem of yeast toxins, there may be a number of other nutritional or genetic problems contributing to inadequate energy wasting.

There also appears to be a problem with thyroid function in people with candidiasis symptoms. Most of the patients we see in the office have many of the characteristic features of those with low thyroid. They are usually cold, with a low body temperature, and frequently have dry hair and skin, fatigue, and constipation. The thyroid function tests are almost always normal, indicating normal circulating levels of thyroid hormone in the bloodstream. There appears to be some defect in the level of thyroid hormone inside the cells. This may be a product of impaired transport of thyroid hormone into the nuclei of the various cells where it can perform its usual functions of regulating the metabolism and controlling body temperature. A consequence of this apparent defect is reduced energy utilization, which contributes to weight gain and interferes with attempts to lose weight.

7. Most people with candidiasis do not exercise effectively. This may be because of the fatigue that is almost always present, which, in turn, may be due to the poor availability of nutrients for muscle action. There may be impairments in the cell membranes of the muscles or in the transport systems that allow nutrients (including oxygen) to get into muscle cells. There may also be impairments in the ability to get waste materials out of the muscle cells, leading to muscle aches, pains, and stiffness. These possible impairments may account for the lack of desire to exercise, the discomfort experienced by those who try it, and the difficulty in getting up to a fitness level conducive to effective weight control.

Effective exercise is necessary for weight loss for a number of reasons:

   a.   It has a direct effect in lowering the level of the fat thermostat.
   b.   It helps to increase the levels of fat-burning enzymes in the muscles.
   c.   It helps to improve the sugar metabolism by somehow reducing insulin resistance and thus insulin levels. (This may be one of the mechanisms by which exercise reduces hunger).
   d.   It also seems to decrease food cravings and burns off some energy that might otherwise be stored as fat.

8. Fluid retention often contributes to the overweight situation. It often makes people feel and look more overweight. The reasons for the fluid retention are not entirely clear, but many patients see ten to fifteen pounds of fluid loss within the first few weeks of treatment for candidiasis.

HEALTH PROBLEMS ASSOCIATED WITH OBESITY

It has long been known that people with excess body fat are at greater risk than thin people for developing a number of serious health problems. A panel of experts from the National Institute of Health recently met regarding the problems of obesity, and gave some interesting statistics. In the obese population, high blood pressure and diabetes are three times as common, high cholesterol is twice as high, and various cancers are also higher than in the thin population. In those twice their normal weight, premature death is twelve times higher than for thin people.[10,11]

It has been thought that the fatness itself is the problem, and great efforts have been made to diet in order to reduce the risks of these diseases. There is very good recent evidence to suggest that reduced-calorie dieting is much more responsible for the health problems than is the excess weight itself.[12,13]

Dr. Paul Ernsberger pointed out that in populations where obesity is not considered to be a social stigma, and dieting is just not done, those who are twice their ideal weight have about the same relative risk of dying as do thin people (compared to twelve times higher death rate referred to by the NIH in a study of those who dieted very rigidly).[14] Ernsberger also demonstrated, in a brilliant scientific study, that experimental animals would develop high blood pressure after being dieted and refed repeatedly (very similar to the pattern followed by many typical dieters).

Heart disease is thought to be higher in the obese population than in normal weight population. A well-known lipid researcher, Dr. Peter Wood, points out that eating less food than average is a predisposing factor for heart disease.[15] In the long-term Framingham study, those men who died ate a daily average of 200 calories less than did survivors.[16] The typical overweight person who cuts down food intake to lose weight also seems to be increasing the risk of heart disease.

A group of grossly obese men who had been on a very restrictive diet were shown, in a long-term follow-up study,[17,18] to develop diabetes ten times more often than a group of men who were just as heavy, but who did not diet.[19]

With the recent understanding of the cancer-preventing role of certain vitamins and vitamin precursors found in foods, it is easy to see why the typical on-and-off dieter, who frequently diets strictly and learns to live on relatively small amounts of food between diets, might not get the cancer-protecting effects of those who eat plenty of good, nutritious food. This cancer risk would appear to be even higher in those who eat much of their food in a refined form with very low or non-existent amounts of protective nutrients.

Restrictive dieting also seems to make people more likely to develop colds, flu, or other infections. This may be just a basic stress effect from dieting, but it is more likely that the greatly reduced nutrient intake associated with restrictive dieting somehow impairs the immune system. This lowered immunity may also be a factor that encourages yeast overgrowth, as does the use of antibiotics to treat the infections.

Being overweight can have a crippling psychological effect on many people. It is bad enough to be overweight in a society that tends to adore thin people, but when society in general (and frequently overweight people themselves) believes that the problem is simply a matter of gluttony, laziness, or lack of self-control, then the guilt, shame, and self-loathing are intensified. A high percentage of the overweight population suffers from depression, irritability, sleep disturbance, fatigue, and preoccupation with food. These problems are even further intensified in those with anorexia and bulimia, two even more extreme forms of dieting. Again, it is now thought to be the dieting efforts more than the excess fat itself that accounts for these psychological problems. Yeast toxins and imbalance of brain chemistry can cause these psychological problems or make them worse.

TREATMENT OF OVERWEIGHT

With these new concepts about obesity, it is understandable why reduced-calorie dieting has been so ineffective for long-term weight control, and how it even seems to make the problem worse. Dieting seems aimed at controlling a symptom of obesity - that of having too much body fat - and has not taken into consideration any of the basic causes of the problem. If a weight management program could be designed to move the fat thermostat to a lower level and correct some of the contributing metabolic problems, then the weight should be controlled naturally and comfortably at a lower level, just as what occurs in thin people.

In 1981, one of the authors (Dennis Remington, M.D.), along with an exercise physiologist (Garth Fisher, Ph.D.), and a Ph.D. in psychology (Edward Parent, Ph.D.), developed such a program. This exciting program involves an entirely new concept of obesity, including an entirely new treatment approach. The book, *How to Lower Your Fat Thermostat*, was written as a guide to help people understand and follow that program. Briefly, the basic principles of that weight control program include the following:

HOW TO LOWER YOUR FAT THERMOSTAT GUIDELINES

1. **Eat a wide variety of wholesome food on a regular basis.** By providing your body with its complete requirements for calories, vitamins, minerals, and other essential nutrients on a regular basis, the starvation defenses (which are triggered by dieting) are not stimulated. In response to the other guidelines, the setpoint of the fat thermostat is free to move downward. These adequate supplies of wholesome nutrients are also invaluable in strengthening the immune system and overcoming many of the nutritional and metabolic problems so often associated with chronic candidiasis.

2. **Eat in harmony with the hunger drives from your fat thermostat. Eat when you are hungry, eat until completely satisfied, then stop eating until you are hungry again. Snacking is not only acceptable, but even encouraged in response to a genuine hunger drive.** Begin to eat at regular intervals, even if you are not very hungry at the usual meal times. This will keep you from going too long without eating, which might trigger starvation defenses. It also encourages you to eat the more appropriate types of food usually available with a regular meal, rather than snacking on food later, which may not be quite as suitable. You will soon get into a pattern of becoming hungry at regular meal times, and should find it easy to establish a healthy pattern of meal eating.

In some cases, especially in those with chronic candidiasis, there may be a problem in distinguishing between hunger resulting from a genuine biological need, and the desire to eat for some other reason. Food addiction, the strong desire to eat specific foods to prevent unpleasant withdrawal symptoms, is a common cause for the desire to eat. If you suspect that you have food addictions, you should read Appendix 2 in detail. Hypoglycemia (low blood sugar) may also contribute to a desire to eat, especially between meals, and is described in detail in Appendix 3.

The problems of food addiction and hypoglycemia seem to be very common in overweight patients who have candidiasis. They may be major factors in the gaining of weight, and it becomes very important to effectively deal with these problems. Fortunately, a good yeast control program usually is very helpful, especially when the specific guidelines for food addiction and hypoglycemia are also followed.

For many chronic dieters, who are used to eating an amount of food dictated by some specific restrictive diet, the concept of eating all the food that is required to produce satisfaction is a hard one to grasp. Many dieters have denied their hunger and starved themselves for so long that they don't even know when they are genuinely hungry, or when they feel satisfied. Some dieters describe being hungry all of the time, and never having a feeling of fullness or satisfaction. Many don't trust their own senses, and are afraid to turn themselves loose for fear of gaining a lot of weight. For those who are living with chronic starvation at a weight level lower than dictated by the fat thermostat, there may indeed be a weight gain after starting this weight control program, but it is usually small and temporary as the proper things are done to naturally lower the fat thermostat.

We have seen some interesting cases in which patients have begun to eat more than they have been able to eat for years, and by following the program, have been able to lose weight in spite of a relatively large food intake. We have been involved in a study where those following the fat thermostat program were assigned the number of calories that should have exactly balanced their energy intake and energy expenditure. In several cases, patients felt full for the entire sixteen weeks of the program. In spite of this, these people all lost weight effectively, presumably because they did the right things to lower the fat thermostat and develop their energy-wasting systems to eliminate the extra calories like thin people do when they overeat.

3. **Decrease your consumption of fats.** Dietary fats are a major factor in raising the fat thermostat. Average people in our society ingest 40 to 45 percent of their calories as fat. This not only keeps people fatter than ideal, but also is generally unhealthy for many other reasons.

Ideally between 10 and 20 percent of your calories should be in the form of fat. The book *How to Lower Your Fat Thermostat* has a number of ways to estimate fat intake. The Table of Food Composition lists the percent of fat within each food item. It becomes easy to eliminate those foods higher than 20 percent fat or to eat them in smaller quantities along with foods less than 20 percent in fat. There is also a unique point system to help evaluate a healthy fat intake without having to measure portions or count grams of fat.

It may be adequate to merely cut down on those foods known to be high in fat, and not worry about the precise amounts. If you are having trouble losing weight effectively, you may have to be more careful and start keeping more accurate track of the amounts of fat in each item.

Restricting fat intake too much is also unhealthy. Certain essential fatty acids and vitamins can be obtained in no other way than through fat-containing foods. Be sure not to restrict fat intake below 10 percent. Keep in mind also that some types of fats are healthier than others, and that the polyunsaturated oils, especially cold-pressed northern oils (like linseed and safflower oil) and fish oils (marine oils, fats in salmon and other seafood, and cod liver oil) are ideal fat sources. These type of fats play a preventive role in heart disease, and help maintain a healthy ratio of prostaglandins, which govern many body processes.

To help reduce fat in the diet try the following:

a.   Use skim milk (all the fat has been removed), or 1% milk.

b. Use low-fat cottage cheese.
c. For cream sauces, use skim milk.
d. Dilute mayonnaise, miracle whip, and other salad dressings with plain low-fat yogurt.
e. Use low-fat salad dressings.
f. Use plain low-fat yogurt, dry onion soup, or low-fat cottage cheese to make your own salad dressings or baked potato toppings.
g. There are two ways to defat gravy drippings, soups, or stews. First put the liquids in the freezer for about forty five minutes then lift off the solid fat and throw away. The other way is to pour the liquids into a four-cup fat strainer, wait one minute, and remove the fat.
h. Use extra lean ground beef. For other beef cuts remove all noticeable fat. Use red meats no more than 2–3 times per week, substitute fish or poultry.
i. Remove the skin from turkey, chicken, and fish.
j. Use water-packed tuna.
k. For recipes using eggs, use the whites only.
l. Reduce butter as a spread or ingredient where possible.
m. Instead of frying beef, poultry, or fish, try baking or broiling.
n. Use fresh fruits and vegetables for desserts and snacks.

4. **Reduce sugar intake.** Experiments have shown that adding refined sugar to the diet of animals causes them to gain about 50 percent more fat than animals eating no sugar. In our society, the average person consumes about 125 pounds of sugar per year. This appears to be a major factor in producing obesity.

It is interesting to speculate on why sugar plays a role in causing obesity when exactly the same number of calories of complex carbohydrates will not. The encouragement of yeast overgrowth and increased yeast toxins may certainly be part of the reason, especially in those with chronic candidiasis, but possibly even in those who have not enough yeast in their intestines to cause other symptoms of candidiasis.

Sugar seems to cause problems for a number of reasons. Because it is highly refined, all the vitamins, minerals, and other complex food molecules have been removed. When much of your caloric intake consists of refined foods, you may feel a need to eat more food to obtain the required nutrients. Sugar is very sweet, and something about sweet foods seems to trigger excessive hunger. We have perhaps all experienced being quite satisfied after a meal, having a bite or two of a sweet dessert, and then feeling a renewed hunger to eat considerably more sugar.

When very sweet things are ingested, a release of insulin occurs even before the sugar gets into the bloodstream, and this may play a role in causing fat gain. Even artificial sweeteners, which are 50 to more than 1,000 times sweeter than table sugar, may cause an abnormal release of insulin, and may be the reason why artificial sweeteners often cause a weight gain (see Appendix 2 for details). As long as refined sugar and artificial sweeteners are regularly consumed, your tastes for sweets will be enhanced, making it difficult to enjoy the taste of the more wholesome foods that are so important for good health. Most people will eat the foods they enjoy the most, and if you are going to eat a healthy diet, it is much better if you can stay away from the excessively sweet things so that you will begin to prefer the healthy foods.

Staying away from refined sugars is even more important if you have candidiasis. Although the refined carbohydrates like white flour are not as healthy as unrefined flour, they at least have some of the nutrients and possibly some of the natural yeast inhibitors, and are thus not quite as much of a problem as refined sugar.

5. **Drink water to satisfy thirst.** Water is essential for life, and we all have a "built-in" thirst mechanism to tell us when we are in need of water. If you answer this thirst drive by drinking soft drinks, alcoholic beverages, juice, milk, or other fluids that contain calories, then you're getting calories you don't need. Unless your energy-wasting systems are functioning well, these unnecessary calories may cause excessive fat gain.

It is particularly important for people with candidiasis to avoid soft drinks, alcoholic beverages, and even fruit juice. Even though fruit juice is not as refined as the sugar in soft drinks, it still may cause problems with weight gain as well as yeast overgrowth. An exception to this rule is milk: if you tolerate milk, you can drink two glasses of low-fat or skim milk daily or get an equal amount of milk substitute in a low-fat form.

It is very important to distinguish between hunger and thirst. If you are hungry, it is best to eat good nutritious food which contains fiber, vitamins, and minerals and which provides some chewing and eating satisfaction. If you are thirsty, it is important to satisfy that need with water. This helps you to get in harmony with the basic hunger and thirst needs of your body.

6. **Exercise effectively.** Although exercise is extremely important for effective weight control, most overweight people simply do not exercise. For the overweight person with candidiasis, this seems particularly true. Almost no one will have the strength, energy, or desire to exercise when dieting or eating food of poor nutritional quality. This should all change, however, with effective yeast management and with eating adequate amounts of wholesome food.

You may need to start exercise at a very low level, and may need to build up very gradually. A great deal of help for patients with chronic candidiasis can be obtained by exercising just twenty to thirty minutes at a time three times a week, but effective weight control may require more exercise. Most people with a weight problem should exercise daily, or at least five times a week, for thirty to sixty minutes at a time. Use rhythmic activities, such as walking, running, swimming, cycling, or aerobic dancing, which use the large muscle groups. Exercise at a moderate pace, enough to cause heavy breathing, but not so hard that you feel breathless to the point of not being able to carry on a conversation.

7. **Reduce stress in your life.** For many people, stress has played a major role in initial weight gain, and it continues to play a role in preventing effective

weight management. Stress seems to raise the setpoint and produce other undesirable biological changes, including interfering with the immune system. In our own clinical experience, most of the people who have problems with weight management are those who experience a great deal of stress in their lives.

Some of this stress may be due to inappropriate levels of stress hormones in the body (which in turn can be a product of yeast toxins), but much of it also comes from the way you have learned to respond to life's problems. For most people, considerable improvement will come through effective exercise, good nutrition, and effective yeast management. For many people, however, additional lifestyle changes will be needed in order to reduce stress to a level that will allow the setpoint to lower and the other biological changes to occur which will allow them to become naturally thin.

The results of following this program to lower the fat thermostat have often been very dramatic. Not only is weight lost effectively, but most of the problems usually associated with obesity are frequently eliminated. Plenty of wholesome food can be eaten to counteract the health problems caused by typical calorie-reduced weight management diets, to ensure plenty of energy, and to guarantee freedom from hunger.

The fat thermostat-lowering program has worked particularly well in patients with candidiasis. This program together with effective yeast control has been a most effective combination. Most people with typical symptoms of candidiasis who are overweight should achieve a remarkable improvement in their weight and their health.

If is important to realize, however, that the changes do not always occur overnight, and weight loss is sometimes rather slow at first. If you are used to evaluating a weight loss program only by how many pounds you can lose in the first week or two, you may be disappointed in this one. You need to understand how the program works, why weight loss may be gradual, and what things other than weight loss indicate success if you want to stay encouraged and committed to the program.

Much invaluable help and detailed information to help you be successful is contained in the book *How to Lower Your Fat Thermostat*. The book *Recipes to Lower Your Fat Thermostat* contains recipes suitable for yeast mangement and weight control as well as meal planning ideas, suggestions for problem times like traveling, eating out, and holidays. *Desserts to Lower Your Fat Thermostat* provides delicious sweet treats without the use of sugar, honey, or artificial sweeteners. After the first month on yeast control, this is ideal for the Candida patient wishing to eat an occasional dessert.. This book has been published by Vitality House International. If you can't find these books in your local bookstore, you may wish to order them directly from the publisher:

Vitality House International
1675 No. Freedom Blvd. Suite 11-C
Provo, Utah 846040
To Order: Call Toll Free: 1-800-637-0708

1. Braitman LE, Adlin EV, Stanton JL. Obesity and caloric intake: the national health and nutrition examination survey of 1971-1975 (Hanes I). J Chron Dis 1985; 38:727-32.

2. Keen H, Thomas BJ, Jarrett RJ, Fuller JH. Nutrient intake, adiposity and diabetes. Br Med J 1979; 1:655-58.

3. Kromhout D. Energy and macronutrient intake in lean and obese middle-aged men (the Zutphen Study). Am J Clin Nutr 1983; 37:295-99.

4. Baecke J, et al. Food consumption, habitual physical activity, and body fatness in young Dutch adults. Am J Clin Nutr 1983; 37:278-86.

5. Garrow JS. Energy Balance and Obesity in Man. New York: Elsevier, 1974; pp 84-85.

6. Wooley SC, Wooley OW, Dyrenforth Sr. Theoretical, practical and social issues in behavioral treatments of obesity. J Appl Behav Analy 1979, 12:3-25.

7. Oscai LB, Brown MM, Miller WC. Effect of dietary fat on food intake, growth and body composition in rats. Growth 1984, 48:415-24.

8. Sclafani A, Xenakis S. Sucrose and polysaccharide induced obesity in the rat. Physiol & Behavior 1984, 32:169-74.

9. Keys A. The Biology of Human Starvation Vol. I. Minneapolis, MN: U of MN Press, 1950; pp. 126-27.

10. Krieger L. MDs urged to treat obesity aggressively. Am Med News March 1, 1985.

11. Health implications of obesity. NIH Consensus Devel Conference Statement 1983; Vol 5 No 9.

12. Petersson B, Trell E, et al. Risk factors for premature death in middle aged men. Brit Med J 1984, 288:1264-68.

13. Rhoads GG, Kagan A. The relation of coronary disease, stroke, and mortality to weight in youth and in middle age. Lancet 1983, i:492-95.

14. Ernsberger PR. Neural mediation of genetic and nutritional effects on blood pressure: role of adrenergic receptor regulation in the kidney, brain, and heart. Dissertation Abstracts - Northwestern University, August 1984.

15. Wood R. The California Diet. Mountain View, CA: Anderson World Books, 1983; p. 27.

16. Sorlie P, Gordon T, Kannel WB. Body build and mortality: the Framingham study. JAMA 1980; 243:1828-31.

17. Drenick EJ. Definition and health consequences of morbid obesity. Surg Clin North Am 1979; 59:963-76.

18. Drenick EJ, Bale GS, Seltzer F, Johnson DG. Excessive mortality and causes of death in morbidly obese men. JAMA 1980; 243:443-45.

19. Waaler HT. Height, weight, and mortality: the Norwegian experience. Acta Med Scand Suppl 1984; 679:1-56.

Appendix Five
CANDIDIASIS AND PREMENSTRUAL SYNDROME

As we have taken careful medical histories from women suffering the symptoms of candidiasis, one thing has become clear: if a woman has candidiasis, there is a good chance that she also suffers from premenstrual syndrome (PMS).

What is PMS?

In her book, *Premenstrual Syndrome: A Clinical Manual*, Dr. Jane Chihal describes it as "the cyclical occurrence of various signs and symptoms beginning near or after ovulation and resolving soon after the onset of menses." Some authorities say that at least one week of the menstrual cycle must be free of symptoms—if symptoms are present throughout the cycle, the condition is not technically PMS.

Knowing something about the physiology of the menstrual cycle helps in understanding PMS. The day that menstrual bleeding begins is considered day one of the menstrual cycle; while the average cycle lasts twenty-eight days, many variations occur and are considered "normal." Ovulation usually occurs fourteen days prior to the onset of menstrual bleeding, regardless of the length of the total cycle.

Immediately following ovulation, the body produces the hormone progesterone, and levels of progesterone in the bloodstream rapidly rise and remain high through the twenty-third day of a twenty-eight-day cycle. Progesterone levels begin to fall fairly quickly on day twenty-four, and by day twenty-eight—when menstrual bleeding begins—little or no progesterone is produced.

Many believe that PMS is related to progesterone: symptoms worsen when progesterone levels are high, and are minimal or absent when progesterone is also absent.

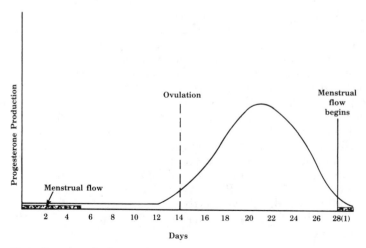

Fig. 1: **Progesterone levels start to increase just before ovulation, and drop rapidly before start of menstrution.**

A strong relationship between candidiasis and PMS is indicated by the following evidence:

1. The symptoms of both conditions are very similar; candidiasis symptoms usually worsen during the premenstrual phase of the cycle.

2. Both conditions are associated with carbohydrate metabolism problems. Both are frequently associated with alcohol intolerance, sugar and sweet cravings, and low blood sugar symptoms, such as dizziness, weakness, and other symptoms relieved by eating[1] (see Appendix 3 for more details).

3. Both have similar predisposing factors, such as multiple pregnancies, chronic dieting, and nutritional deficiencies.[2]

4. A very similar diet has been successful in treating both conditions; avoiding refined sugars seems especially important for both.

5. Similar vitamin, mineral, and fatty acid supplements seem to help the symptoms of both conditions.

6. There is a high incidence of allergy in both conditions.

7. There is usually a significant improvement in PMS symptoms with effective candidiasis management; in some cases, PMS symptoms have been completely eliminated. Some women have reported that their menstrual period caught them unprepared—there were none of the usual unpleasant warning symptoms!

CAUSES OF PMS

We do not know exactly what causes PMS; a number of complex and interrelated factors are undoubtedly involved. In at least some cases, candidiasis seems to be the cause of PMS. The following theories help explain the relationship between candidiasis and PMS:

1. **Progesterone seems to enhance yeast growth and activity.** At times when progesterone levels are high—such as during pregnancy or when a woman is taking progesterone-containing birth control pills—vaginal "yeast infection" is common, and many symptoms of candidiasis are worse. The same thing happens during the premenstrual phase of the cycle.

Here's how it works. With women who have a controlled population of yeast, the amounts of toxins produced is small and can be "detoxified" or destroyed before they cause any problems. Even when more yeast and more toxins are produced premenstrually, there are still no symptoms. If yeast become more numerous, there are enough toxins produced during some days of the cycle to cause mild symptoms. As the disease progresses, the symptoms become more severe and last longer. If the condition gets bad enough, symptoms may occur all month long, although worse premenstrually.

When PMS symptoms begin to occur all month long, some experts would no longer accept a diagnosis of PMS, even though symptoms are much worse premenstrually. We still believe it is the same syndrome as it was during milder stages, and we still call it PMS, for lack of a better name. The following diagram explains this theory.

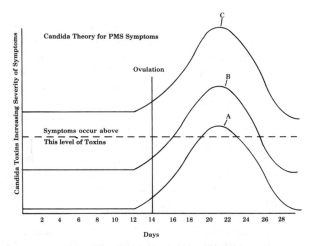

Fig. 2   Candida and Candida toxins increase in last half of menstrual cycle in response to progesterone level. Line A represents modest levels of yeast toxins; enough to produce mild symptoms for only a few days. Line B represents more yeast toxins with more severe symptoms lasting most of the time between ovulation and menstruation. Line C represents more yeast toxins with constant symptoms becoming more severe premenstrually.

2. **Toxins produced by Candida may interfere with the transport of progesterone and other hormones into the various cells.** Most hormones must act on some internal part of the cells, and can only do their job if they get inside. There may be adequate progesterone in the bloodstream, but if it doesn't get into the cells, the result will be the same as if there was a progesterone deficiency.

There may also be a relative imbalance between estrogen and progesterone. Some theorists believe that PMS is the result of too much estrogen and not enough progesterone.[3,4]

3. **Candida produce many metabolic by-products and hormones, some of which are extremely similar to human estrogens.** Candida in controlled numbers are no problem, but in large numbers can produce enough estrogen-like hormones to upset the estrogen-progesterone balance in the body. Candida by-products can also interfere with the ability of cells to receive estrogen, in a sense "competing" with the estrogen. Other by-products can compete with the body's hormone actions in many ways, which may explain the irregular menstrual periods, infertility, and miscarriages suffered by many candidiasis patients.

Candida also have receptor sites on their cell walls for steroid hormones, and may tie up hormones which normally would be used by the body. The imbalances that could result from Candida producing some female hormones and tying up others could be a major factor in causing PMS.

4. **Candidiasis victims generally have a high number of allergies**—and recent research has shown that some women produce antibodies that result in an "allergic reaction" to ovarian tissue and the female hormones produced by the ovaries. The result can be interference with the body's hormone production. If a woman becomes allergic to her own progesterone, she would react to it when it is produced, and then have symptoms during the premenstrual phase of the cycle. This often happens and the medical literature has described a "startlingly rapid and effective clearing of symptoms" with an allergy treatment technique called neutralization[5] (described in more detail in Appendix 2).

Elizabeth was an attractive, vivacious, productive young lady in her mid-twenties who was happy, energetic, and full of life during most of the month. For about ten days during her cycle, she developed a severe, dark, suicidal depression so severe that she had been hospitalized on a number of occasions for her own safety. Various antidepressant drugs were of little value, and even her good times were severely affected by fear and dread of the inevitable episode of hopeless despair before her next cycle. Similar symptoms could be triggered even in the good phases of the cycle by eating certain foods or being exposed to certain chemicals.

Elizabeth came to our office for allergy treatment, and while she was here, went into a severe depression, typical of her PMS pattern. She was found to be sensitive to progesterone, was given sublingual drops of progesterone at a neutralizing dosage, and within a few minutes, noticed improvement. Within two hours, she was completely over her depression and other PMS symptoms. She remained free of symptoms by using the sublingual drops three times a day, and from then on felt completely well throughout the entire menstrual cycle.

DIAGNOSING PMS

PMS is usually very easy to diagnose. If various unpleasant symptoms consistently are present or become worse within two weeks of menstruation, then you have PMS. Some women realize that their symptoms come and go, but have never related them specifically to the time of the cycle. Women who have had their uterus removed through hysterectomy but who still have their ovaries may not be aware of the cyclical nature of their symptoms. Detailed daily tracking of symptoms through at least two menstrual cycles can help determine a diagnosis. Following are several forms that you may want to use to track your own symptoms for the next few cycles.

PMS SYMPTOM CALENDAR

The PMS Calendar is essential for the diagnosis of PMS. In addition, it is the only way to monitor your response to treatment. The PMS Calendar should be completed according to the following instructions:

1. Mark the date of the first day of your menstrual period that corresponds to the first day of your cycle (the first day of bleeding). If you do not have periods simply begin with the first day of each month.

2. Each morning before arising, take your temperature orally with an oral thermometer. With a red pencil put a dot below the appropriate date and opposite the temperature.

3. Weigh your self unclothed each morning before you eat or drink and after you empty your bladder and, if possible, your bowels. Record the results.

4. Note any medications taken or dietary changes made under the heading, "Treatment." Write the name and dose of medication (e.g. progesterone suppositories 200 mg). Note the number of times that medication was taken on a given day by writing the appropriate number in the box opposite the medication and below the date.

5. Choose the most common or severe physical and emotional symptoms that you experience with PMS from the symptom list below and write them in the blanks on the PMS Calendar. (Remember, the list below is not complete. Add any other recurring symptoms you can identify to your calendar.)

6. Note at the end of each day if you have experienced any of the physical or mental symptoms during that day. If you have experienced a symptom, estimate the severity of that symptom from 1 (mild) to 7 (severe) and write the number in the box opposite the symptom and below the appropriate date.

7. Also, keep a written description of how severe your PMS was during the month, how effective the treatment was and suggestions or any questions you have.

PHYSICAL SYMPTOMS

Abdominal Bloating
Headache
Breast Swelling
Chest Pain
Decreased Alcohol Tolerance
Seizures
Sensitivity to Light
Incoordination "Clumsiness"
Acne
Hives or Rash
Itching
Herpes "Cold Sores"
Dizziness
Craving for Sweets or Salty Foods
Backache
Increased Thirst

Breast Tenderness
Leg Cramps
Heart Palpitations
Sharp One-Sided Ovarian Pain
Increased Alcohol Consumption
Increased Appetite
Joint Pain
Constipation
Eye Problems
Sinusitis
Sensitivity to Noise
Nasal Congestion
Fainting Spells
Leg Heaviness or Swelling
Accidents
Vaginal Itching

MENTAL SYMPTOMS

Intolerant
Depression
Fatigue

Hostility
Anger
Sadness

Paranoia	Fear
Panic	Restlessness
Inability to Cope	Tearfulness
Decreased Self-Esteem	Physical Aggression
Mental Aggression	Decreased Sex Drive
Forgetfulness	Loneliness
Poor Concentration	Insecurity
Sense of Being Out of Control	Inefficiency
Guilt Feelings	Desire to Stay at Home
Dissatisfaction with Appearance	Poor Judgement
Indecision	Insomnia
Desire to be Alone	Suicidal Thoughts
Mania	Desire to Leave Home
Weakness	Increased Sex Drive
Irritability	Physical Violence
Absent from Work	

PMS Calendar
Used by permission of William R. Keye, M.D.
University of Utah PMS Center
Copyright 1982

TREATING PMS

Since many factors seem to be involved in PMS, no specific treatment measure works for everyone. Many drugs and supplements have been tried with mixed results. In our clinical experience, the following measures are the most important:

1. Use an effective candidiasis management program if it seems even moderately likely that you might have candidiasis. Follow the guidelines provided in the main text.

2. A good, wholesome diet is probably the single most important treatment measure. This not only involves avoiding refined foods and eating healthy foods, but also eating plenty of them. You are unlikely to get well by continued scanty food intake, even if you are eating good food.

3. A good exercise program involving thirty to sixty minutes of aerobic activity per session at least three times a week is very important. Follow the guidelines in the main text. If you can, exercise every day.

4. Take nutritional supplements, especially vitamin B_6,[6,7,8] magnesium,[9] and certain essential fatty acids. The general guidelines provided in the main text should be adequate. Although a number of fatty acid supplements (including marine oil and various cold-pressed oils) may be effective, the one most tested seems to be Efamol primrose oil;[10,11,12] take two to three capsules daily. Certain vitamins and minerals are needed to make the primrose oil optimally effective, but these are provided with the general nutritional recommendations in the main text.

5. If these measures by themselves do not produce reasonable control of symptoms, then you may need to take progesterone under your doctor's supervision. Tiny doses of progesterone can be given in a provocative-neutralizing technique,[13] but it may be difficult to find a doctor who will use this technique. Progesterone may be given in large doses by various routes. Large doses of synthetic progesterone do not seem to work well and, in fact, may aggravate the situation. Natural progesterone is inactivated by the stomach. and so cannot be used orally; it must be given by injection or in vaginal suppositories. The most comfortable route appears to be suppositories, and they are usually available in 200 or 400 mg. strength. They are used at a dosage that will control symptoms, and may need to be increased up to 4,000 mg. daily. The dosage often needs to be continually increased from time to time to produce the desired effect.

There is an apparent conflict here. If progesterone causes Candida overgrowth, which contributes to PMS, and if allergic responses to progesterone account for some PMS symptoms, then wouldn't progesterone make the situation worse? In some cases, it does make PMS worse. In most cases, however, it provides relief, and there's a logical explanation why: progesterone is very similar in structure to another hormone called cortisol—which is known for its ability to relieve allergy symptoms—and may even have some cortisol-like activity. Furthermore, progesterone is converted into cortisol as part of its normal metabolism. Large amounts of progesterone, then, have cortisol-like effects. In other words, progesterone might help control allergic reactions, even to itself! Large doses of an allergic substance may also overpower the immune system, and somehow reduce the reactions to that substance. Progesterone in large doses may also reverse an imbalance between estrogen and progesterone. If that was part of the problem contributing to PMS, then we would expect relief of symptoms.

When more specific information is available about the pathological processes involved in PMS, more effective means of control will be found. It is very unlikely, however, that any drug will be able to control PMS symptoms completely in the presence of poor diet. We are convinced that nutrition plays a major role, so start now to improve your diet while researchers continue their quest for improved medication.

1. Reid RL, Yen SSC. Premenstrual syndrome. Am J Obstet Gyn 1981; 139:85-104.
2. Goei GS, Ralston JL, Abraham GE. Dietary patterns of patients with premenstrual tension. J App Nutr 1982; 34:4-11.
3. Backstrom T, Mattsson B. Correlation of symptoms in premenstrual tension to estrogen and progesterone concentrations in blood plasma. Neuropsychobiology 1975; 1:80-86.
4. Varma TR. Hormones and electrolytes in premenstrual syndrome. Int J Gyn Obstet 1984; 22:51-58.
5. Mabray CR, Burditt ML, et al. Treatment of common gynecologic-endocrinologic symptoms by allergy management procedures. Obstet & Gyn 1982; 59:560-64.
6. Abraham GE, Hargrove JT. Effect of vitamin B-6 on premenstrual symptomatology in women with premenstrual tension syndromes: a double blind crossover study. Infertility 1980; 3:155-65.
7. Kerr GD. The management of the premenstrual syndrome. Curr Med Research & Opinion 1977; 4:29-34.
8. Barr W. Pyridoxine supplements in the premenstrual syndrome. The Practitioner 1984; 228-425-27.
9. Abraham GE, Lubran MM. Serum and red cell magnesium levels in patients with premenstrual tension. Am J Clin Nutr 1981;34:2364-66.
10. Puolakka J, Makarainen L, et al. Biochemical and clinical effects of treating the premenstrual syndrome with prostaglandin synthesis precursors. J Reproductive Med 1985;30:149-53.
11. Pye JK, Mansel RE, Hughes LE. Clinical experience of drug treatments for mastalgia. Lancet Aug 17, 1985;373-77.
12. Horrobin DF, Phil D. The role of essential fatty acids and prostaglandins in the premenstrual syndrome. J Reproductive Med 1983;28:465-68.
13. Mabray CR. Obstetrics and gynecology and clinical ecology. Clin Ecology Fall-Winter 1982-83; 1:103-13.

PMS CALENDAR

Name _____

Month _____

	1	2	3	4	5	6	7	8	9	10	11	12	13	14	15	16	17	18	19	20	21	22	23	24	25	26	27	28	29	30	31	32	33	34	35
Date																																			
Day of Menstrual Cycle																																			
Weight																																			

Treatment

1. _____
2. _____
3. _____

Physical Symptoms

1. _____ 98.8
2. _____ 98.6
3. _____ 98.4
5. _____ 98.2
6. _____ 97.8
7. _____ 97.6
8. _____ 97.4
9. _____ 97.2

Mental Symptoms

1. _____
2. _____
3. _____
4. _____
5. _____
6. _____
7. _____
8. _____
9. _____
10. _____

PMS CALENDAR

Name _____

Month _____

	1	2	3	4	5	6	7	8	9	10	11	12	13	14	15	16	17	18	19	20	21	22	23	24	25	26	27	28	29	30	31	32	33	34	35
Date																																			
Day of Menstrual Cycle																																			
Weight																																			

Treatment

1. _____
2. _____
3. _____

Physical Symptoms

1. _____ 98.8
2. _____ 98.6
3. _____ 98.4
5. _____ 98.2
6. _____ 97.8
7. _____ 97.6
8. _____ 97.4
9. _____ 97.2

Mental Symptoms

1. _____
2. _____
3. _____
4. _____
5. _____
6. _____
7. _____
8. _____
9. _____
10. _____

Copyright 1982 by
Dr. William R. Keye, M.D.

Appendix Six
YEAST-FREE MENU SUGGESTIONS

Wish you had help in planning delicious meals that provide complete nutrients—and are legitimate on the yeast control diet?

This appendix provides that help! Below you'll find a list of the recipes in Appendix 7 next to each, in parentheses, are the items you'll need to add to make each a complete meal. Some recipes are complete meals by themselves, so no additional items are listed. Dilled Chicken Fricassee is a complete meal by itself, for example; Breast of Chicken Creole would be a complete meal if you served brown rice and a green vegetable with it. And remember: any of the bread substitutes would be a great addition to any of the main dishes!

Specific recipes that are listed after main dishes are found in the Meal Accompaniments or Vegetable sections of the recipe collection. To make it even easier, we've listed some green and yellow vegetables at the end of the Vegetable Section; use a variety, and have fun with your meals.

MAIN DISHES/CHICKEN

Dilled Chicken Fricassee (complete meal)

Roast Chicken (Dinner: Sweet Potato Patties and green veg)
(Lunch: Lettuce Salad and a Muffin)
(Lunch: Whole Wheat Tortilla as a sandwich)

Breast of Chicken Creole (brown rice and green veg)
Chicken Cacciatore (whole wheat spaghetti and salad)
Stuffed Chicken Thighs (baked potato and green veg)
Chicken with Dumplings (brown rice and salad)
Brunswick Stew (salad)
Lemon Chicken (brown rice and salad)
Herb-Roasted Chicken Breasts (baked potato and green or yellow veg)
Creole Chicken and Zucchini (brown rice and salad)
Chicken and Noodles (salad)
Chicken Rolls (green veg and salad)

MAIN DISHES/FISH

Cod and Potato Dinner (green or yellow veg)
Tuna Vegetable Pilaf (complete meal)
Tuna and Zucchini Cakes (Oven-Baked Fries and yellow veg)
Fish Cakes (brown rice and green or yellow veg)
Halibut Steaks (baked potato and green or yellow veg)

Fish and Shrimp Creole (brown rice and green veg)
Baked Halibut (baked potato and green veg)
Baked Salmon (brown rice and green or yellow veg)
Halibut Paprika (baked potato and green veg and/or salad)

MAIN DISHES/LAMB

Lamb Patties with Vegetables (complete meal)
Roast Leg of Lamb (Barley Oven Pilaf and green or yellow veg)
Lamb Chop Skillet Dinner (green or yellow veg)

MAIN DISHES/BEEF

London Broil (Herbed Potatoes and green veg)
Spaghetti Pie (green veg and salad)
Beef Stew (salad)
Bean Stew (salad)
Chili (salad)
Chili Con Carne (salad)
Meat Loaf (baked potato and green or yellow veg)
Spaghetti Sauce (whole wheat spaghetti and salad)
Vegi-Burgers (Barley Oven Pilaf and green veg)
Oven Steak and Vegetables (salad)
Chili Skillet Supper (green veg and salad)
Easy Goulash (salad)
Stuffed Peppers (salad)
Vegetarian Chili (salad)

MAIN DISHES/TURKEY

Turkey Spaghetti Sauce (whole wheat spaghetti and salad)
Turkey Creole (brown rice and salad)
Turkey Tetrazzini (brown rice or whole wheat noodles and salad)
Enchilada Casserole (salad)

VEGETABLE RECIPES

Herbed Potatoes
Oven-Baked Fries
Italian-Style Zucchini
Vegetable Delight
Gvetch
Stovetop Beans
Herbed Green Beans
Simple Summer Squash
Golden Yam Puff
Sweet Potato Patties

Tomato Sauce (for a meatless
   spaghetti sauce)

GREEN VEGETABLES
Green beans
Peas
Broccoli
Spinach
Asparagus
Green peppers
Turnip greens
Beet greens
Collards
Brussels sprouts
Kale
Okra

YELLOW VEGETABLES
Carrots
Squash
Yams
Sweet Potatoes

OTHERS
Cabbage
Eggplant
Cauliflower
Parsnips

BREAKFAST IDEAS

Vegetable Omelet (bread substitute)
Pop-Up Eggs
Three-Grain Waffles
Annette's Oatmeal Waffles
Pear Buckwheat Waffles
Wheat Pancake Mix
Hearty Pancakes with Corn Fritter Variation
Yogurt-Blueberry Pancakes
Sweet Potato Pancakes

Note: Any of the muffin recipes make a nice breakfast addition.

BREAD SUBSTITUTES

Banana Nut Muffins
Whole-Grain Pumpkin Muffins
Pumpkin Nut Muffins
Bran Muffins
Honey Bran Banana Muffins
Bran Buttermilk Muffins
Apple Oatmeal Muffins
Applesauce Muffins
Cinnamon Nut Muffins
Pineapple Bran Muffins
Yogurt Muffins
Apple Whole Wheat Muffins
Tropical Muffins
3-Grain Muffins
Wheat-Free Muffins
Irish Soda Bread
Irish Whole Wheat Oatmeal Bread
Whole Wheat Flat Bread
Rye Flat Bread
Poppy Seed Crackers
Jolene's Rye Crackers
Whole Wheat Tortillas

Note: If you have a wheat sensitivity, you can substitute the flour in a recipe with rye flour, rice flour, corn flour, or oat flour (simply process oats in a blender until they are of flour consistency). Oat bran can be substituted for wheat bran.

MEAL ACCOMPANIMENTS

Barley Oven Pilaf

SOUPS

Cream of Zucchini Soup
New England Clam Chowder
Potato Soup
Cream of Tomato Soup
Turkey Chowder
Hamburger Soup
Vegetable Soup
Chicken and Corn Soup
Minestrone Soup
Chicken and Vegetable Soup

Note: Any of these soups would make a hearty lunch or dinner with the addition of a bread substitute.

DIPS AND SALAD DRESSINGS

Cottage Cheese Dip
Vegetable Dill Dip
Guacamole

Note: Serve the above dips with fresh raw vegetables or use as a salad dressing by thinning it down.

Norma's Salad Dressing
French Dressing

Note: Serve these dressings on green salad garnished with any fresh raw vegetables you'd like.

Appendix Seven

YEAST-FREE RECIPES

The following recipes have been adapted to fit the guidelines of the yeast control diet. Many recipes that you are now using can be adapted. For example, if your meatloaf calls for bread cubes, substitute rolled oats; if your recipe says white flour, substitute a whole grain flour. Some dishes that are dependent upon cheese for their flavor will be better if you leave them alone for awhile. If the recipe merely says sprinkle with parmesan cheese or cheddar cheese, then you will be able to successfully leave that part off without changing the original recipe taste too much. Mushrooms are easily left out of a recipe and the taste isn't dramatically altered. If you want to stir-fry, instead of using soy sauce use fresh garlic and ginger for added flavor.

Following each recipe is nutritional information. **RCU** and **FU** indicate refined carbohydrate units and fat units (designations used for the scoring system in *How to Lower Your Fat Thermostat*). **Cal** represents the number of calories in each serving, and **%F** represents the percentage of the total calories in that recipe derived from fat sources. **P, F,** and **C** represent the grams of protein, fat, and carbohydrate respectively for each serving of the recipe. **Na** represents the number of milligrams of sodium in each serving.

If you are trying to lose weight, you may also modify the higher fat recipes by reducing the fat-containing items (especially cooking oils, butter, egg yolks, nuts, etc.) By serving vegetables, brown rice, or other low-fat items along with a recipe, you can lower the ratio of fat. You might also want to try some of the suggestions for lowering the fat content in your diet as suggested in Appendix 4.

Yeast-free cooking will require a little more of your time since most prepared items can't be used (they usually have too much sugar or refined carbohydrates). Plan ahead, make double recipes, and freeze the extra. If you work outside the home, try making an extra meal or two on your day off and freeze it. You then have a quick meal that just needs to be heated up. For lunches away from home, freeze meal-size portions and microwave at your job site. For children's lunches, try making a sandwich in a whole wheat tortilla; serve meat slices along with a muffin, carrot and celery sticks; put soup, stew, or spaghetti in an insulated thermos and include a muffin.

Become familiar with the guidelines given in Chapter 7 and learn to adapt. Bon appetit!

MAIN DISHES/CHICKEN

DILLED CHICKEN FRICASSEE

⅓	C	whole wheat flour
1	tsp.	salt
½	tsp.	paprika
4		chicken breasts
2	T	cold-pressed oil
2	C	chicken broth
1	T	dried dill weed
8		small new potatoes (12 oz)
12	oz.	fresh or frozen green beans
1	T	lemon juice, or to taste

1. Mix flour, salt and paprika; coat chicken. Reserve leftover flour mixture.

2. Heat oil, add chicken, skin side down, cook 3 minutes, until well browned; turn chicken.

3. Stir reserved flour mixture into pan drippings. Gradually stir in chicken broth, 1 Tbsp dill; bring to a boil.

4. Add potatoes and green beans, reduce heat, cover, simmer 20 minutes or until chicken and vegetables are tender.

5. Stir in lemon juice and sprinkle with dill (if desired, for a stronger dill flavor).

Yield: 4 servings

	RCU	FU	Cal	%Ft	P	F	C	Na
Per Serving	0	1	347	23	33	9	30	755

ROAST CHICKEN

| 4–5 | lb. | roasting chicken |
| to taste | | salt and pepper |

1. Rinse off whole chicken.

2. Sprinkle chicken with salt and pepper.

3. Place chicken on rack in uncovered roaster breast up. Bake in 300 degree oven for 30 minutes per pound or until fork tender.

4. For dinner: slice chicken and serve with Sweet Potato Patties (recipe included) or a baked potato and a vegetable.

5. For lunch: remove chicken from the bones and serve with a salad and a muffin. OR dice deboned chicken and place in a lettuce salad. OR serve sliced deboned chicken as a sandwich in a whole wheat tortilla (recipe included).

Yield: 4 servings

Per 3 oz.	RCU	FU	Cal	%Ft	P	F	C	Na
serving	0	1	181	34	26	6	0	582

BREAST OF CHICKEN CREOLE

½	C	ground oat flour*
1½	tsp.	thyme leaves, crushed
1½	tsp.	garlic powder
1		egg
2		whole chicken breasts, boned, skinned, split
3	T	cold-pressed oil
¼	C	water
1	8-oz.	tomato sauce OR
	can	Tomato sauce recipe in Vegetable section
¼ to ½C		sliced green onions

1. In shallow plate, combine ground oat flour, thyme, and garlic powder.

2. Place egg in separate shallow dish and beat with 2 Tbsp water.

3. Pound each chicken breast half between sheets of wax paper to even thickness. Dip into dry ingredients, then egg, and again into dry ingredients, coating well.

4. Sauté chicken in oil over medium heat about 12 to 15 minutes, or until chicken is cooked through, turning once. Remove chicken to serving platter.

5. Turn heat to high and add the water, stirring to scrape brown bits. Add tomato sauce and green onions; heat through. Pour over chicken.

(*To make ground oat flour, place ¾ cup oats in blender; cover and blend about 1 minute, stopping occasionally to stir oats. Makes ½ cup oat flour).

Yield: 4 servings

	RCU	FU	Cal	%Ft	P	F	C	Na
Per Serving	0	2	276	42	20	13	18	306

CHICKEN CACCIATORE

3		whole chicken breasts, split and skinned
¼	C	olive oil
1	C	sliced onion
½	C	diced green pepper
1	clove	garlic, crushed
½	tsp.	crushed oregano
½	tsp.	crushed basil
¼	tsp.	ground black pepper
1	16-oz. can	tomatoes
2	T	whole wheat flour
		Chopped parsley

1. Heat oil, sprinkle chicken with salt, and brown both sides of chicken.

2. Remove chicken and add onion, green pepper, and garlic to skillet. Sauté until the onion is tender.

3. Stir in seasonings and tomatoes.

4. Add chicken. Bring to a boil. Cover; reduce heat and simmer 1 hour, turning chicken halfway through cooking.

5. Remove chicken to serving platter.

6. Blend together flour and small amount of sauce from skillet; stir into mixture in skillet.

7. Cook until thickened, about 3 minutes. Pour over chicken. Garnish with parsley.

Yield: 6 servings

	RCU	FU	Cal	%Ft	P	F	C	Na
Per Serving	0	1	256	53	30	15	110	78

STUFFED CHICKEN THIGHS

6		chicken thighs, boned and flattened
to taste		salt and pepper
¼	C	minced onion
⅓	C	minced carrots
½	C	minced celery

⅛	tsp.	ground thyme
½	tsp.	crushed basil
½	tsp.	garlic salt
1		egg
½	C	cooked brown rice
		whole wheat flour to dredge thighs
¼	C	butter
⅓	C	water
1	C	chicken broth
1	T	whole wheat flour for thickening

1. Bone chicken—cut on one skinless side, push meat away and remove bone and gristle end. Open and pound well to flatten. Season with salt and pepper.

2. Combine vegetables and seasonings. Mix in egg and rice.

3. Fill thighs with mixture, fold, and secure with string or skewers. Dredge with flour.

4. Melt butter in skillet and brown thighs. Place thighs in oven-proof dish. Add water.

5. Bake at 350 degrees for 50 to 60 minutes until done.

6. Remove drippings and heat in skillet. Blend in 1 Tbsp flour and cook 1 minute. Slowly add chicken broth and stir until smooth and thick.

7. Season to taste. Place chicken on serving dish and pour sauce over it.

Yield: 6 servings

	RCU	FU	Cal	%Ft	P	F	C	Na
Per Serving	0	2	239	38	22	10	13	546

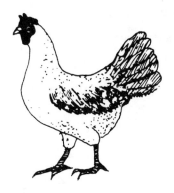

CHICKEN WITH DUMPLINGS

1		whole chicken, quartered
1	med.	onion, quartered
6		carrots, cut into 1-inch pieces
3	stalks	celery, cut into 1-inch pieces
1	can	chicken broth
1	tsp.	salt
$\frac{1}{8}$	tsp.	pepper
$\frac{1}{4}$	tsp.	thyme
1	T	lemon juice
6	T	whole wheat flour

1. Put washed chicken in 6-quart pan. Add all ingredients except flour and dumplings.

2. Add 3 cups water. Bring to a boil and simmer, covered, 45 minutes or until chicken and vegetables are tender.

3. Remove chicken and vegetables. Strain broth into a bowl and measure—you should have 5 cups—and return to pan. Bring to boiling.

4. In a small bowl, blend flour and ½ cup water until smooth, pour mixture into boiling broth, stirring constantly. Boil until broth thickens.

5. Return chicken and vegetables to pan. Return to a boil and cover. You may serve this over brown rice or whole wheat noodles or you can make the following dumpling recipe:

Dumplings:

2	C	whole wheat flour	$\frac{1}{4}$	C	butter
1	T	baking powder	1	C	milk

1. Combine flour and baking powder.

2. Cut in butter and add milk and stir.

3. Drop dough by rounded Tbsp onto the top of the boiling mixture.

4. Cook, uncovered, 10 minutes. Cover and cook 10 minutes longer until dumplings are puffed and a toothpick inserted comes out clean.

Yield: 6 servings

	RCU	FU	Cal	%Ft	P	F	C	Na
Per Serving	0	1	452	22	46	11	41	983

BRUNSWICK STEW

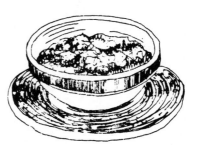

18		peppercorns
6		whole cloves
2		garlic cloves
2		bay leaves
3		sprigs parsley
¼	tsp.	thyme
2	qts.	chicken stock
1		chicken, quartered
1	lg.	onion, chopped
3	med.	onions, chopped
3		potatoes, cubed
1	28-oz. can	tomatoes or 1 quart tomatoes
1	can	corn, drained; reserve ⅓ cup corn kernels
½	tsp.	salt
¼	tsp.	freshly ground pepper

1. Combine first 6 ingredients in piece of cheesecloth and tie with a string. Add to a 8-quart pot with stock and bring to simmer.

2. Add chicken and 1 chopped onion. Simmer, covered, until chicken is tender, about 1½ to 2 hours.

3. Remove chicken, discard skin and bones, and cut meat into bite-size pieces. Set aside.

4. Add remaining ingredients to stock. Cover and simmer about 40 minutes.

5. Stir in chicken and corn.

6. Bring stew to simmer, then drop dumpling batter in by tablespoons. Cover securely and simmer until puffed and a toothpick comes out clean (about 15 minutes).

Corn Dumplings:

1	C	whole wheat flour	2	tsp.	baking powder
1	T	cornmeal	½	tsp.	salt

1. Combine ingredients and cut in 1 Tbsp butter.

2. Add up to ⅔ cup cold milk and ⅓ cup corn kernels and stir until moistened.

Yield: 6–8 servings

	RCU	FU	Cal	%Ft	P	F	C	Na
Per Serving	0	0	338	30	43	10	19	715

LEMON CHICKEN

4		chicken breast halves
1		egg, slightly beaten
2	T	water
1	C	whole wheat flour
¼	C	cold-pressed oil
2	T	butter
½	C	onion, finely minced
2	tsp.	basil
2	cloves	garlic, finely minced
½	C	lemon juice
1	C	water
½	tsp.	grated lemon rind
4		lemon slices, ¼ inch thick
		Cooked brown rice

1. Remove bones and skin from chicken breasts.

2. Combine egg and water, beat slightly. Dip chicken breasts in mixture and coat with flour. Repeat dipping and coating.

3. Fry chicken in heated oil until golden brown. Drain on paper towel.

4. Melt butter over low heat in skillet; add onion, basil, and garlic; sauté onion until translucent and garlic is tender.

5. Combine lemon juice, water, and lemon rind; add to onion mixture.

6. Return chicken breasts to skillet. Attach a lemon slice to each with a toothpick. Simmer, covered, for 25 minutes.

7. Serve chicken and lemon sauce over cooked brown rice.

Yield: 4 servings

	RCU	FU	Cal	%Ft	P	F	C	Na
Per Serving	0	3	565	38	37	24	48	159

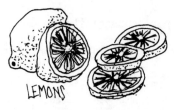

LEMONS

HERB-ROASTED CHICKEN BREASTS

2   whole large broiler fryer breasts, split and boned
1½ T   minced parsley

1. Wipe breasts dry. Turn in herb basting sauce (see recipe below) to coat.

2. Tuck edges under, to form compact shape—about 1½" thick.

3. Place skin side up in baking dish. Roast at 425 degrees and baste occasionally with pan drippings—just until nearly opaque to center—about 15 minutes.

4. Remove to warm plate and spoon pan juice over chicken. Sprinkle with parsley.

Herb Sauce:

3   T   butter, melted
1   T   finely chopped onion
1   large garlic clove, crushed and minced
1   tsp.   crumbled thyme
½   tsp.   each, salt and pepper
½   tsp.   rosemary, crumbled
¼   tsp.   ground sage
⅛   tsp.   marjoram, crumbled
dash hot pepper sauce (optional)

Stir together ingredients until well blended. Add one cup apple juice.

Yield: 4 servings

	RCU	FU	Cal	%Ft	P	F	C	Na
Per Serving	0	2	394	28	56	12	5	487

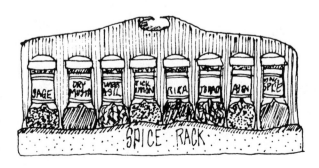

CREOLE CHICKEN AND ZUCCHINI

4		fryer chicken quarters
		vegetable cooking spray
½	C	chopped green pepper
¼	C	chopped celery
1		onion, diced
1	lb.	(about 3) zucchini squash, diced.
1	tsp.	celery salt
½	tsp.	pepper
½	tsp.	curry powder
½	tsp.	basil
1		bay leaf
1	28-oz. can	tomatoes, undrained
¼	C	water

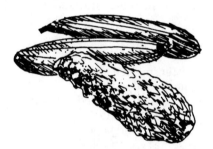

1. Spray Dutch oven with vegetable cooking spray; heat to medium high temperature and add chicken. Cook, turning, about 10 minutes or until brown on all sides. Remove chicken.

2. Add green pepper, celery, and onion and cook, stirring, about 5 minutes. Drain and discard any excess oil; add zucchini.

3. Sprinkle celery salt, pepper, curry powder, and basil over the vegetable mixture.

4. Add bay leaf, tomatoes, and water.

5. Arrange chicken over all and simmer over medium-low heat about 30 minutes or until chicken is fork tender and liquid is reduced. Serve over brown rice.

Yield: 4 servings

	RCU	FU	Cal	%Ft	P	F	C	Na
Per Serving	0	1	393	41	41	18	18	447

CHICKEN AND NOODLES

1		fryer chicken, cooked, boned, skinned and broken into pieces
1½	C	thinly sliced carrots
2	C	chicken broth
1	16-oz.	low-fat small curd cottage cheese
2	T	lemon juice
1	8 oz.	spinach or whole wheat noodles, cooked and drained
¼	tsp.	pepper
½	tsp.	salt

1. In a Dutch oven, place carrots and chicken broth; bring to a boil over high temperature. Reduce heat to low and simmer until carrots are just tender, about 5 minutes.

2. In blender, place cottage cheese and lemon juice; blend until smooth, about 1 minute.

3. Pour off broth from carrots and with blender running, slowly add warm broth to cottage cheese-lemon juice mixture.

4. Blend 1 more minute and then return contents of blender to pan with carrots.

5. Stir in chicken and cooked noodles; sprinkle with pepper and salt.

6. Over low heat, simmer, uncovered, about 20 minutes (keep temperature low so sauce does not separate).

Yield: 4–6 servings

	RCU	FU	Cal	%Ft	P	F	C	Na
Per Serving	0	0	277	19	22	6	33	502

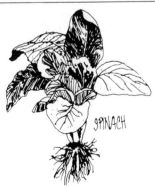

SPINACH

CHICKEN ROLLS

2	C	low-fat cottage cheese
3		eggs
6	T	whole wheat flour

1. Combine all ingredients in a blender and beat until smooth.

2. Lightly brown each pancake on a lightly oiled grill or frying pan. Each pancake should be about 4-inches in diameter.

3. While warm, put a spoonful of filling on each pancake and roll. Place smooth side up in a flat baking dish.

4. Before baking, cover with white sauce. Bake at 350 degrees for 20 minutes.

5. Chicken rolls may be prepared ahead and stored in the refrigerator or freezer without the white sauce.

Filling: Sauté 1 cup diced, cooked chicken, a small can of sliced ripe olives, and 2 Tbsp chopped chives or green onions until warm.

White Sauce:

1	T	whole wheat flour
1	T	butter
Dash of salt		
1	C	milk
¼	tsp.	dill weed (optional)

1. Melt the butter and add the flour and salt over low heat and mix well.

2. Add the milk and stir until smooth and thick.

3. Add ¼ tsp. dill weed or more if desired.

Yield: 4 servings

	RCU	FU	Cal	%Ft	P	F	C	Na
Per Serving	0	1	381	45	36	19	17	805

MAIN DISHES/FISH

COD AND POTATO DINNER

3	T	whole wheat flour
1	tsp.	salt
1	tsp.	thyme
4	T	cold-pressed oil
1	16-oz. pkg.	frozen cod fillets, cut crosswise into 4 pieces
5	C	hashed-brown potatoes
1	med.	red or green bell pepper, cut into ¼ inch strips
¼	C	plain yogurt

1. Mix flour with ½ tsp. each salt and thyme. Heat 2 Tbsp oil over medium heat.

2. Coat fish well in flour mixture. Add to skillet and cook 5 minutes per side or until lightly browned. Remove from skillet and keep warm.

3. Add remaining 3 Tbsp oil to pan drippings and heat over medium heat.

4. Add potatoes; cover and cook 10 minutes. Turn potatoes and stir in pepper strips and cook 4 minutes or until tender.

5. Season with remaining salt and thyme.

6. Arrange fish on potato mixture, top each piece with plain yogurt.

Yield: 4 servings

	RCU	FU	Cal	%Ft	P	F	C	Na
Per Serving	0	3	782	49	40	43	63	920

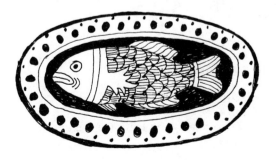

TUNA-VEGETABLE PILAF

1	12-oz. can	tuna, drained
2	T	cold-pressed oil
1	tsp.	minced garlic
1	C	uncooked long-grain brown rice
3	C	chicken broth
1	C	sliced celery
2		green onions, sliced
1	C	frozen or fresh green peas
1	lg.	tomato, cut in wedges

Fresh ground pepper to taste

1. Heat oil and add garlic and cook 1 minute.

2. Add rice and stir constantly about 2 minutes.

3. Stir in 2 cups broth; bring to a boil. Reduce heat, cover, and simmer 10 minutes or until most of the liquid is absorbed.

4. Add remaining 1 cup broth, the celery, and green onions. Cover and simmer 25 minutes longer.

5. Fold in peas and tuna. Cover and cook 5 minutes longer.

6. Remove from heat and let stand 5 minutes before serving.

7. Garnish with tomato and season with pepper (if desired).

Yield: 4 servings

	RCU	FU	Cal	%Ft	P	F	C	Na
Per Serving	0	1	331	21	30	8	69	342

TUNA AND ZUCCHINI CAKES

½	C	chopped onion
1	T	butter
1	6½-oz. can	water-pack tuna, drained and flaked
1	C	shredded zucchini
3		slightly beaten eggs
½	C	whole wheat (non-yeast-containing) cracker crumbs
¼	C	finely chopped parsley
⅛	tsp.	pepper

½   tsp.   salt
2   T   cold-pressed oil

1. Cook the onion in the butter until tender but not brown.

2. Remove from the heat and, in a bowl, combine onion mixture, tuna, zucchini, eggs, ¼ cup cracker crumbs, parsley, and pepper. Stir until combined.

3. Shape into six ½-inch-thick patties; coat with remaining cracker crumbs.

4. Cook over medium heat about 3 minutes per side, or until golden brown.

Yield: 3 servings

	RCU	FU	Cal	%Ft	P	F	C	Na
Per Serving	0	3	342	53	26	20	38	512

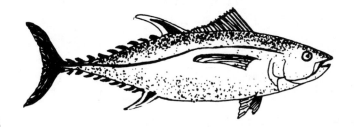

FISH CAKES

2   C   cooked, flaked fish (any canned or leftover fish)
1   C   cold mashed potatoes
¼   C   minced onion
2   tsp.   lemon juice
2   eggs, beaten
½   tsp.   salt
¼   tsp.   pepper
½   C   oat flour
oil

1. Combine the first 7 ingredients, mix well.

2. Shape into patties and coat with oat flour.

3. Cook in a small amount of hot oil unil brown on both sides.

Yield: 4 servings

	RCU	FU	Cal	%Ft	P	F	C	Na
Per Serving	0	2	390	32	45	14	73	312

HALIBUT STEAKS

2		halibut steaks
2	T	lemon juice
½	tsp.	salt
2		tomatoes, chopped
1		carrot, shredded
2	T	green onion, chopped
2	T	parsley, finely chopped
2		lemon wedges

1. Place fish in baking dish; sprinkle with lemon juice and salt.

2. Combine tomato, carrot, green onion, and parsley; sprinkle over fish.

3. Cover and bake at 350 degrees for 25 to 30 minutes.

4. Serve fish with a lemon wedge.

Yield: 2 servings

	RCA	FU	Cal	%Ft	P	F	C	Na
Per Serving	0	1	285	28	32	9	19	663

FISH AND SHRIMP CREOLE

1	7-oz. pkg.	frozen shrimp
1	16-oz. pkg.	cod fillets
1	T	butter
1½	C	chopped onions
½	C	chopped green pepper
2		cloves garlic, minced
4	med.	ripe tomatoes, peeled and chopped
2	T	chopped parsley
2	tsp.	paprika
1		bay leaf
1	T	cornstarch
1	T	water
3	C	hot cooked brown rice

1. Melt butter in a large saucepan. Add onions, green pepper, and garlic; sauté until tender.

2. Add tomatoes, parsley, paprika, and bay leaf; bring to a boil. Reduce heat; cover and simmer 30 minutes.

3. Cut cod into 1-inch square pieces.

4. Add sauce with shrimp. Cook about 5 minutes, stirring occasionally, until shrimp turns pink and fish flakes easily with a fork.

5. Blend together cornstarch and water. Add to creole and cook, stirring until slightly thickened. Serve over brown rice.

Yield: 6 servings

	RCU	FU	Cal	%Ft	P	F	C	Na
Per Serving	0	1	338	18	33	7	38	160

BAKED HALIBUT

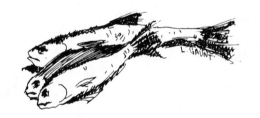

4 halibut steaks
butter
salt
pepper
paprika
lemon wedges
chopped fresh parsley

1. Place halibut in greased pan; dot with butter.

2. Sprinkle with salt, pepper and lightly with paprika.

3. Bake at 350 degrees for 15 to 20 minutes, approximately 6 to 8 minutes for each ½ inch of filet.

4. Serve with lemon wedges and garnish with fresh parsley.

Yield: 4 servings

	RCU	FU	Cal	%Ft	P	F	C	Na
Per Serving	0	1	261	24	48	7	0	428

BAKED SALMON

1		whole salmon
1		lemon, sliced
1	sm.	onion, sliced
2	T	butter, melted

1. Rub butter on salmon and place in a baking dish.

2. Put slices of onion and lemon inside the cavity of the fish.

3. Sprinkle with salt and cover with aluminum foil.

4. Bake at 325 degrees for about an hour, until done (fish should be fork tender). Serve with lemon wedges.

Yield: 4–6 servings

	RCU	FU	Cal	%Ft	P	F	C	Na
Per Serving	0	1	147	37	21	6	3	88

HALIBUT PAPRIKA

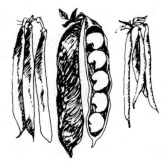

2		halibut steaks
to taste		salt and pepper
1	lb.	small new potatoes, parboiled
1	T	butter
½	C	water
⅓	C	plain yogurt
1	tsp.	lemon juice
½	tsp.	paprika

Cooked whole green beans

1. Sprinkle halibut with salt and pepper, place with potatoes in greased baking dish.

2. Dot with butter, sprinkle with water.

3. Bake at 425 degrees until fish flakes easily when tested with a fork. Remove fish and potatoes to platter, keep warm.

4. Drain juices from pan into saucepan; combine with yogurt, lemon juice, paprika and ⅛ tsp. pepper. Cook and stir until hot; do not boil.

5. Serve over halibut and potatoes. Serve with cooked whole green beans.

Yield: 2 servings

	RCU	FU	Cal	%Ft	P	F	C	Na
Per Serving	0	2	470	29	36	15	46	732

MAIN DISHES/LAMB

LAMB PATTIES WITH VEGETABLES

1	lb.	ground lamb
1		egg
2	T	rolled oats
1¼	tsp.	salt
1	tsp.	crumbled rosemary
1	dash	of hot-pepper sauce
1	T	olive oil
1	med.	onion, sliced into rings
2	cloves	garlic, crushed
8	oz.	zucchini, cut into ¼ inch slices
1	16-oz. can	tomatoes, broken up
1	16-oz. can	small whole potatoes, drained

1. Mix lamb, egg, oats, 1 tsp. salt, ¾ tsp rosemary, and the hot pepper sauce in a bowl. Shape into 8 patties.

2. Heat oil and add lamb patties and cook about 2 minutes per side, or until done as desired. Remove patties from skillet.

3. Add onion and garlic to pan drippings. Cook over medium heat until onion is golden.

4. Stir in zucchini and tomatoes. Season with remaining ¼ tsp. salt and rosemary. Cover and simmer about 10 minutes, until zucchini is tender.

5. Stir in potatoes; put lamb patties on top of vegetables. Cover and heat through.

Yield: 4 servings

	RCU	FU	Cal	%Ft	P	F	C	Na
Per Serving	0	4	668	65	30	48	30	725

ROAST LEG OF LAMB

1		leg of lamb (5 to 9 lbs.)
2	cloves	garlic, thinly sliced
2	T	lemon juice
1½	tsp.	salt
¼	tsp.	pepper
2	T	cold-pressed oil

1. With point of a sharp knife, cut many small slits in surface of lamb. Push a garlic sliver into each slit.

2. Combine lemon juice, salt, pepper and oil. Rub mixture into slits and over surface of lamb.

3. Place lamb on rack in roasting pan and roast in 325 degree oven until internal temperature reaches 140 for rare (20-25 minutes per pound), 160 for medium (25-30 minutes per pound) and 170 (30-35 minutes per pound) for well done.

4. Allow lamb to rest 20 minutes before carving.

Yield: 6–8 servings

Per 3 oz. Serving	RCU	FU	Cal	%Ft	P	F	C	Na
	0	4	270	63	22	19	1	453

LAMB CHOP SKILLET DINNER

4		lamb shoulder chops, about ¾ inch thick
4	T	cold-pressed oil
2	med.	onions, sliced
½	tsp.	minced garlic
1	C	chicken broth
¼	tsp.	rosemary, crumbled
½	tsp.	salt
4	med.	potatoes, sliced ¼ inch thick

1. Brown chops on both sides in 2 Tbsp oil. Remove chops.

2. Add remaining 2 Tbsp oil to skillet; stir to loosen browned pan drippings.

3. Add onions and garlic; cook and stir 2 minutes until lightly browned.

4. Stir in broth, rosemary, and salt; arrange layer of potatoes, then chops on top.

5. Cover, simmer 35 minutes or until chops and potatoes are tender, adding more broth if needed to prevent scorching.

Yield: 4 servings

	RCU	FU	Cal	%Ft	P	F	C	Na
Per Serving	0	4	573	60	19	38	41	585

MAIN DISHES/BEEF

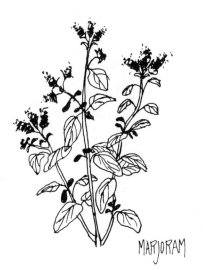

LONDON BROIL

¼	C	olive oil
¼	C	lemon juice
¼	C	water
2	T	chopped parsley
1	T	grated onion
1	tsp.	dried marjoram
1	tsp.	dried thyme
1	tsp.	salt
1	tsp.	minced garlic
½	tsp.	hot pepper sauce
1	lb.	boneless beef top round

MARJORAM

1. Mix all ingredients except meat in a shallow glass baking dish. Add beef; turn to coat.

2. Cover; refrigerate overnight, turning meat several times.

3. Drain and reserve marinade. Turning and basting once, broil or grill over medium heat 4 to 5 inches from heat source, 20 minutes (rare).

4. Let meat stand 5 minutes before carving. Slice on the diagonal.

Yield: 4 servings

	RCU	FU	Cal	%Ft	P	F	C	Na
Per Serving	0	3	341	71	22	27	2	607

SPAGHETTI PIE

6	oz.	whole wheat spaghetti
1	T	butter
2		well-beaten eggs
1	C	low-fat cottage cheese
1	lb.	lean ground beef
½	C	chopped onion
¼	C	chopped green pepper
1	C	tomatoes, cut up
1	6-oz. can	tomato paste
1	tsp.	dried oregano, crushed
½	tsp.	garlic salt

1. Cook the spaghetti according to directions; drain.

2. Stir butter into hot spaghetti. Stir in eggs.

3. Form spaghetti mixture into a "crust" in a buttered 10-inch pie plate. Spread cottage cheese over bottom of spaghetti crust.

4. Cook ground beef, onion and green pepper until vegetables are tender and meat is browned. Drain off excess fat.

5. Stir in undrained tomatoes, tomato paste, oregano, and garlic salt; heat through.

6. Turn meat mixture into spaghetti crust. Bake at 350 degrees for 20 minutes.

Yield: 6 servings

	RCU	FU	Cal	%Ft	P	F	C	Na
Per Serving	0	2	350	33	28	13	32	336

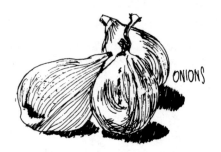

ONIONS

BEEF STEW

1	lg.	onion, chopped
1	clove	garlic, finely minced
2	T	cold-pressed oil
2	lbs.	lean stew beef, cut into 1-inch cubes
½	C	whole wheat flour
1	C	tomato juice
2		beef bouillon cubes
1	28-oz. can	tomatoes or 1 quart tomatoes
1	8-oz. can	whole-kernel corn, drained
1	C	potatoes, diced
1	C	carrots, sliced
½	C	celery, chopped
1¼	tsp.	salt
½	tsp.	freshly ground black pepper

1. Sauté onion and garlic in oil. Remove onion and garlic and set aside. Reserve drippings.

2. Coat meat in flour. Brown meat in reserved pan drippings and add more oil if necessary. Set meat aside.

3. Bring tomato juice to a boil, remove from heat, and add bouillon cubes, stirring until dissolved.

4. Combine onion and garlic, meat, tomato juice mixture, tomatoes, corn, potatoes, carrots, celery, salt and pepper in a 3-quart casserole; stir until well blended.

5. Cover and bake at 325 degrees for 2½ to 3 hours, stirring once.

Yield: 8 servings

	RCU	FU	Cal	%Ft	P	F	C	Na
Per Serving	0	4	491	57	33	31	19	511

BEAN STEW

1. Wash and drain 2 cups of mixed beans (use any combination of beans such as navy beans, great northern beans, baby lima beans, dried peas, pinto beans, black-eye beans, etc.).

2. Add 3 quarts of water, one pound cooked lean ground beef (well browned) 1 bay leaf, a large pinch each of basil and thyme, and 1 tsp salt. Simmer until nearly tender.

Add:

1	lg.	onion, chopped
3	stalks	celery, chopped
3	lg.	carrots, diced
1	16-oz. can	tomatoes, diced
1	6-oz. can	tomato paste
1	T	parsley flakes
2	T	beef bouillon

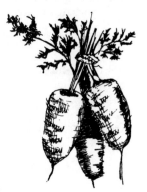

salt and pepper to taste

Adjust the liquids and seasonings as needed.

Yield: 8 servings

	RCU	FU	Cal	%Ft	P	F	C	Na
Per Serving	0	1	271	23	23	7	29	765

CHILI

1	lb.	dried pinto beans
2	½-qts.	water
2	28-oz. cans	tomatoes or 2 quarts tomatoes, undrained
1½	lbs.	lean ground beef
1	lb.	lean ground pork (NOT sausage)
3	med.	green peppers, chopped
1	lg.	onion, chopped
2	cloves	garlic, crushed
½	C	chopped fresh parsley
⅓	C	chili powder (or less if desired)
1½	tsp.	cumin seeds
1	tsp.	salt
1½	tsp.	pepper

1. Wash beans; place in a large pan, add water, and let soak overnight.

2. Bring to a boil. Reduce heat; cover and simmer 2½ hours or until beans are tender.

3. Add tomatoes; cover and simmer for 15 minutes.

4. Sauté meat, green pepper, onion, garlic, salt, and pepper until vegetables are tender.

5. Stir in parsley and chili powder; simmer for 20 minutes.

6. Add meat mixture to beans, stir in cumin. Bring to a boil.

7. Reduce heat; cover and simmer ½ hour. Uncover and cook over medium heat 30–60 minutes, to desired thickness.

Yield: 1 gallon or 12 (1½ cup) servings

	RCU	FU	Cal	%Ft	P	F	C	Na
Per Serving	0	2	328	30	25	11	33	809

CHILI CON CARNE

1	tsp.	cold-pressed oil
1	med.	onion, chopped
1	clove	garlic, minced
½	C	green pepper, chopped
1	lb.	lean ground beef
1	28-oz. can	tomatoes or 1 quart tomatoes
1	15-oz. can	kidney or pinto beans, drained
2	tsp.	chili powder
1	tsp.	oregano
½	tsp.	pepper
½	tsp.	salt

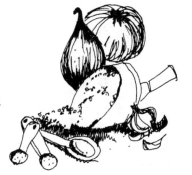

1. Heat oil and add next three ingredients.

2. Add ground beef and cook until browned.

3. Add remaining ingredients; bring to a boil, reduce heat, and simmer 30 minutes, stirring occasionally.

Yield: 4 servings

	RCU	FU	Cal	%Ft	P	F	C	Na
Per Serving	0	2	409	33	40	15	27	454

MEAT LOAF

1	lb.	lean ground beef
¾	C	rolled oats
¼	C	grated carrot
¼	C	finely chopped celery
¼	C	finely chopped onion
¼	C	finely chopped green pepper
2		eggs, slightly beaten
1	tsp.	parsley flakes
1	tsp.	salt
¼	tsp.	pepper
1	8-oz. can	tomato sauce

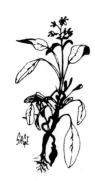

SAGE

1. Combine all ingredients.

2. Bake at 350 degrees for 1 hour or until done.

Yield: 6 servings

	RCU	FU	Cal	%Ft	P	F	C	Na
Per Serving	0	2	252	39	25	11	11	549

SPAGHETTI SAUCE

1½	lbs.	lean ground beef
1	med.	onion, chopped
1	C	chopped celery
½	C	chopped green pepper
2	cloves	garlic, minced
1	15-oz. can	tomato sauce
1	6-oz. can	tomato paste
¾	C	water
1½	tsp.	dried whole oregano
1	tsp.	salt
½	tsp.	pepper
1	tsp.	basil
½	tsp.	rosemary, crushed
2	T	parsley, finely chopped

Cooked whole wheat spaghetti

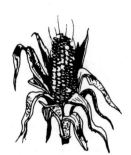

1. Cook ground beef with onion and garlic until browned.

2. Add all other ingredients except spaghetti and stir well.

3. Cover, reduce heat, and simmer for 1½ hours, stirring occasionally.

4. Serve sauce over cooked spaghetti.

Yield: 6 servings

	RCU	FU	Cal	%Ft	P	F	C	Na
Per Serving	0	2	412	39	38	18	12	600

VEGI-BURGERS

1	lb.	lean ground beef
1		potato, grated
1		carrot, grated
1	sm.	onion, finely chopped
½	tsp.	oregano
½	tsp.	garlic powder
2		eggs

salt and pepper to taste

1. Combine all ingredients and form into patties. If mixture is too moist, add rolled oats to take up some of the moisture.

2. Cook in a skillet until browned.

Yield: 4 servings

	RCU	FU	Cal	%Ft	P	F	C	Na
Per Serving	0	3	449	44	51	22	8	638

OVEN STEAK AND VEGETABLES

1–1½lbs.		beef round steak
2	T	whole wheat flour
1	tsp.	salt
⅛	tsp.	pepper
¼	C	olive oil
1	8-oz. can	tomato sauce
2	T	whole wheat flour
3–4		fresh tomatoes, cut up, or 1 pint canned tomatoes
1	med.	onion, chopped
2	T	fresh chopped parsley
4		carrots, cut into strips
2	C	sliced zucchini
½	tsp.	basil

Hot cooked brown rice

1. Cut meat into serving pieces.

2. Combine 2 Tbsp flour, salt, and pepper. Coat meat in flour mixture.

3. Brown meat in oil. Transfer meat to baking dish. Reserve drippings in skillet.

4. Combine 2 Tbsp flour and tomato sauce; stir into pan drippings in skillet.

5. Stir in tomatoes, onion, and parsley. Cook and stir until thickened. Pour over meat.

6. Add carrots. Cover and bake at 325 degrees for one hour.

7. Add zucchini. Cover and continue baking 15 to 20 minutes or until meat and vegetables are tender.

8. Season with salt and pepper. Serve with hot brown rice.

Yield: 4–6 servings

	RCU	FU	Cal	%Ft	P	F	C	Na
Per Serving	0	3	545	38	38	23	46	572

CHILI SKILLET SUPPER

½	C	chopped onion
⅓	C	chopped green pepper

1	lb.	lean ground beef
1	28-oz. can	whole tomatoes or 1 quart tomatoes
1½	tsp.	salt
2	tsp.	chili powder
⅛	tsp.	black pepper
¾	C	whole wheat elbow macaroni, uncooked

1. Brown onion, green pepper, and beef lightly.

2. Add tomatoes, salt, chili powder, and pepper, mixing well.

3. Bring food to a boil. Stir in macaroni.

4. Cover and reduce heat to simmer for approximately 25 minutes.

Yield: 6 servings

	RCU	FU	Cal	%Ft	P	F	C	Na
Per Serving	0	1	300	42	26	14	7	635

EASY GOULASH

1½	lbs.	lean ground beef
1	bunch	green onions, chopped
1	sm.	clove garlic, minced
2		green peppers, chopped
to taste		salt and pepper
1	28-oz. can	tomatoes, chopped or 1 quart of tomatoes
½	lb.	whole wheat noodles, cooked

1. Brown beef and add onion, green pepper, garlic, salt, and pepper. Cook briefly.

2. Add tomatoes and juice. Simmer 30 minutes.

3. Add cooked and strained noodles.

Yield: 6 servings

	RCU	FU	Cal	%Ft	P	F	C	Na
Per Serving	0	2	381	43	36	18	6	497

STUFFED PEPPERS

6–8		green peppers
1	lb.	lean ground beef
½	lg.	onion, chopped
1	C	bulgur wheat, OR barley OR brown rice
1	28-oz. can	tomatoes, undrained or 1 quart tomatoes
1	20-oz. pkg.	frozen cut corn

1. Cut green peppers in half lengthwise and seed. Boil peppers in slightly salted water approximately 15 minutes; drain and arrange cut side up in 9"x13" baking dish.

2. Cook meat and onion until browned; add tomatoes. (If not enough liquid, add more tomatoes)

3. Add corn and bulgur wheat, OR barley OR brown rice. Cook slowly, stirring, until wheat, barley or rice is tender.

4. Pour meat mixture over peppers and bake at 350 degrees for 30 minutes.

Yield: 6–8 servings

	RCU	FU	Cal	%Ft	P	F	C	Na
Per Servings	0	1	269	23	16	7	37	338

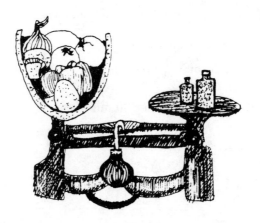

VEGETARIAN CHILI

1	lb.	dried kidney beans
7	C	water
1	C	tomato juice
1	C	bulgur or cracked wheat
2	T	cold-pressed oil
2	cloves	garlic, crushed
1½	C	chopped onion
2	C	chopped tomatoes
2	C	water
1	C	chopped carrot
1	C	chopped celery
4	C	chopped green pepper
1	6-oz. can	tomato paste
2	T	lemon juice
1½	tsp.	ground cumin
1½	tsp.	chili powder
1	tsp.	dried basil
½	tsp.	salt
¼	tsp.	pepper

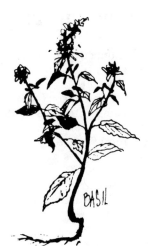

BASIL

1. Wash beans and place in 3 cups water in a large pan.

2. Bring to a boil and cook 3 minutes. Remove from the heat, cover, and let soak 1 hour.

3. Add remaining 4 cups water; bring to a boil. Cover, reduce heat, and simmer 1 hour. Set aside.

4. Bring tomato juice to a boil; pour over bulgur. Stir well and set aside.

5. Heat oil; add garlic and onion; saute until onion is tender.

6. Add remaining ingredients; cover and simmer 20 minutes.

7. Add vegetable mixture and bulgur mixture to beans. Cook until heated.

Yield: 3 quarts (8 servings)

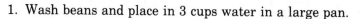

	RCU	FU	Cal	%Ft	P	F	C	Na
Per Serving	0	0	239	19	11	5	42	422

MAIN DISHES/TURKEY

TURKEY SPAGHETTI SAUCE

1	C	chopped onion
1	clove	garlic, minced
2	T	olive oil
1½	lbs.	ground uncooked turkey
1	28-oz. can	whole tomatoes, undrained and chopped
2	6-oz. cans	tomato paste
1	C	water
1		bay leaf
1½	tsp.	dried oregano
¾	tsp.	salt
¼	tsp.	pepper
1	tsp.	dried basil

Hot cooked whole wheat spaghetti

1. Sauté onion and garlic in olive oil until onion is tender.

2. Add turkey and cook until done.

3. Stir in next 8 ingredients; simmer, uncovered, 1 hour.

4. Remove bay leaf and spoon sauce over cooked spaghetti.

Yield: 6 servings

	RCU	FU	Cal	%Ft	P	F	C	Na
Per Serving	0	1	278	31	12	10	114	365

TURKEY CREOLE

½	C	onions, finely diced
¼	C	diced green pepper
½	C	sliced celery
1	T	butter
1½	C	canned tomatoes
1		bay leaf
½	tsp.	celery salt

¼   tsp.   dried basil
1   C   chopped cooked turkey
½   C   cooked peas
brown rice, cooked

1. Sauté onions, green pepper, and celery in butter until tender.

2. Add remaining ingredients (except rice). Season to taste with salt and pepper.

3. Serve over cooked brown rice.

Yield: 4 servings

	RCU	FU	Cal	%Ft	P	F	C	Na
Per Serving	0	1	191	33	7	7	216	60

TURKEY TETRAZZINI

¼   C   butter
¼   C   whole wheat flour
1   tsp.   salt
¼   tsp.   white pepper
1   C   turkey or chicken broth
1   C   milk
3   C   cooked turkey, cut into bite-sized pieces
¼   C   green pepper, finely chopped
½   C   slivered almonds
Paprika

PEPPERS

1. Melt butter in saucepan; add flour, salt, pepper; blend.

2. Add broth and milk, stirring while cooking until thickened.

3. Add remaining ingredients except paprika. Simmer a few minutes.

4. Serve over brown rice or whole wheat noodles. Garnish with paprika.

Yield: 6 servings

	RCU	FU	Cal	%Ft	P	F	C	Na
Per Serving	0	2	317	40	11	14	126	498

ENCHILADA CASSEROLE

2	T	butter
½	C	onion, chopped
¼	C	celery, diced
¼	C	green pepper, diced
1	16-oz. can	tomato sauce
½–1	tsp.	chili powder
¼	tsp.	dried basil
¼	tsp.	dried oregano
1	pkg.	7-inch corn tortillas
1	C	cooked turkey (beef pot roast or chicken may be substituted)

1. Melt butter; add onion, celery, and green pepper and cook until tender.

2. Add tomato sauce, chili powder, basil, and oregano.

3. Place a tortilla in the bottom of a buttered 7-inch casserole; add a thin layer of turkey, then sauce. Repeat for all ingredients.

4. Bake at 350 degrees for 20 to 30 minutes or until hot.

Yield: 4 servings

	RCU	FU	Cal	%Ft	P	F	C	Na
Per Serving	0	2	272	29	6	9	84	811

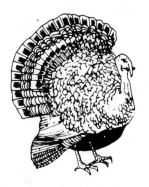

VEGETABLES

HERBED POTATOES

2½	lbs.	baking potatoes, peeled and thinly sliced
¼	C	cold-pressed oil
2	T	finely chopped fresh parsley
2	T	minced fresh chives (or green onion tops)
1	med.	garlic clove, finely minced

salt and freshly ground pepper

1. Heat oven to 350 degrees.

2. Soak potatoes in cold water to cover for 5 minutes, changing water once.

3. Combine oil, herbs, garlic, salt, and pepper in a bowl.

4. Drain potatoes and pat dry. Add to bowl, turning to coat well.

5. Place in baking dish. Bake until edges are golden brown, about 1 hour.

Yield: 6 servings

	RCU	FU	Cal	%Ft	P	F	C	Na
Per Serving	0	1	193	42	3	9	24	319

OVEN BAKED FRIES

2	med.	potatoes

1. Scrub potatoes. Bake potatoes at 400 degrees for 15 minutes.

2. Remove from oven and cool slightly.

3. Cut each potato lengthwise into 8 julienne sticks. Place on baking sheet sprayed with non-stick coating.

4. Bake at 400 degrees for 25 to 30 minutes or until the potato sticks are golden brown.

Yield: 2 servings

	RCU	FU	Cal	%Ft	P	F	C	Na
Per Serving	0	0	80	0	2	0	18	3

ITALIAN STYLE ZUCCHINI

1	lb.	zucchini
1	T	olive oil
1	sm.	clove garlic, finely chopped
1/4	C	onion, finely chopped
1	tsp.	salt
1		tomato, peeled and quartered
1/2	tsp.	oregano

1. Slice zucchini into thin slices.

2. Saute the garlic and onion in oil 1 minute.

3. Stir in zucchini and remaining ingredients; cover and cook over low heat 15 minutes.

Yield: 4 servings

	RCU	FU	Cal	%Ft	P	F	C	Na
Per Serving	0	1	64	56	2	4	8	538

VEGETABLE DELIGHT

1	C	coarsely diced potatoes
1	C	sliced carrots
1	C	cauliflower flowerets
1 1/2	C	broccoli flowerets
1	C	sliced celery
1/4	C	diced onions
1/4	C	water

Seasoning salt

1. Put all vegetables and water in a Dutch oven.

2. Add seasoning salt to taste.

3. Cover and steam on low heat for approximately 40 minutes.

Yield: 6 servings

	RCU	FU	Cal	%Ft	P	F	C	Na
Per Serving	0	0	61	0	1	0	13	129

GVETCH

1	lg.	eggplant, diced into 1-inch cubes
2	med.	zucchini, sliced into ½-inch rounds
1	lg.	onion, coarsely chopped
1	clove	garlic, minced
1		green pepper, cut into squares
2	T	olive oil
1	lg.	potato, cut into large chunks
4		carrots, sliced into rounds
3		tomatoes, chopped

juice of 1 lemon
1   tsp.   salt
⅛   tsp.   pepper
½   tsp.   basil
½   tsp.   oregano

1. Heat oven to 350 degrees.

2. In a Dutch oven, heat the olive oil and sauté onion, garlic, and green pepper until they are tender.

3. Stir in eggplant, zucchini, potato, and carrots; sauté several more minutes.

4. Add tomato, lemon, salt, pepper, basil, oregano, and 2 Tbsp of water.

5. Bake in a covered dish for 45 minutes.

6. Serve with brown rice or bulgur wheat.

Yield: 8 servings

	RCU	FU	Cal	%Ft	P	F	C	Na
Per Serving	0	1	112	32	3	4	18	258

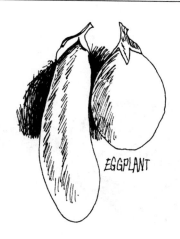

EGGPLANT

STOVETOP BEANS

1	16-oz. pkg.	dried pinto beans
2	qts.	water
1½	C	tomato juice
3	lg.	ripe tomatoes, peeled, seeded and chopped OR
1½	C	canned and drained tomatoes, chopped
2		onions, chopped
2	cloves	garlic, crushed
1	T	chili powder
1½	tsp.	garlic salt
2	tsp.	cumin seeds
1½	tsp.	salt
½	tsp.	pepper

1. Place beans in a large saucepan. Cover with water 3 inches above beans; let soak overnight.

2. Drain beans and return to saucepan; add 1½ cups tomato juice.

3. Slowly bring to a boil. Reduce heat; simmer, uncovered, 30 minutes or until most of tomato juice has been absorbed.

4. Add remaining ingredients, stirring well. Bring to a boil. Reduce heat; cover and simmer 1 hour.

5. Uncover and continue to simmer 2 hours or until beans are tender.

Yield: 8 servings

	RCU	FU	Cal	%Ft	P	F	C	Na
Per Serving	0	0	137	2	8	0	27	451

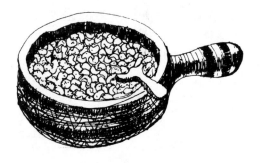

HERBED GREEN BEANS

1	lb.	fresh green beans
1		onion, chopped
1	T	olive oil
1	lg.	stalk celery, finely chopped
½	C	chopped green pepper
¼	C	water
½	tsp.	dried tarragon
¼	tsp.	lemon-pepper seasoning

1. Remove strings from beans; wash beans, cut into 2-inch pieces.

2. Heat oil and sauté onion until tender.

3. Add celery and green pepper, cover and cook over low heat 5 minutes.

4. Add green beans and remaining ingredients; cover and cook 20 minutes or until beans are tender.

Yield: 4 servings

	RCU	FU	Cal	%Ft	P	F	C	Na
Per Serving	0	1	104	35	3	4	14	32

SIMPLE SUMMER SQUASH

1	T	butter
1	med.	onion, chopped
1	lb.	yellow summer squash, sliced ¼-inch thick (about 4 ½ cups)
1	lg.	ripe tomato, chopped (1 cup)
½	tsp.	salt

1. Melt butter in skillet and add onion and cook about 3 minutes until tender. Stir in remaining ingredients.

2. Cover and simmer, stirring occasionally, 20 minutes or until squash is tender.

Yield: 4 servings

	RCU	FU	Cal	%Ft	P	F	C	Na
Per Serving	0	1	79	34	3	3	10	311

GOLDEN YAM PUFF

4	med.	yams or sweet potatoes
½	C	milk
½	stick	butter, melted
4		eggs, beaten
1	tsp.	baking powder
½	tsp.	dried marjoram, crumbled
¼	tsp.	dried thyme, crumbled
¼	tsp.	salt

1. Cook yams in boiling water to cover for 20 minutes, until soft. Peel.

2. In a large bowl, mash yams until smooth.

3. Add milk, butter, eggs, baking powder, marjoram, thyme, and salt; beat until light and fluffy.

4. Turn mixture into buttered 2-quart casserole.

5. Bake at 350 degrees for 45 to 50 minutes, until golden brown and a knife inserted in center comes out clean.

Yield: 4–6 servings.

	RCU	FU	Cal	%Ft	P	F	C	Na
Per Serving	0	2	230	47	6	12	25	217

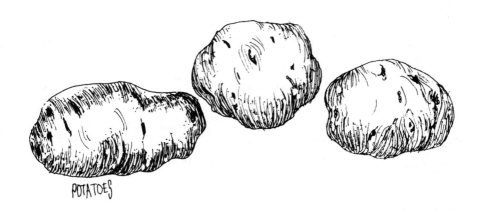

POTATOES

SWEET POTATO PATTIES

2	C	cooked, mashed sweet potatoes
⅓	C	minced celery
¼	tsp.	salt
1	tsp.	milk
2	T	butter, melted
¾	C	crushed corn flakes

1. Combine sweet potatoes, celery, and salt; mix well, and stir in milk.

2. Shape into 12 balls; dip in melted butter, roll each in corn flakes and flatten to make a patty shape.

3. Place patties on a broiler pan. Broil 6 to 7 inches from the heat for 3 minutes. Turn and broil for 3 additional minutes on the other side.

Yield: 6 servings

	RCU	FU	Cal	%Ft	P	F	C	Na
Per Serving	0	1	124	29	2	4	20	97

TOMATO SAUCE

1	T	olive oil
1	med.	onion, diced
2	cloves	garlic, finely minced
2	tsp.	basil
2	tsp.	oregano
2	T	parsley, finely chopped
1	qt.	finely chopped tomatoes
to taste		salt and pepper

1. Heat olive oil and sauté onion.

2. Add garlic, basil, oregano, parsley, and ground tomatoes. Simmer 45 minutes.

3. Season to taste. Serve on cooked whole wheat pasta.

Yield: 4 servings

	RCU	FU	Cal	%Ft	P	F	C	Na
Per Serving	0	1	99	36	3	4	15	660

BREAKFAST IDEAS

OMELET WITH VEGETABLES

1	med.	zucchini, thinly sliced
¼	C	sliced green onion
¼	C	chopped green pepper
2		tomatoes, cut up
½	tsp.	basil, crushed
½	tsp.	salt
1	T	cold water
2	tsp.	cornstarch
8		eggs
¼	C	water
½	tsp.	salt
⅛	tsp.	pepper
2	T	butter

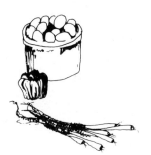

1. For filling: in a saucepan, cook zucchini, green onion, and green pepper in a small amount of boiling salted water about 5 minutes, or until vegetables are crisp-tender. Drain well.

2. Add tomatoes, basil, ½ tsp. salt, and bring to boiling; reduce heat.

3. Combine the 1 Tbsp cold water and cornstarch and add to tomato mixture.

4. Cook and stir until thickened.

5. For omelets: beat together eggs, water, ½ tsp. salt, and pepper until blended.

6. In a skillet heat ¼ of the butter until slightly brown. Coat sides of pan with butter.

7. Add ¼ of the egg mixture and cook over medium heat. As eggs set, remove from heat.

8. Spoon ¼ of the filling mixture across the center.

9. Fold ⅓ of the omelet over center. Overlap the remaining third atop filling. Serve warm. Repeat to make 3 more omelets.

Yield: 4 servings

	RCU	FU	Cal	%Ft	P	F	C	Na
Per Serving	0	3	270	60	15	18	13	630

POP-UP EGGS

1	C	whole wheat flour
1	C	milk
4		eggs
½	cube	butter

1. Melt butter in a 9 x 13 pan.

2. Mix the flour, milk and eggs well and pour batter over the melted butter.

3. Bake at 350 degrees for 25 minutes or until eggs pop up.

Yield: 6 servings

	RCU	FU	Cal	%Ft	P	F	C	Na
Per Serving	0	2	201	54	8	12	17	146

THREE-GRAIN WAFFLES

3		eggs
1	C	milk
½	C	cooked brown rice
¼	C	plain yogurt
2	T	lemon juice
2	T	cold-pressed oil
¾	C	whole wheat flour
¼	C	cornmeal
1½	tsp.	baking soda
¼	tsp.	ground cinnamon
¼	tsp.	ground ginger
½	tsp.	salt

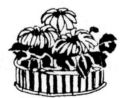

1. Separate eggs. Beat yolks well.

2. Combine yolks, milk, rice, yogurt, lemon juice, and oil.

3. Combine remaining ingredients; add to rice mixture. Stir just until combined well.

4. Beat egg whites till soft peaks form; fold into batter. Do not overmix.

5. Bake according to waffle iron directions.

Yield: 6 servings

	RCU	FU	Cal	%Ft	P	F	C	Na
Per Serving	0	1	175	42	7	8	18	362

ANNETTE'S OATMEAL WAFFLES

3	C	rolled oats
3	C	warm milk
2		eggs
4	T	cold-pressed oil
1	dash	salt

1. Whip eggs and oil together in blender until thoroughly mixed.

2. Add warm milk and rolled oats. Blend in blender until smooth.

3. Place in preheated, lightly oiled waffle iron. Bake approximately 10 minutes.

Yield: 6 7-inch waffles or 6 servings

	RCU	FU	Cal	%Ft	P	F	C	Na
Per Serving	0	2	305	41	12	14	33	87

PEAR BUCKWHEAT WAFFLES

2	C	buckwheat flour
2	tsp.	baking powder
1	tsp.	baking soda
2	tsp.	sugar
1	tsp.	salt
2		egg yolks, beaten
¼	C	melted butter
2	C	buttermilk
2		egg whites
3		fresh Bartlett pears, cored and sliced
¼	C	butter

1. Combine flour, baking powder, soda, sugar, and salt.

2. Mix together yolks, melted butter, and buttermilk. Stir in dry ingredients.

3. Whip whites until stiff but not dry. Fold them into batter until just blended.

4. Bake as desired in waffle iron.

5. Melt remaining butter and lightly sauté pear slices until warm, about 1 minute.

6. Arrange on waffles and serve.

Yield: 6 servings

	RCU	FU	Cal	%Ft	P	F	C	Na
Per Serving	0	3	363	42	7	17	43	496

WHEAT PANCAKE MIX

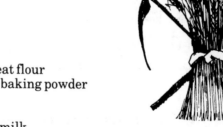

8	C	whole wheat flour
4	T	plus 2 tsp. baking powder
¼	C	sugar
4	tsp.	salt
2½	C	powdered milk
1½–2C		cooking oil

Mix all ingredients together. Store in a covered container in a cool place.

To make pancakes: Mix 1½ cups wheat mixture, 1 egg, and enough water to make the right pancake consistency. Cook on lightly oiled hot griddle.

Yield: 12–24 pancakes per recipe

	RCU	FU	Cal	%Ft	P	F	C	Na
Per Serving	0	1	192	47	5	10	23	346

HEARTY PANCAKES

3	C	flaked whole-grain sugar-free cereal, crushed to fine crumbs (to crush, place in blender one cup at a time)
1½	C	whole wheat flour
4	tsp.	baking powder
½	tsp.	salt
1	T	sugar
2		eggs
¼	C	cold-pressed oil
2¼	C	milk

1. In small mixing bowl, stir together cereal, flour, baking powder, salt, and sugar. Set aside.

2. In large bowl, beat eggs until foamy. Stir in oil and milk.

3. Add cereal mixture, mixing until batter is smooth. Let stand about 2 minutes.

4. Pour pancakes onto lightly oiled hot griddle. Cook, turning once, until golden brown on both sides. Serve warm.

Corn Fritter Variation: add 1 16-oz can whole-kernel corn, drained.

Yield: 5 cups batter or 48 pancakes

	RCU	FU	Cal	%Ft	P	F	C	Na
Per Cup	1	2	360	37	12	15	46	605

YOGURT-BLUEBERRY PANCAKES

1½	C	whole wheat flour
1	T	sugar
1	tsp.	baking powder
½	tsp.	baking soda
½	tsp.	salt
1		egg
1	C	plain yogurt, room temperature
¼	C	cold-pressed oil
¼	C	water or milk
1	C	or more blueberries, fresh or frozen
½	C	chopped nuts, if desired

1. Heat griddle while mixing batter.

2. Combine dry ingredients, set aside.

3. Beat egg and yogurt mixture well.

4. Add oil and dry mixture. Beat well.

5. Fold in blueberries carefully. Add chopped nuts, if desired.

6. Pour batter onto lightly greased griddle. Brown both sides.

Yield: 24 pancakes

	RCU	FU	Cal	%Ft	P	F	C	Na
Per Pancake	0	1	86	52	3	5	8	64

SWEET POTATO PANCAKES

1	C	whole wheat flour
¼	tsp.	salt
½	tsp.	baking soda
1		egg, separated
1	C	buttermilk
1	T	butter, melted
¾	C	shredded pared sweet potatoes or yams (1 medium)

1. Combine flour, salt, and soda.

2. In mixing bowl, beat egg yolk and buttermilk until well blended.

3. Stir in flour mixture, melted butter, and sweet potato.

4. In small mixing bowl, beat egg white until stiff; fold into batter.

5. Using 2 Tbsp batter for each pancake, drop batter onto a hot greased griddle. Cook until cakes are puffy, full of bubbles, and edges are cooked. Turn and cook other side.

Yield: 24 medium pancakes.

	RCU	FU	Cal	%Ft	P	F	C	Na
Per Pancake	0	0	32	23	1	1	5	41

BREAD SUBSTITUTES

For weight control, substitute unsweetened applesauce for the amount of oil in each muffin recipe.

BANANA NUT MUFFINS

1¼	C	whole wheat flour
2	T	honey
2½	tsp.	baking powder
½	tsp.	salt
¼	tsp.	soda
¾	C	oats
1		egg, beaten
3	T	cold-pressed oil
½	C	milk
1	C	mashed very ripe bananas
⅓	C	chopped nuts

1. Combine flour, baking powder, salt, soda, and oats.

2. Add egg, oil, milk, honey, bananas, and nuts.

3. Stir only until dry ingredients are moistened.

4. Fill greased muffin cups 2/3 full. Bake at 400 degrees for 15 minutes or until done.

Yield: 12 muffins

	RCU	FU	Cal	%Ft	P	F	C	Na
Per Muffin	½	1	178	40	5	8	21	171

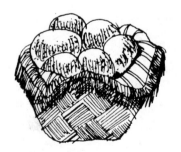

WHOLE GRAIN PUMPKIN MUFFINS

1¼	C	whole wheat flour
½	C	toasted wheat germ
2	T	honey
2½	tsp.	baking powder
½	tsp.	salt
¾	tsp.	ground cinnamon
¾	tsp.	ground nutmeg
2		eggs
¾	C	milk
½	C	canned pumpkin
¼	C	cold-pressed oil
1	tsp.	vanilla

1. Stir together the flour, wheat germ, baking powder, salt, cinnamon, and nutmeg. Make a well in the center.

2. Combine egg, honey, milk, pumpkin, oil, and vanilla; add all at once to dry ingredients. Stir just until moistened.

3. Spoon into greased muffin cups.

4. Bake at 400 degrees for 15 to 20 minutes.

Yield: 12 muffins

	RCU	FU	Cal	%Ft	P	F	C	Na
Per Muffin	½	1	149	42	6	7	17	175

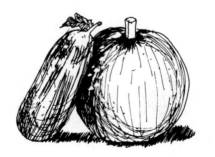

PUMPKIN-NUT MUFFINS

1¾	C	whole wheat flour
1	tsp.	baking soda
½	tsp.	baking powder
1	tsp.	ground cinnamon
1	tsp.	ground nutmeg
½	tsp.	ground ginger
2		eggs, slightly beaten
⅔	C	buttermilk
⅓	C	butter, melted
½	tsp.	vanilla
2	T	honey
1	C	canned pumpkin
½	C	chopped pecans, optional

NUTMEG

1. Heat oven to 375 degrees. Grease 18 muffin pan cups.

2. Combine flour, baking soda, baking powder, cinnamon, nutmeg, and ginger.

3. Beat together eggs, buttermilk, melted butter, honey, vanilla, and pumpkin in large bowl.

4. Stir in dry ingredients, all at once, just until moistened. Fold in nuts.

5. Spoon into prepared muffin cups filling almost to the top. Bake 15 to 20 minutes. Remove muffins from cups and cool on racks. Serve warm.

Yield: 18 muffins

	RCU	FU	Cal	%Ft	P	F	C	Na
Per Muffin	½	1	94	38	3	4	12	105

BRAN MUFFINS

2		eggs
2	T	honey
1	C	milk
3	T	cold-pressed oil
1½	C	unprocessed bran flakes
½	C	oat bran
½	C	whole wheat flour
2	tsp.	baking powder

1. Heat oven to 375 degrees. Grease muffin cups.

2. Beat eggs and honey until smooth.

3. Whisk in milk and oil.

4. Stir in bran flakes. Let soak 10 minutes.

5. Mix oat bran, flour, and baking powder in a large bowl.

6. Add soaked bran mixture and fold in just until moistened. Scoop batter into muffin cups.

7. Bake for 15–20 minutes or until firm in center.

Yield: 12 muffins

	RCU	FU	Cal	%Ft	P	F	C	Na
Per Muffin	½	1	109	41	4	5	12	155

HONEY BRAN BANANA MUFFINS

2	C	unprocessed bran flakes
1	C	buttermilk
½	C	well-mashed ripe banana
¼	C	cold-pressed oil
2	T	honey
1		egg, slightly beaten
¾	C	whole wheat flour
1	tsp.	soda
⅛	tsp.	salt

1. Combine bran cereal and buttermilk; let stand 10 minutes.

2. Stir in banana, oil, honey, and egg.

3. Add flour, soda, and salt; blend well.

4. Spoon batter into muffin tins, ⅔ full. Bake 15 minutes at 425 degrees.

Yield: 12 muffins

	RCU	FU	Cal	%Ft	P	F	C	Na
Per Muffin	½	1	125	43	3	6	16	204

BRAN BUTTERMILK MUFFINS

1½	C	buttermilk
1½	C	unprocessed bran flakes
2	T	honey
2	T	cold-pressed oil
1		egg, beaten
1¼	C	whole wheat flour
2	tsp.	baking powder
½	tsp.	baking soda
½	tsp.	salt

1. Add buttermilk to bran flakes and let stand until absorbed.

2. Beat together honey, oil, and egg and add to buttermilk mixture.

3. Add flour, baking powder, soda, and salt; blend until dry ingredients are just moistened.

4. Fill greased muffin cups ⅔ full and bake at 400 degrees for 15 to 20 minutes.

Yield: 12 muffins

	RCU	FU	Cal	%Ft	P	F	C	Na
Per Muffin	½	0	90	30	4	3	12	260

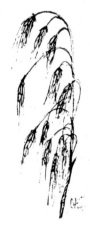

APPLE OATMEAL MUFFINS

1¼	C	whole wheat flour
1	C	quick-cooking oats
2	tsp.	baking powder
1½	tsp.	cinnamon
1	tsp.	baking soda
½	tsp.	salt
2		eggs
¼	C	cold-pressed oil
2	T	honey
½	C	milk
2	C	finely diced apples

1. Heat oven to 350 degrees. Grease 12 muffin pans.

2. Combine flour, oats, baking powder, cinnamon, baking soda, and salt; set aside.

3. Beat eggs and add oil, honey, and milk; mix well.

4. Add liquids to dry ingredients and stir until just combined; stir in apples.

5. Fill muffin tins ⅔ full with batter. Bake about 15 to 20 minutes.

Yield: 12 muffins

	RCU	FU	Cal	%Ft	P	F	C	Na
Per Muffin	½	1	167	32	4	6	24	175

APPLESAUCE MUFFINS

2	C	whole wheat flour
1	T	baking powder
¼	tsp.	baking soda
½	tsp.	cinnamon
¼	tsp.	salt
1	C	applesauce
½	C	milk
1		egg, slightly beaten
2	T	honey
2	T	cold-pressed oil

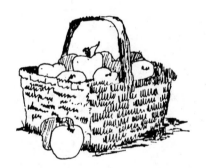

1. Combine first 5 ingredients. Make a well in the center.

2. Combine applesauce, milk, egg, honey, and oil and add to dry ingredients, stirring just until moistened.

3. Grease muffin pans and fill ⅔ full. Bake at 400 degrees for 15 to 20 minutes.

Yield: 12 muffins

	RCU	FU	Cal	%Ft	P	F	C	Na
Per Muffin	½	0	111	24	3	3	18	155

CINNAMON NUT MUFFINS

1¾	C	whole wheat flour
1	T	baking powder
½	tsp.	salt
2	T	honey
½	C	chopped pecans, optional
2		eggs, beaten
½	C	milk
¼	C	cold-pressed oil
1	tsp.	cinnamon

1. Combine dry ingredients. Make a well in the center.

2. Combine eggs, milk, and oil. Pour into the center of the well.

3. Stir until just moistened. Cook at 400 degrees for 15 minutes or until done.

Yield: 12 muffins

	RCU	FU	Cal	%Ft	P	F	C	Na
Per Muffin	½	1	127	43	4	6	16	168

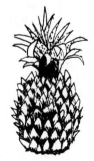

PINEAPPLE BRAN MUFFINS

1	C	unprocessed bran flakes
½	C	milk
1	C	unsweetened crushed pineapple (not completely drained)
¼	C	cold-pressed oil
1		egg
1	C	whole wheat flour
2	tsp.	baking powder
¼	tsp.	salt
¼	tsp.	soda
1	T	honey

1. Soak cereal in milk. Add other liquids.

2. Combine all dry ingredients and combine until moistened.

3. Bake at 400 degrees for 15 to 20 minutes.

Yield: 12 muffins

	RCU	FU	Cal	%Ft	P	F	C	Na
Per Muffin	0	1	102	53	3	6	11	167

YOGURT MUFFINS

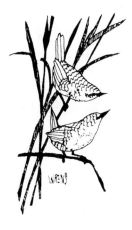

2	C	whole wheat flour
2	tsp.	baking powder
½	tsp.	baking soda
¾	tsp.	cinnamon
¾	tsp.	nutmeg
½	C	chopped pecans
1		egg, beaten
¼	C	cold pressed oil
⅓	C	milk
2	T	honey
1	8 oz.	carton plain yogurt

1. Combine flour, baking powder, soda, salt, cinnamon, and nutmeg in large bowl. Stir in pecans; make a well in center of mixture.

2. Combine egg, oil, milk, honey, and yogurt; add to dry ingredients and stir until moistened.

3. Spoon into greased muffin pan, filling two thirds full. Bake at 400 degrees for 20 minutes or until golden brown.

Yield: 12 muffins

	RCU	FU	Cal	%Ft	P	F	C	Na
Per Muffins	½	1	164	49	4	9	18	89

APPLE WHOLE WHEAT MUFFINS

⅓	C	butter
2	T	brown sugar
2		eggs
1¾	C	whole wheat flour
1	T	baking powder
¾	tsp.	ground cinnamon
¼	tsp.	baking soda
¼	tsp.	salt
⅛	tsp.	ground ginger
1	C	plain yogurt
1½	C	cored and finely chopped apples

1. Cream butter and brown sugar until light and fluffy.

2. Beat in eggs one at a time, beating well after each addition.

3. Combine flour, baking powder, cinnamon, baking soda, salt, and ginger.

4. Add dry ingredients and yogurt alternately to creamed mixture.

5. Fold in chopped apples.

6. Spoon batter into 12 greased or paper lined muffin cups. Muffin cups will be full.

7. Bake at 425 degrees for 15–20 minutes or until a toothpick inserted near center comes out clean.

Yield: 12 muffins

	RCU	FU	Cal	%Ft	P	F	C	Na
Per Muffin	0	1	141	38	4	6	18	148

TROPICAL MUFFINS

2½	C	unprocessed bran flakes
1⅓	C	whole wheat flour
2½	tsp.	baking soda
½	tsp.	salt
1	C	unsweetened shredded coconut
2		eggs
¾	C	buttermilk
¼	C	cold-pressed oil

| 1⅓ | C | unsweetened applesauce |
| 2 | T | honey |

1. Combine first 5 ingredients, mix to blend.

2. In another bowl beat eggs; add buttermilk, oil, applesauce, and honey; add to dry ingredients. Mix just until blended.

3. Spoon batter into 18 greased muffin cups.

4. Bake at 375 degrees for 15 to 20 minutes.

Yield: 18 muffins

	RCU	FU	Cal	%Ft	P	F	C	Na
Per Muffin	½	1	134	54	3	8	14	206

3 GRAIN MUFFINS

1	C	rolled oats
½	C	whole wheat flour
½	C	cornmeal
2	tsp.	baking powder
¼	tsp.	salt
1	tsp.	cinnamon
½	C	milk or water
¼	C	cold-pressed oil
2		eggs
2	T	honey
1	C	firmly-packed shredded carrots

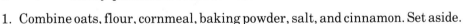

1. Combine oats, flour, cornmeal, baking powder, salt, and cinnamon. Set aside.

2. In a large bowl, beat milk, oil, eggs, and honey until blended.

3. Add flour mixture, stir only until moistened. Lightly stir in carrots.

4. Spoon into greased muffin cups filling ⅔ full.

5. Bake in a 400 degree oven 15–20 minutes.

Yield: 12 muffins

	RCU	FU	Cal	%Ft	P	F	C	Na
Per Muffin	½	1	137	39	4	6	18	107

WHEAT-FREE MUFFINS

1	C	rolled oats
1½	C	oat bran
½	C	chopped nuts
¼	tsp.	salt
1	T	baking powder
1		mashed banana
2		eggs, lightly beaten
3	T	cold-pressed oil
2	T	honey
¾	C	milk

1. Combine the dry ingredients in a bowl.

2. Mix together the mashed banana, eggs, oil, honey, and milk.

3. Add this mixture to the dry ingredients and combine only until moistened.

4. Fill greased or paper lined muffin cups ⅔ full. Bake at 400 degrees for about 20 minutes.

Yield: 12 muffins

	RCU	FU	Cal	%Ft	P	F	C	Na
Per Muffin	½	1	133	47	4	7	12	104

IRISH SODA BREAD

4	C	whole wheat flour
½	tsp.	salt
1	tsp.	baking soda
2	tsp.	baking powder
2	tsp.	cream of tartar
½	C	butter
3	T	honey
1½-1¾C		buttermilk

1. Blend together flour, salt, baking soda, baking powder, and cream of tartar.

2. Cut in butter with a pastry blender.

3. Make a well in center of flour mixture; add honey and buttermilk. Add enough buttermilk to make a soft dough.

4. Form with floured fingers into a round shape and place smooth side up on lightly floured baking sheet. Cut an X on top. This keeps the crust from splitting.

5. Bake at 350 degrees for 35–45 minutes until a rich brown. Tap bottom of loaf. If it sounds hollow, the bread is done.

Yield: 16 slices

	RCU	FU	Cal	%Ft	P	F	C	Na
Per Slice	½	1	173	36	5	7	26	233

IRISH WHOLE WHEAT OATMEAL BREAD

¾	C	buttermilk
1		egg, beaten
1	T	butter, melted
1¾	C	whole wheat flour
1	C	quick-cooking oats
2	T	honey
1½	tsp.	baking powder
½	tsp.	baking soda
½	tsp.	salt

1. Heat oven to 350 degrees. Grease large baking sheet.

2. Combine buttermilk, honey, egg, and melted butter in small bowl and blend well.

3. Mix remaining ingredients in large bowl. Make well in center of dry ingredients. Pour buttermilk mixture into well.

4. Gradually draw flour from inner edge of well into center until completely incorporated.

5. Transfer dough to floured work surface and knead lightly for 3 minutes. Shape dough into disc.

6. Transfer to prepared baking sheet. Make an X on top using sharp knife.

7. Bake until tester inserted in center comes out clean, 40 to 50 minutes. Serve warm.

Yield: 12 slices

	RCU	FU	Cal	%Ft	P	F	C	Na
Per Slice	½	0	110	16	4	2	19	164

WHOLE WHEAT FLAT BREAD

2	T	honey
½	C	shortening
1	qt.	buttermilk
1	tsp.	salt
6	C	whole wheat flour
2	tsp.	baking powder
2	tsp.	soda

1. Cream sugar and shortening in a bowl. Gradually add buttermilk; mix well.

2. Stir in salt and 3 cups of the whole wheat flour; beat thoroughly.

3. Mix the rest of the flour with the baking powder and soda. Add to mixture, stirring until dough leaves sides of bowl.

4. Roll on lightly floured surface until nearly paper thin. Lift carefully onto greased cookie sheets.

5. Bake at 375 degrees for 12 minutes until brown and crisp. Serve hot.

Yield: 48 slices

	RCU	FU	Cal	%Ft	P	F	C	Na
Per Slice	0	0	75	31	2	3	11	81

RYE FLAT BREAD

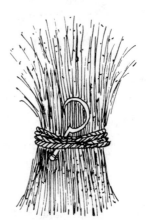

2	C	rye flour
¾	C	instant non-fat dry milk
½	C	sesame seed
½	C	sunflower seeds
1	dash	salt
3	T	cold-pressed oil
1	C	water
1		egg, well beaten

1. Combine rye flour, dry milk, sesame seeds, sunflower seeds, and salt; mix well.

2. Stir in oil and 1 cup water; mix well.

3. Fold in egg.

4. Spoon out evenly on well-greased and floured baking sheet. Flatten ⅓ to ½ inch thick with oiled hands; the dough will be very sticky.

5. Bake at 450 degrees for 10 to 12 minutes. Brown under broiler. Best if served hot.

Yield: 16 slices

	RCU	FU	Cal	%Ft	P	F	C	Na
Per Slice	0	1	188	48	7	10	18	45

POPPY SEED CRACKERS

⅓	C	poppy seed
2	C	whole wheat flour
1½	tsp.	salt
½	tsp.	soda
¼	tsp.	pepper
⅓	C	cold-pressed oil
1	T	honey
1		egg, slightly beaten
⅓	C	minced onion

1. Combine poppy seed with ⅓ cup boiling water; cool.

2. Place flour, salt, soda, and pepper into bowl. Stir in remaining ingredients and poppy seed mixture, mixing well.

3. Knead lightly on floured surface until smooth.

4. Roll out half the dough at a time to ⅛-inch thickness. Cut with 1½-inch biscuit cutter.

5. Place on baking sheet; prick with fork. Bake at 425 degrees for 10 minutes or until lightly browned. Store in airtight container.

Yield: 8 dozen crackers

	RCU	FU	Cal	%Ft	P	F	C	Na
Per Cracker	0	0	16	56	0	1	2	30

JOLENE'S RYE CRACKERS

½	C	rye flour
½	C	quick cooking oats
½	C	walnuts
1	tsp.	baking powder
2		eggs
1	tsp.	vanilla
1	T	honey
⅓	C	cold-pressed oil

1. Mix dry ingredients; add remaining ingredients, stir well.

2. Pour into greased 9 x 9 square pan.

3. Bake at 350 degrees for 30–35 minutes.

4. Cut into squares while warm.

Yield: 16 crackers

	RCU	FU	Cal	%Ft	P	F	C	Na
Per Cracker	0	1	125	65	3	9	7	31

WHOLE WHEAT TORTILLAS

4	C	whole wheat flour
¼	tsp.	baking powder
¼	C	cold-pressed oil
1	C	warm water
1½	tsp.	salt

1. Combine all ingredients and knead for 5 minutes. You may need a little more water, but the dough should be very stiff. Let stand for 10 minutes.

2. Shape into balls and let stand for 10 minutes more. The ball will be a bit dry.

3. Roll very thin to form a circle. Cook on a hot griddle.

Yield: 12 tortillas

	RCU	FU	Cal	%Ft	P	F	C	Na
Per Tortilla	0	1	158	28	5	5	25	245

MEAL ACCOMPANIMENTS

BARLEY OVEN PILAF

3	C	water or chicken broth
1	C	quick-cooking barley
½	tsp.	salt
1	C	finely chopped onion
½	C	shredded carrot
½	C	chopped green onions
2	T	olive oil
¼	C	toasted wheat germ
¼	tsp.	garlic powder
2	T	finely chopped parsley

1. In saucepan, bring water to boiling. Add barley and salt; return to boiling.

2. Reduce heat; cover and simmer for 12 to 15 minutes or until barley is tender. Do not drain.

3. Meanwhile, in another saucepan, cook onion, carrot, and green onions in oil until tender.

4. In a greased 1½-quart casserole, combine undrained barley, vegetables, wheat germ, and garlic powder.

5. Bake, uncovered, at 350 degrees for 25 to 30 minutes or until light brown.

6. Fluff with a fork to serve. Sprinkle with parsley.

Yield: 8 servings

	RCU	FU	Cal	%Ft	P	F	C	Na
Per Serving	0	1	167	22	5	4	28	276

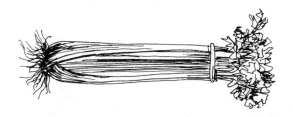

SOUPS

CREAM OF ZUCCHINI SOUP

2	med.	onions
1½	lbs.	zucchini
½	C	milk
1	pinch	cayenne pepper
2	T	butter
3	C	chicken broth
⅛	tsp.	black pepper
⅛	tsp.	salt

1. Chop and cook onion in butter until clear and soft, but not browned.

2. Wash and slice zucchini.

3. Combine onion, zucchini, and chicken broth in saucepan and bring to a boil, then simmer for 15 minutes or until the squash is tender.

4. Add seasonings and put mixture into blender to puree until smooth.

5. Add milk. Adjust seasonings to taste.

Yield: 4 servings

	RCU	FU	Cal	%Ft	P	F	C	Na
Per Serving	0	1	113	45	4	6	13	451

NEW ENGLAND CLAM CHOWDER

2	T	butter
1	sm.	onion, diced
½	C	diced celery
3	C	cubed potatoes
		water
½	tsp.	salt
¼	tsp.	pepper
2	C	milk
1	7½-oz. can	minced clams, drained; reserve liquid

1. Melt butter. Add onion and celery and cook until tender, but not browned.

2. Add potatoes, clam juice plus water to make 2 cups, salt, and pepper.

3. Cover; simmer until potatoes are tender, about 15 minutes.

4. Add milk and clams; heat through.

Yield: 4 servings

	RCU	FU	Cal	%Ft	P	F	C	Na
Per Serving	0	1	258	24	16	7	33	475

POTATO SOUP

5	med.	potatoes, peeled and cubed
1	med.	onion, chopped
½	C	celery, chopped
3	C	water
1	C	milk
1	tsp.	salt
1	tsp.	chicken bouillon
2	tsp.	chives, chopped
⅛	tsp.	white pepper

1. Combine potatoes, onion, celery, and water in a 3-quart pan. Bring to a boil; cover, reduce heat, and simmer until potatoes are tender.

2. Drain, and reserve 1½ cups cooking liquid and set vegetables aside.

3. Mash vegetable mixture and add to reserved cooking liquid, along with the milk, salt, bouillon, chives, and pepper.

4. Cook, stirring constantly, until heated.

Yield: 4–6 servings

	RCU	FU	Cal	%Ft	P	F	C	Na
Per Serving	0	0	138	0	6	0	29	629

CREAM OF TOMATO SOUP

1	qt.	tomatoes, put into blender until smooth
3	slices	onion
3	T	butter, melted
3	T	whole wheat flour
¼	tsp.	baking soda
1	tsp.	salt
1	dash	pepper
1	qt.	milk

1. Boil tomatoes and onion together for 10 minutes. Discard the onion.

2. Mix together melted butter, flour, soda, salt, and pepper. Add to tomatoes and stir until thick.

3. Then add 1 quart cold milk. Heat, but do not boil.

Yield: 4–6 servings

	RCU	FU	Cal	%Ft	P	F	C	Na
Per Serving	0	1	157	40	8	7	19	793

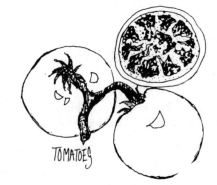

TOMATOES

TURKEY CHOWDER

2	T	butter
2	T	whole wheat flour
2	C	milk
2	C	chopped cooked turkey
1½	C	diced cooked potatoes
1	10-oz. pkg.	frozen mixed vegetables, cooked
1	tsp.	chicken flavored bouillon granules
½	tsp.	dried minced onion
⅛	tsp.	white pepper

1. Melt butter over low heat; add flour, stirring until smooth. Cook 1 minute, stirring constantly.

2. Gradually add milk and cook over medium heat, stirring constantly until mixture thickens.

3. Add remaining ingredients and mix well. Cook over low heat, stirring constantly, until heated.

Yield: 6 servings

	RCU	FU	Cal	%Ft	P	F	C	Na
Per Serving	0	1	165	22	8	4	69	184

HAMBURGER SOUP

1	lb.	lean ground beef
1	28-oz. can	tomatoes or 1 quart tomatoes
1	lg.	onion, chopped
1		green pepper, chopped
2	cans	kidney beans, drained
3	C	water
2	C	potatoes, diced
1½	tsp.	seasoned salt
½	tsp.	thyme
1½	tsp.	chili powder
1		bay leaf
½	tsp.	garlic salt
⅛	tsp.	pepper

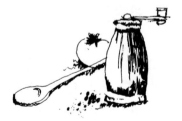

1. Brown hamburger and onions, remove any fat drippings.

2. Add rest of ingredients. Simmer 2–3 hours.

Yield: 8 servings

	RCU	FU	Cal	%Ft	P	F	C	Na
Per Serving	0	1	230	47	21	12	175	388

VEGETABLE SOUP

¼	C	butter
½	C	peeled and diced carrot
½	C	diced onion
½	C	diced celery
¼	tsp.	oregano, crumbled
¼	tsp.	Italian seasoning, crumbled
⅛	tsp.	basil, crumbled
⅛	tsp.	thyme, crumbled
⅛	tsp.	rosemary, crumbled
1		diced garlic clove
1		bay leaf
7	C	beef stock
2	C	whole tomatoes, drained
⅔	C	diced potato
1	C	cooked kidney beans
1	C	cooked navy beans
½	C	whole wheat macaroni
1	T	fresh parsley, chopped
¼	C	barley
½	C	split peas
¼	C	lentils
to taste		salt and pepper
1	C	chopped spinach
½	C	chopped cabbage

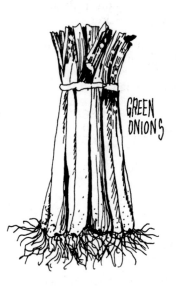

GREEN ONIONS

1. Heat butter and add the next 10 ingredients and cook until the vegetables soften, stirring frequently about 10 minutes.

2. Add the next 10 ingredients. Season with salt and pepper.

3. Cover and cook about 1 hour.

4. Add spinach and cabbage. Cook 10 minutes. Adjust seasonings.

Yield: 10 servings

	RCU	FU	Cal	%Ft	P	F	C	Na
Per Serving	0	1	187	39	7	8	85	361

CHICKEN AND CORN SOUP

1		whole chicken fryer
6	C	chicken stock
1	can	creamed corn
1	T	minced dry onion
4		chicken bouillon cubes
1	tsp.	dried parsley
½	tsp.	salt
¼	tsp.	black pepper
4	T	cornstarch

1. Cook the chicken until tender in 6½ cups of water. Remove the chicken and return the chicken stock to a large pan.

2. Chop the chicken into cubes. Add to the stock along with the creamed corn, dry onion, bouillon cubes, parsley, salt, and pepper. Bring mixture to a boil.

3. Combine cornstarch and ¼ cup water; stir into chicken stock mixture, cooking and stirring until the mixture boils and thickens.

Yield: 6 servings

	RCU	FU	Cal	%Ft	P	F	C	Na
Per Serving	0	0	182	15	25	3	11	971

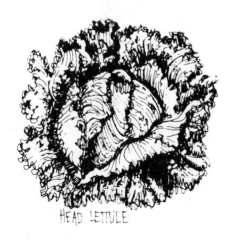

HEAD LETTUCE

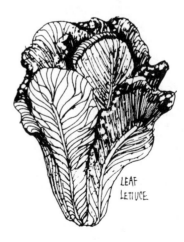

LEAF LETTUCE

MINESTRONE SOUP

¼	C	olive oil
3	C	diced onions
2	C	diced carrots
2	C	diced celery
2	C	diced canned or bottled tomatoes
1	16-oz. can	green beans
1	15-oz. can	kidney beans
2	C	chopped cabbage
2	tsp.	salt
1	tsp.	white pepper
1½	tsp.	garlic powder
3	T	beef bouillon
2	T	chicken bouillon
1½	tsp.	basil
2	tsp.	oregano
8	C	water
1	can	tomato sauce
½	C	barley
1	15-oz. can	garbanzo beans
1	C	whole wheat macaroni

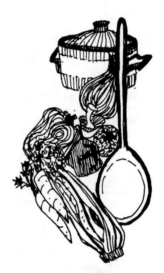

1. Heat olive oil. Sauté diced onions, carrots, and celery.

2. Add tomatoes, green beans, kidney beans, cabbage, salt, pepper, garlic powder, bouillons, basil, oregano, water, tomato sauce, and barley. Simmer 45 minutes.

3. Stir in garbanzo beans and macaroni, and simmer until macaroni is tender.

Yield: 12 servings

	RCU	FU	Cal	%Ft	P	F	C	Na
Per Serving	0	1	216	33	8	8	79	424

CHICKEN AND VEGETABLE SOUP

1		chicken
		Water
4	C	diced carrots
4	C	diced celery
1	C	diced green pepper
2	lg.	onions, diced
3	C	diced fresh or canned tomatoes, with liquid
½	C	snipped parsley

Juice of 1 lemon
to taste   salt and pepper
1   tsp.   curry powder
1–2 C   dried potato flakes, depending on thickness desired

1. Cover chicken with water and cook for about 1 hour, until tender. Remove chicken from water; cool.

2. Retain liquid; refrigerate overnight. Remove fat from chilled liquid; discard fat.

3. Cut chicken into small pieces. Discard skin and bones.

4. Add water to liquid, if necessary, to make two quarts. Heat to boiling.

5. Add carrots, celery, green pepper, onions, tomatoes, parsley, lemon juice, salt, pepper, and curry powder. Bring to a boil.

6. Cover and simmer for two hours, stirring often.

7. Add dried potato flakes; heat to boiling.

Yield: 15 one cup servings

	RCU	FU	Cal	%Ft	P	F	C	Na
Per Serving	0	0	96	28	11	3	73	145

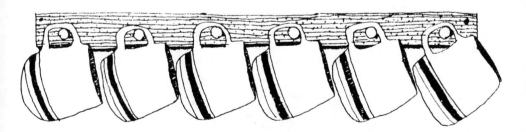

DIPS AND SALAD DRESSING RECIPES

COTTAGE CHEESE DIP OR SALAD DRESSING

1	lb.	low-fat creamed cottage cheese
2	T	buttermilk (For Dip) OR
4	T	buttermilk (For Salad Dressing)
2	tsp.	dill weed
1	tsp.	onion powder
1	pinch	salt
½	tsp.	Beau Monde Seasoning

1. Place cottage cheese and buttermilk in a blender; blend until smooth.

2. Stir in spices.

Yield: 12 servings

	RCU	FU	Cal	%Ft	P	F	C	Na
Per Serving	0	0	35	26	5	1	2	15

VEGETABLE DILL DIP

1	C	plain yogurt
2	T	minced onion
2	tsp.	Bon Appetit
1	C	mayonnaise
1	T	parsley flakes
2	tsp.	dill weed

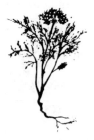

1. Mix all ingredients until well blended.

2. Chill to enhance flavor.

3. Use dip with raw carrots, celery, radishes, cucumbers, cauliflower, broccoli, and other raw vegetables.

Yield: 12 servings

	RCU	FU	Cal	%Ft	P	F	C	Na
Per Serving	0	1	131	96	1	14	1	111

GUACAMOLE

2	med.	avocados, mashed
1	T	finely chopped onion
½	tsp.	chili powder (or more if preferred)
1	dash	salt
1	T	lemon juice
1	tsp.	cold-pressed oil
1	clove	garlic, finely minced
2		tomatoes, peeled and chopped
2	T	mayonnaise

1. Mix together all ingredients. Chill.

2. Serve as a dip with raw vegetables or corn chips or use as a salad dressing.

Yield: 12 servings

	RCU	FU	Cal	%Ft	P	F	C	Na
Per Serving	0	1	58	78	1	5	3	14

NORMA'S SALAD DRESSING

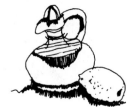

¾	C	olive oil
juice from 1 lime		
1	clove	garlic, minced finely
½	tsp.	basil
¼	tsp.	oregano
freshly ground pepper		

1. Blend together.

2. Shake well before using.

Yield: 6 servings

	RCU	FU	Cal	%Ft	P	F	C	Na
Per Serving	0	4	251	100	0	28	0	0

FRENCH DRESSING

½	C	olive oil
4	T	lemon juice
⅛	tsp.	cayenne pepper
⅛	tsp.	basil
⅛	tsp.	parsley flakes
⅛	tsp.	oregano
1	clove	garlic, crushed

1. Combine first 6 ingredients in a jar with lid and shake well.

2. Add crushed garlic clove and shake well again.

3. Let the jar stand for 30 minutes and then remove the garlic clove. Shake well before using.

Yield: 6 servings

	RCU	FU	Cal	%Ft	P	F	C	Na
Per Serving	0	3	171	100	0	19	0	0

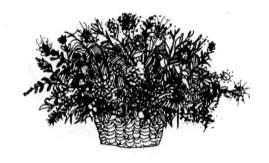

Appendix Eight
INFORMATION FOR PHYSICIANS

CHRONIC CANDIDIASIS

Over the last number of years, a greatly expanded concept of illness caused by Candida albicans has emerged. Improved treatment techniques have also evolved, and thousands of doctors across the world have collectively treated millions of people for disease believed to be caused by Candida. Remarkable improvements in a wide range of health problems have been reported in the medical literature. A number of articles appearing in various magazines[1,2,3,4,5] and a variety of books[6,7,8,9,10,11,12] written for the lay public have been written. Some other doctors have not only refused to accept these reports, but have been very vocal in denouncing them as unproven, unscientific, illogical and impossible.

The purposes of this appendix are to present the current concept of Candida-induced illness, present possible theories to explain observations, present findings from the scientific literature to support the observations and theories, and to discuss possible reasons for the controversy.

ADVANCING CONCEPTS OF INFECTIOUS DISEASES

In the early days of medicine, doctors described various clinical syndromes without understanding what caused them. After bacteria were discovered, there was a tremendous explosion of knowledge relating specific bacteria to specific clinical syndromes. Later, a similar phenomenon occurred with the discovery of viruses. After the advent of antibiotics, bacterial infections could be cured. Symptoms or signs which improved with treatment were then attributed to the bacteria, and gave further proof that bacteria caused those problems. The concept of disease caused by infectious microbes was relatively simplistic at first--the organism invaded the tissues, the host got sick, the antibiotic got rid of the organism, and the host completely recovered.

Besides direct invasion of tissues, other ways were discovered by which bacteria could cause disease. Various toxic substances were found excreted by bacteria which created clinical problems. These toxins have been associated with much of the pathology associated with bacterial-induced diseases such as diphtheria, tetanus, gas gangrene, and toxic shock syndrome. A variety of fungi have also been shown to produce mycotoxins, which induce various symptoms in humans.

Humans have been long known to have mechanisms for fighting off infections, and developing resistance to further infections. The nutritional status of the host is known to be important for disease resistance (although largely ignored in modern medicine), and deficiency of specific vitamins is clearly linked with disease susceptibility.

Various immunoglobulins, antibodies, and a variety of other immune mediated substances, were discovered to influence host immunity, and a much more expanded concept of microbe-induced illness was formulated. One of the first of these findings was the role of auto-antibodies formed in response to beta hemolytic streptococcus in causing rheumatic heart disease. A wide range of auto-immune diseases have been identified, and many of the common diseases have been linked to this pathological process. The initiating cause for many of these autoimmune processes has been shown to be a specific microorganism. Insulin-dependent diabetes is now thought to be caused by an immune response to various virus infections such as coxsackie virus B, rubella, and measles.[13] Further proof comes with the ability to cause an early remission with the immune-suppressing drug, cyclosporine.[14,15] There is also some evidence that chronic diseases such as multiple sclerosis may be initiated by viral exposure.[16,17]

Bacteria have also been shown to be initiators for chronic, autoimmune diseases. Antibodies to the common pathogen Klebsiella have been thought to be instrum-ental in causing ankylosing spondylitis,[18] and antibodies to Proteus has been thought be a cause for rheumatoid arthritis.[19,20] Some of the autoimmune - endocrine diseases are thought to be initiated by particular organisms, including Yersinia causing Grave's disease.[21] Yersinia can cause a chronic enterocolitis, and has also been linked to cases of rheumatoid arthritis.[22]

Although some **chronic illnesses** such as syphilis and tuberculosis have been long known, most infectious diseases have been thought to cause acute illness only. It has also been thought that the immune system quickly brought the infect-ious agents under complete control. It is now clear that various organisms can cause chronic illness, often lasting for many years, and often for the life of the patient. For example, those afflicted with polio may, decades later, develop "post-poliomyelitis progressive muscular atrophy."[23]

Diseases caused by viral and bacterial pathogens may also cause **multi-system disease**. These illnesses may be a consequence of many factors, including presence of living organisms, autoimmune responses to those organisms, permanent dam-age to various components of endocrine systems, and central nervous system pathology. Chronic Fatigue Syndrome is an example of a chronic, multi-system illness thought to be caused by a virus. Lyme's disease is a good example of a bacteria causing chronic, multi-system disease. A November 1990 study described treating a group of patients who had chronic multi-system symptoms up to 14 years after acute infection with B. burgdorferi, that improved with specific antibiotic therapy.[24] Both diseases are characterized by an acute febrile illness, followed by a variety of symptoms in various body systems including fatigue, disturbed memory, depression, headaches, muscle pains, arthritis, etc., often lasting for many years.

As new information emerges, it is reported to doctors in the various medical journals. Reports may be of one or more cases of patients in which a previously unreported symptom or sign was associated with a particular microbe. For in-stance, a relationship was reported in a patient with cluster headache associated with a Herpes virus infection, which cleared on two occasions with acyclovir treatment.[25] Other reports include new theories or mechanisms that may account for well known features of an existing disease. The literature may report results of various new treatments for well known diseases, and various treatments methods may be compared for efficacy. Most doctors continue to update their knowledge base and improve their ability to treat diseases by reading the medical literature, and applying the suggested principles. Doctors also learn from other doctors who have developed some skill in treating a particular disease. Learning may come by direct one-on-one contact, or through teaching sessions at hospital rounds, or conferences.

Modern medicine is certainly not a static thing, and in fact, there has almost been an explosion of information in recent years regarding the role of viruses and bacteria in causing illness. Likewise, there has been a rapidly expanding body of information regarding the role of Candida albicans (and related species) in causing human illness. Just like viruses and bacteria, Candida species produce a number of toxins, and are capable of inducing a variety of immune mediated problems. Literally thousands of articles have been printed from around the world in various scientific and medical journals describing various facets of Candida. Several AMA approved conferences have been held in recent years dealing specifically with new findings related to Candida and human illnesses. [26,27,28,29,30] Various university-based clinicians and researchers from around the world presented new information about diagnosing and treating Candida at these conferences.

From this expanding body of information about Candida, we would next like to present the current concept of Candida-induced illness. The information for this appendix comes from approximately 3,000 references (abstracts or full articles) obtained from several comprehensive searches of the world scientific and medical literature. Information also comes from attendance at or from the tapes of several Yeast/Human Interaction Symposia dealing exclusively with Candida-induced health problems. Much has been learned from close observation of over 5,000 patients who have started on a "trial of therapy" for suspected Candida-related health problems. All of these patients evaluated their symptoms before treatment began, and each visit after treatment was started, using a comprehensive symptom check list containing 157 items. We now have literally millions of individual pieces of data from which to evaluate clinical response to therapy.

The term **chronic candidiasis** is not completely adequate to described the expanded range of health problems induced by Candida, since that name merely implies an infection. Other names including chronic candidosis, Candida-induced illness, candidiasis hypersensitivity syndrome, Candida-related complex, and the yeast connection have also been used. All these names have limitations, and so we would like to stick to "chronic candidiasis" (CC), but have the reader keep in mind that we are referring to not only the infective component, but a range of other features as well. A formal definition will be given later.

The current concepts mainly arise from attempts to explain the improvements repeatedly observed in patients who undergo therapy for suspected CC. Whether these attempted explanations are correct or not matters very little. They are based on currently accepted medical theories, and if some of these theories are incorrect, then the concepts will also likely prove to be incorrect. The most important issue is this: thousands of doctors from around the world have treated millions of people suspected of having CC with a multifaceted treatment program. A great number of health problems often clear up completely and dramatically.

CURRENT CONCEPTS IN CHRONIC CANDIDIASIS

Candida albicans appears to cause disease in humans as a consequence of a number of factors.

1. Candida can invade various tissues directly.
2. Candida can produce various specific toxins and toxic metabolites.
3. Candida may provoke inappropriate host immunological responses.
4. Candida may contribute to nutrient deficiencies.
5. Candida may interfere with endocrine function.

1. CANDIDA INFECTIONS

Candida albicans has been shown to have the ability to invade virtually every tissue in the human body. (Other Candida species have similar properties, but the focus of this discussion will be mainly on the more common albicans species.) Infection of the mouth in babies and the vagina in women has been known and described in the medical literature for many years. Invasion of other tissues including the esophagus,[31,32] stomach,[33] small and large intestines, gall-bladder,[34] liver,[35] peritoneum,[36,37] urinary bladder,[38] kidney, prostate,[39] epididymis,[40] throat, mouth,[41] gums, tongue, lungs,[42] nose, ears,[43] sinuses,[44] thyroid,[45] heart,[46,47,48,49] pericardium,[50] muscles,[51] skin,[52,53] finger and toe nails, bones,[54] various parts of the eye,[55,56] and even the brain[57,58,59,60] have also been described. These infections run the gamut from acute, mild, self-limiting, localized infections to fulminating, rapidly fatal infestation of virtually all body tissues.

Part of the Candida controversy centers around the issue of acute versus chronic infections. Although the two extremes mentioned above are fairly well accepted by most physicians, many doctors have expressed disbelief that Candida infections can become chronic.

Chronic mucocutaneous candidiasis has been described in the literature for many years. In this condition, Candida invades mucous membranes, skin and nails, and stays for literally years, if untreated. Some types appear to be genetic, and others appear to be the result of some form of acquired immune suppression (such as AIDS). Every dentist deals with patients who have chronic candidiasis in the mouth,[61] especially when dentures or other appliances harbor these organisms and seem to interfere with natural host defenses. Every dermatologist deals with patients who have chronic onchymycoses, or chronic skin infections around the nails, in the groin, intertriginous areas under the breasts, perianal, or perineal area.

Acute and chronic infections of the esophagus have been described, particularly in immuno-compromised patients. Candidal esophagitis has been described as the most frequent infection of the esophagus.[62] Much of the research for the new anti-Candida drug Fluconazol has been done with **chronic esophagitis. Chronic gastritis and peptic ulcers** have been reported to be the consequence of Candida infections.[63] In a number of studies, they have been identified in the biopsies of ulcer craters in a high percentage of patients.[64,65,66,67] **Chronic diarrhea** and **colitis** caused by Candida infections have also been described. **Chronic perianal itching** has also been reported to be caused by Candida infections.

Candida has been long known to cause **chronic vaginal infections**. Every primary care physician has seen many patients who complain of persistent vaginal itching, burning, and discharge which responds only temporarily or partially to topical treatment. A recent study in the New England Journal of Medicine showed no significant difference in the cultures before treatment versus after treatment with up to 24 weeks of treatment with Nystatin.[68] Even after 16 weeks of continuous treatment, another eight-week block of treatment produced further improvement. This and other studies now suggest the ability of Candida to survive in the vagina in spite of rather prolonged therapy.

Although most bladder and urinary tract infections are thought to be caused by bacteria, it is now clear that **chronic kidney and bladder infections** can also be caused by Candida.[69,70,71,72,73,74] Much of the recent Fluconazol research has been done on those with chronic urinary tract infections.[75] These patients, often with a history of problems going back many years, who often fail to respond to oral Nystatin and other Candida control measures, responded well to systemic Fluconazol treatment.

To understand chronic infections with Candida, it is necessary to understand something about their structural characteristics. Candida can exist in a simple yeast form, living mainly on mucous membrane surfaces (superficial candidiasis). In more severe cases, Candida can produce "hyphae", which can invade between the cells and even into the cells of the host epithelium (invasive candidiasis).[76] Hyphae invasion of the deep tissues may explain the resistance of chronic vaginitis and other chronic Candida infections to convention topical therapy. Candida may also be spread to various parts of the body through blood-borne "chlamydospores" (disseminating candidiasis).[77] There is some controversy as to which form of Candida is more virulent. When both the yeast and mycelial form of Candida are injected into experimental animals, the yeast form is more lethal, probably due to toxin content.[78] Some particularly invasive strains of Candida appear to be more prone to occur in the hyphae phase.[79]

Candida albicans, then, can exist in the human body in a wide spectrum of states. Candida can exist as a commensal organism, merely a part of the normal flora causing no disease at all. Candida can cause acute, superficial, regional, self-limiting infections. It can become invasive and chronic, causing deep, resistant infections of various mucous membrane structures. It can disseminate widely to cause infection in almost every tissue of the body. It can become very fulminating, and cause rapid death through extensive tissue damage and toxin production.

Factors influencing Candida "infections"

The human intestinal tract, skin, and various mucous membranes, sterile at birth, quickly become colonized with various microorganisms picked up during passage through the birth canal, and by various other human contacts. A particular balance of microorganisms is achieved by a number of interrelated host versus parasite factors:

a. **Many microorganisms produce anti-microbial chemicals** that inhibit the growth of other organisms that would otherwise compete for living space and nutrients.[80,81] Most microorganisms seem to have this capacity,[82] and most of our antibiotics, including penicillin, tetracycline, cephalosporin, and erythromycin, are produced by various fungal and bacterial species. Lactobacilli in particular has been shown to produce a number of chemicals toxic to other organisms, and particularly to Candida species.

b. **Toxic by-products from various metabolic processes** may produced conditions (like altered pH levels) that favor the growth of some microorganisms, while inhibiting the growth of others[83]. Toxins like ethanol,[84,85] lactic acid,[86] and hydrogen peroxide[87,88] may be lethal to certain organisms, but not others. Various toxins may also suppress immunity, allowing Candida to become more numerous.

c. **The type of food available in the gut may greatly affect the ratio of microorganisms. Breast milk appears to enhance the growth of various strains of Lactobacillus bacteria.**[89,90] Some theorize that there is a specific growth-enhancer in breast milk; others suggest that the Lactobacilli are actually transmitted through the milk. Lactobacilli appear to be species specific, and cow's milk may not support the growth of a healthy Lactobacilli population in humans as well as does breast milk.

d. **All plants appear to manufacture chemicals that keep them from being consumed by various microorganisms in the soil and air.**[91,92,93,94,95] For example, modern strains of mold-resistant soybeans have levels of phenylisothiocyanate many times higher than that of strains grown thirty years ago. **This anti-fungal chemical,**[96] **and others produced by different plants that we eat for food, may inhibit intestinal Candida species.**[97,98,99,100] **Refined sugars, which have no fungal inhibitors, encourage the rapid growth of various fungi, including Candida.** Refined carbohydrates in the diet may encourage rapid growth of Candida, in a similar way to the rapid growth of baker's yeast when sugar water is added. Adding refined carbohydrates to cow's milk in baby formulas (to more closely simulate breast milk) may further contribute to the difference in gut microorganism balance between breast-fed and cow's milk-fed babies.

A number of studies have shown that refined sugar added to the culture media in which Candida is grown will increase their growth rate[101,102] or increase their virulence when experimental animals are inoculated with those organisms.[103,104] With Candida albicans grown on various culture media, "the sucrose medium in every case produced the greater proportion of filaments",[105] or hyphae, which are the invasive form of Candida thought to be more pathogenic.

Candida seems to grow more optimally and induce infection in humans when blood and tissue glucose levels are higher than normal.[106] This is perhaps the explanation for the strong tendency for diabetics to develop Candida infections. Several authors have theorized that those who are pregnant or taking oral contraceptives, who are well known to have a propensity for vaginitis, may be more vulnerable because of disturbed glucose metabolism and higher blood sugar levels, as well as higher glucose levels in vaginal secretions.[107,108] It has been shown that an "application of glucose to the vulva or vagina increase an established mycosis, or in the case of 'carriers' precipitate a mycosis."[109] Refined sugar has been shown to increase Candida adherence to mucous membrane surfaces.[110,111]

Clinical experience in literally hundreds of patients with a favorable response to Candida treatment measures, has repeatedly shown a rapid return of vaginal infection and many other unpleasant symptoms with the reintroduction of refined sugar into the diet.

e. **A competent immune system is necessary to keep various microorganisms (including Candida) from becoming too numerous and causing dis-**

eases.[112,113,114,115] Candida albicans, as well as other organisms, produce a variety of chemical substances (to be discussed later) that protect themselves from the human immune system, which might otherwise completely eradicate them. A balance between the various organisms and their human host is thus achieved. When a person's immune system is severely compromised, however, Candida albicans can cause severe invasion of tissues, and even rapid death.

Other microbes also have the ability to adversely affect the human immune system, the most notable being the HIV virus, which is thought to cause AIDS, in which the immune systems ability to control infections is severely impaired. In those with AIDS, even normal flora, with very low virulence, can become lethal.

f. **Vitamin deficiency may increase vulnerability to candidiasis.** A healthy immune system is dependant on a nutritious diet, with adequate levels of specific vitamins and other nutrients. Malnourishment has been shown to be a major cause of impaired immunity.[116,117,118] The medical literature frequently describes serious Candida infections in those who are debilitated or poorly nourished.[119,120] It has been shown that a deficiency in a variety of vitamins can promote Candida growth in animals.[121] Vitamin C deficient cient diet produces an increased susceptibility to candidiasis.[122,123] Vitamin B deficiency has also been reported to be associated with candidiasis.[124] Most of the patients seen in our office have either been on a number of calorie-reduced weight-reduction diets or have consistently eaten a nutritionally inadequate diet with high levels of refined or highly processed foods.

g. **Antibiotics, especially the broad-spectrum antibiotics, kill competing bacteria,** thus allowing opportunistic Candida to overgrow.[125,126,127,128,129,130] Many antibiotics may also have some direct effect on inhibiting the immune system. Some antibiotics, particularly tetracycline, have been shown to promote Candida overgrowth even in vitro, presumably by providing nitrogen or some other nutrients required for optimal Candida growth.[131] All experienced physicians have seen cases of thrush, diaper rash, or diarrhea in babies, or vaginitis in women after antibiotic use. These acute infections may clear quickly after stopping the antibiotic, in people with reasonably competent immune systems (if their immune system were functioning perfectly, they would likely have not developed the infection for which they were treated with an antibiotic in the first place). If the immune system is impaired significantly, however, Candida over-growth in the vagina and in the intestines may become chronic.

h. **Corticosteroids** are also well known to promote Candida overgrowth. Systemic steroid therapy given either orally or by injection has been long associated with immune impairment and candidiasis. Even corticosteroid sprays have been shown to promote Candida growth in areas of direct contact, including the pharynx and esophagus.[132] Many investigators have been able to produce an experimental animal model of chronic candidiasis by giving the animal corticosteroids[133,134] or other immune suppressing drugs. The best animal models for chronic candidiasis are created by giving them both corticosteroids and antibiotics.[135,136,137]

i. **Chemotherapeutic agents, radiation, and other immune suppressing drug regimes** may also impair immunity, and thus encourage chronic Candida overgrowth in a similar fashion to corticosteroids. In the past, it was hard to produce an experimental animal model of chronic gastrointestinal candidiasis in healthy animals. Such a model with chronic, invasive lesions in the tongue, esophagus, stomach, vagina, or other area that can be examined under the microscope, is very useful to study the effectiveness of various anti-Candida drugs. Candida inoculated into a healthy animal will, if not fatal initially, be fairly quickly eradicated by the animal's local and general immune defenses. A number of ways have now been discovered that create a chronic candidiasis condition. A good way is to give the animals either an antibiotic or corticosteroids (or both) prior to Candida exposure. This regime allows the Candida to invade various tissues, and establish a clear-cut infection. The immune suppressing properties of the established Candida organisms now maintain the infection indefinitely, long after the initiating drugs are stopped. Other immune suppressing drugs have also been instrumental in promoting chronic candidiasis, including Cyclosporin, etc. Some strains of animals have been found that are genetically vulnerable to Candida, and can easily be given a chronic, invasive infection.[138] Producing nutrient deficiencies can also make animals vulnerable to infection. Repeated exposure to Candida, even in a healthy animal, also seems to work.[139]

   The combination of broad-spectrum antibiotics and corticosteroids (a favored regime of the conventional allergists and infectious disease specialists) has also been described many times in patients we have seen prior to developing features of CC. Other drugs, poor diet, repeated exposure, and various other conditions found to produce chronic Candida infection in animals are often found in humans, setting them up for chronic Candida infections.

j. **H2 blockers** suppress the production of stomach acids. These acids are effective barriers to prevent microorganisms from entering the gut. Candida often thrive in those digestive systems made more hospitable by lowering the stomach acids.[140,141,142] Spermicidal products have been shown to increase the adherence of Candida, contributing to infections.[143] Other drug regimes may also contribute to CC.

k. **Estrogen appears to play a role in creating a host environment more favorable for Candida growth.** Most physicians are familiar with the higher rate of vaginal candidiasis during or after pregnancy[144] and in association with female hormones used as contraceptives or in replacement therapy.

l. **Stress is well known to enhance susceptibility to viral infections like Herpes simplex. Stress seems to also contribute to the development of candidiasis symptoms.** Whether stress interferes with the immune system and allows more yeast growth, or whether stress merely adds to stress hormone excess already present in many candidiasis sufferers is unknown. In either event, stress increases the symptoms that Candida therapy will usually reduce, and stress management is an important part of treatment in some patients.

m. **Other infections seem to be contributors to candidiasis.** Infections that produce diarrhea may well produce an imbalance in intestinal microorganisms, which may allow the opportunistic Candida to overgrow. Viral infections caused by Epstein-Barr virus and Cytomegalovirus virus may interfere with the immune system enough to allow Candida overgrowth. Subtle changes have been shown in the white cells in those with chronic fatigue syndrome thought to be caused by these viruses and perhaps many other organisms. The "Friend Leukemia Virus" has also been shown to induce a "profound immunosuppression" with "an increased susceptibility to subse-quent infection with the opportunistic pathogen Candida albicans."[145] HIV virus causes obvious white cell changes and severely compromised immun-ity. AIDS has frequently been shown to be a contributing factor to over-growth with Candida organisms.

n. **Virulence characteristics of Candida organisms** contribute to their growth and invasion of tissues. Strains that possess higher degrees of adherence[146,147,148,149,150] and proteinase production[151,152] have been shown to be more virulent. A theoretical role for phenotypic switching[153,154,155] and molecular mimicry[156,157,158] have also been described to help Candida evade host immune surveillance systems.

2. CANDIDA TOXINS

It has long been known that Candida species produce very toxic substances. Dead Candida cells[159] and even a cell-free supernatant from a Candida suspension when injected into experimental animals produces the same type of clinical features, including vascular collapse and death, as caused by living Candida inoculations. Many of these specific toxic substances have been identified, and their role in causing disease has been elucidated.

These toxins specifically manufactured by Candida to kill or inhibit competing microorganisms[160] may also be toxic to man.[161] Other fungi also produce toxins, perhaps the best known being aflatoxins produced by Aspergillus species.[162] Aflatoxins have been implicated in deaths of livestock that have eaten contaminated feed. These aflatoxins have been isolated and concentrated by the Russians, and apparently serve as the active agents in the "yellow rain" chemical warfare used in the recent devastating Afghanistan occupation.[163]

Volatile organic compounds produced by mold, and responsible for the characteristic mold or mildew odor, have been implicated in causing health problems, both acute and chronic. "Headaches, eye and throat irritation, nausea, dizziness, and fatigue in subjects occupying contaminated interiors" has been described.[164] This article, appearing in the November 1990 issue of the Journal of Allergy and Clinical Immunology, describes precisely the same type of symptoms associated with Candida. It is interesting that the American Academy of Allergy and Immunology would accept this information into their official journal, while denying that similar problems could occur from toxins produced by Candida.

A variety of toxic by-products and wastes from Candida metabolic processes have also been identified. Various chemical compounds which appear to be an integral part of Candida cellular structure have also been described. Among the more important of the various Candida toxins are the following:

ethanol
acetaldehyde
glycoprotein toxins
polysaccharide protein complexes
tyramine
Canditoxin
mannan
proteinase

Japanese researchers report that certain strains of Candida albicans in the gut produce ethanol which is absorbed hematogenously in amounts sufficient to cause clinical and legal intoxication after ingestion of high levels of carbo-hydrate.[165,166] Acetaldehyde, even more toxic than ethanol, can also be produced in relatively large amounts.[167] Acetaldehyde has a strong affinity for binding to sulfhydryl and amine groups,[168] and may thus produce a wide range of problems to be described later.

A great deal has been written in the scientific literature regarding Candida toxins.[169,170,171,172] Some of these toxins have been identified as being glyco-proteins,[173,174,175,176,177] polysaccharide-protein complexes,[178] tyra-mine,[179] and a specific compound called "canditoxin".[180,181,182] The physical properties and activities of various other toxic substances produced by Candida albicans have also been described.[183,184,185] Mannan will be described later. Candida species have recently been shown to produce **proteinase**.[186] Candida variants that produced higher levels of proteinase were shown to be more viru-lent.[187,188]

The concept of toxin-induced diseases is an old one in medicine. Food poisoning from the exotoxins produced by Staphylococcus and Clostridium species (botulism) is well understood. Intestinal colonization of Clostridium botulinum has recently been shown to occur after antibiotic use, with resulting toxins-induced chronic illness--a dysbiosis closely paralleling candidiasis.[189,190] Bacterial-induced disease states like tetanus, diphtheria, and toxic shock syndrome involve toxin production. Toxins from "bacterial overgrowth" in a jejunal loop were shown to cause a clinical picture of skin eruptions, myalgia, and arthralgia,[191] features similar to those observed with Candida overgrowth.

Heavy metal poisoning, pesticide toxicity, and various industrial chemical contamination all produce symptoms caused, in part, by interference with enzymatic actions. Mercury reportedly has a strong affinity for enzyme sulf-hydryl groups.[192] The widely varied symptoms described recently due to pent-aborane intoxication[193] were attributed in part to affinity for amine groups.[194] Symptoms caused by these various toxins very closely parallel those observed in candidiasis.

3. CANDIDA INTERFERENCE WITH THE IMMUNE SYSTEM:

a. **Candida albicans appears to interfere with the ability to resist infections.**
    Carlson has shown that the Staph. aureus bacteria thought to be responsible for toxic shock syndrome can be given to newborn mice in relatively large numbers (several million organisms) before causing death. After infesting

mice with Candida albicans, a very small number of Staph. aureus (less than 10 organisms) are rapidly lethal.[195,196,197] Candida produce glycoprotein toxins[198,199] and other chemical inhibitors[200] that interfere with cell mediated immunity as well as other immune system functions.[201,202,203,204,205,206] A person infected with Candida may then be unable to adequately control them, and may also have impaired ability to control other microorganisms as well.[207] The precise mechanisms by which Candida species, their toxic metabolites, and Candida antigen-antibody immune complexes produce immune suppression have been extensively studied. Some of the more well known mechanisms include the following.

1. Decreased numbers of peripheral lymphocytes.[208]
2. Decreased number of T-cells.[209]
3. Decreased number of natural killer cells.[210]
4. Leukocyte migration inhibition.[211]
5. Decreased phagocytosis of Candida cells.[212,213,214,215]
6. Decreased neutrophil attachment to Candida hyphae and bacteria.[216,217]
7. Impaired lymphocyte transformation or blastogenesis.[218,219]
8. Increased suppressor cell population with production of suppressor factor.
9. Interference with polymorphonuclear leukocyte activity.[220,221,222,223,224,225,226,227]
10. Decreased production of complement.[228]
11. Activation of suppressor T-cells.[229,230]

Witkin from Cornell pointed out that lymphocytes from women with chronic vaginitis failed to proliferate when exposed to Candida antigens, although they responded normally to other antigens.[231] Lymphocytes from normal women did proliferate in response to Candida antigen, although this response could be arrested by incubating these cells with serum from patients with chronic vaginitis. It has been shown that mannan from the Candida cell wall was one agent that could account for this cell-mediated immune suppression.[232,233,234,235]

Although the **initial** vaginal infection with Candida may be precipitated by antibiotics, corticosteroids, or other factors, Witkin expressed the belief that the Candida organisms themselves produce further immune suppression and are likely to be the predominant reason that these infections become chronic. Other workers have also demonstrated that chronic Candida infections can be the result of Candida-induced suppression of cellular immunity.[236,237,238,239]

b. **Candida may contribute to autoimmunity and endocrinopathy.** Besides interfering with a person's ability to fight off infection, **Candida-induced immune damage may cause other important immunological problems.** Witkin states that Candida infections may lead to "subsequent endocrinopathies and autoantibody formation,"[240] and refers to 3 other sources to substantiate this belief.[241,242,243] Candida infections have long been known to be associated with immune system abnormalities in **autoimmune** polyendocrinopathy-candidiasis-ectodermal dystrophy syndrome (APECED),[244] or also referred to as **APICH syndrome** (autoimmunity, polyendocrinopathy, immune dysregulation, candidiasis, hypersensitivity).[245] The predominant defect appears to be a T-cell abnormality allowing Candida overgrowth.[246] The Candida may then cause or contribute to the autoimmunity and polyendocrinopathy.

Although candidiasis has been thought by some workers to merely be a consequence of the immune dysfunction associated with the disorder,[247] there is good evidence for Witkin's theory that Candida is responsible for the endocrinopathy and autoimmunity, including the following:

1. Immunological and endocrine abnormalities have been reversed following successful antifungal antibiotic therapy for Candida infections.[248,249,250]

2. Women with chronic Candida vaginitis also have a higher incidence of endocrine dysfunction and autoimmunity similar to those found with APICH, suggesting that the Candida organisms contribute to these defects.[251]

3. Some patients with chronic mucocutaneous candidiasis were successfully treated and their immunosuppression reversed with transfer factor.[252,253] This transfer factor was derived from the lymphocytes of patients with delayed-hypersensitivity skin tests to Candida. The fact that this anti-Candida substance improved the immunosuppression as well as the Candida infection is suggestive that Candida caused the immunosuppression.

4. A group of patients with "visceral candidiasis" were studied and found to have a high incidence of "parathyroid, thyroid, pancreatic, and adrenocortical dysfunctions." Antimycotic medication seemed to help the endocrinopathy.[254] A wide range of allergy or sensitivity to foods, chemicals, hormones, and other antigens are often present in those suspected of having CC. These intolerances usually improve and often disappear entirely with treatment for Candida. The pathological processes involved with these allergies are closely related to those involved with autoimmunity.

    This chemical inhibition of the immune system by Candida has a close parallel. The drug **cyclosporine** (derived from a fungal species that presumably produced this chemical to enhance its own survival) strongly suppresses immunity, particularly suppressing rejection responses to transplanted organs.

c. **Candida appears to cause a sensitivity to chemical odors, foods, and other allergic disorders.**[255,256,257] At this point, an important issue needs to be raised; the issue of allergy definition. Originally, the term referred to "a condition of unusual sensitivity to a substance or substances which, in like amounts, do not affect others" (Webster dictionary definition). Conventional allergists, in their quest for mechanisms and legitimacy, have narrowed their definition of allergy to include only IgE mediated, classical allergy responses to proteins. They have tended to deny the existence of reactions where no causative mechanism can be found. Conflict over such issues eventually resulted in several other allergy groups being formed, including The American Academy of Environmental Medicine, the Pan American Allergy Society, and the American Academy of Otolaryngic Allergy. These groups have developed a much broader concept of allergy. Almost every conceivable adverse response to almost every known substance has been reported by members of these other groups. They have also pioneered the development of much improved allergy testing and treatment techniques. Both the concepts and improved treatment techniques developed by other allergy groups have been widely criticized and denounced in formal position papers published by The American Academy of Allergy and Clinical Immunology. For the purposes of this paper, we will use the original, broader definition of allergy.

A great deal of work has been done showing that Candida is highly antigenic, and that allergy to Candida organisms cause such conditions as asthma, eczema, chronic urticaria, seborrheic dermatitis, and psoriasis. Yeast glycoprotein toxins cause histamine release, which in turn can cause a number of chronic "allergic" problems.[258,259,260,261] Histamine may be one of the factors that produce increased gut permeability often reported with Candida growth in the gut. This increased permeability has been thought to allow incompletely digested food particles to enter the circulation, causing immune system response to those amino acid sequences in the food. These reactions may or may not be typical IgE mediated allergic responses. Rea has reported an altered T lymphocyte helper/suppressor ratio in chemically sensitive patients.[262] Candida also produce similar immune system changes.

The suppressor system may then fail to control responses to substances that are not a threat. It's highly probable that at least some of these chemically sensitive patients have immune system damage triggered by Candida.

Prostaglandins have been implicated a number of times in adverse reactions to foods.[263,264] Witkin also showed that the macrophages from women with chronic vaginitis produced increased amounts of prostaglandins, which could account for the immune system defects and allergies associated with Candida.[265] Other vaso-active substances, such as tyramine, produced by Candida or by the host response to Candida, may also be triggers for symptoms associated with Candida infections. Some of the symptoms may be caused by non-immunological responses.

Although the role of Candida in causing IgE mediated classical allergy has been well known for many years, the relationship of Candida to "nonclassical allergy" has been more recently described. In 1962, a study was done on two groups of people who showed a delayed hypersensitivity to Candida antigen, but no other reactions on skin testing.[266] One group had classical allergy, such as asthma and hay fever. The second group was described as "chronically ill and were treated for many years by physicians including specialists in the various branches of medicine. They were given symptomatic treatment according to the signs and symptoms with which they presented themselves. The results of this kind of symptomatic treatment proved to be a complete failure." After hyposensitization injections with Candida albicans antigen, thirteen out of eighteen got complete relief, and five showed a "remarkable improvement." Included in the chronic, resistant health problems shown to clear with Candida allergy treatment were conditions such as migraine headaches, various gastrointestinal problems, non-asthmatic bronchial manifestations, blepharoconjunctivitis, and vulvitis.

Russian doctors working with antibiotic plant workers infected with Candida noted that "often the diseases are accompanied by an allergy."[267] The relationship between Candida infection and food and chemical allergy was described again by Truss in the late 1970's. Many other workers who have tried his treatment principles have also noted a strong tendency for food and chemical allergies to improve along with many other features in those with a positive response to Candida therapy. Members of the American Academy of Environmental Medicine have embraced this concept, and many papers have been presented at their meetings regarding the relationship of Candida to allergy.

Although a great deal of work has been done on the effect of Candida on the immune system, the important thing to remember is not how it happens, but that **Candida albicans does in fact cause immune system damage leading to chronic and invasive infections with Candida and other organisms, autoimmunity, endocrinopathy, and food and chemical intolerance.** We have now treated thousands of patients who had allergies that improved with treatment for Candida. Many patients, even after 20 or more years of daily chronic suffering with asthma, eczema, urticaria, allergic rhinitis, and many non-classical allergy symptoms, are now completely free of these problems. Former asthmatic cripples can now run and be exposed to cold with not a trace of bronchospasm with no medication of any kind. Many other doctors who have treated Candida using Truss's technique report similar observations.

4. CANDIDA RELATED NUTRIENT DEFICIENCIES

The nutritional status of someone with CC may be impaired in a number of ways:

a. Those who are nutritionally depleted because of digestive disturbances, poor dietary habits, or restrictive dieting often become immune impaired and vulnerable to various infections, including Candida infections. (Recently, we have seen dozens of patients who developed all the features of CC after powdered protein, starvation dietary regimes.) Their nutritional status can further be worsened by the Candida.

b. Lactobacillus species in the human gut manufacture a variety of vitamins (especially B vitamins) which can be absorbed and utilized by the host. They also reportedly help the host to produce certain digestive enzymes. If antibiotics reduce the number of these organisms, and Candida species then predominate, keeping Lactobacillus numbers down, the host loses the benefit of those organisms. Vitamin deficiency may result.

c. Candida organisms may utilize some of the vitamins and minerals contained in the ingested food, and thus further deplete the nutritional status of the host.

d. Candida-induced gut inflammation may cause diarrhea, and thus loss of nutrients. Loss of Lactobacillus-produced digestive enzymes may further interfere with digestion and nutrient utilization.

Several researchers have indicated that chronic intestinal candidiasis leads to B vitamin deficiency.[268,269] A parallel situation has been demonstrated in an experimental colony of cockroaches who became infected with intestinal yeast. The yeast competed with the host for nutrients to the point that these insects died of malnourishment.[270] Various human parasites, including tape worms, are also known to cause malnourishment in their host.

Truss, Crook, and others who have described CC have pointed out the tendency for nutrient deficiency, and have made specific suggestions for nutrient replacement. Russian antibiotic-plant workers with candidiasis were treated with vitamins, presumably because their doctors knew about Candida-induced nutrient deficiency.[271]

5. CANDIDA RELATED ENDOCRINE ABNORMALITIES

A great number of endocrine problems have now been attributed to autoimmunity. Autoantibodies may attack various endocrine glandular tissues, receptor sites for various endocrine hormones, or specific hormones themselves. Endocrine dysfunction may come about as a consequence of cell damage to endocrine organs, binding of secretory products of the endocrine glands, or dysfunction of the receptor sites for these various endocrine hormones.

A November 1990 New England Journal of Medicine article outlined the latest evidence that autoimmune processes causing endocrinopathies are frequently triggered by various microbes.[272] Both hypofunction and hyperfunction of endocrine systems have been described on this autoimmune basis. Autoantibodies to various viruses have clearly been shown to cause decreased insulin production in type 1 diabetes.[273] Hyperthyroidism associated with Grave's disease has been shown to be associated with antibodies to Yersinia, a gram-negative bacillus.[274,275] Pseudomonas and E. coli have also been implicated in autoimmune endocrinopathies.[276]

The relationship between chronic mucocutaneous candidiasis and various autoimmune endocrinopathies is very clear and extensively described in the literature.[277,278] IgE from those with candidiasis blocked cortisol secretion, leading to speculation that Candida may be a trigger for Addison's disease.[279] Other workers also related candidiasis to Addison's disease.[280] Candidiasis has also been shown to be associated with hypothyroidism, hypoparathyroidism, and often with multiple endocrinopathies.[281,282,283,284,285,286,287] Studies in women with chronic vaginal candidiasis have shown similar endocrine disturbances, especially ovarian antibodies and menstrual disturbances.[288,289,290]

Receptors for estrogen and corticosteroids have been found on the cell wall of Candida. These receptors and other molecular sequences on the cell wall have been shown to be identical to those in their human hosts.[291,292] This "molecular mimicry" may cause antibodies formed against these Candida components to attack host receptor sites and other tissues, interfering with endocrine function, and perhaps accounting for a lot of other symptoms.

Besides immune-induced endocrine problems, these receptors may also tie-up estrogen and corticosteroids, and thus cause relative deficiencies or imbalances of adrenal and ovarian hormones. Candida have been shown to produce various steroid substances, including estrogen. This estrogen, very close structurally to human estrogen, may attach to host estrogen receptor sites, and either activate them or competitively inhibit human estrogen activity. These activities may account for the high incidence of menstrual irregularity, dysmenorrhea, premenstrual syndrome, endometriosis, and infertility reported by Truss, Crook and others in patients with CC. Effective treatment of the vaginitis has been shown by Mathurs to improve the menstrual irregularities.[293]

Perhaps the best proof for the relationship between candidiasis and menstrual irregularities is found in the results of a recent New England Journal of Medicine article in which women with Candida vaginitis and other problems were treated with various protocols of oral and vaginal nystatin and placebo. In three different comparisons of active to placebo treatment, nystatin improved menstrual irregularities with a significance of P=.005, .002, and .001. In other words, there were only 5 chances out of a thousand, 2 chances out of a thousand, and 1 chance out of a thousand respectively that these improvements were not from the active treatment.

A relationship between Candida and endometriosis has been theorized, and many convincing case reports and theories by various doctors are given for that relationship in a chapter of a book produced by the Endometriosis Association.[294]

Infertility has also been associated with candidiasis by Truss, Crook, and other workers. One study showed conception to occur in a significant number of formerly infertile women when they were treated for Candida.[295] Frequent spontaneous miscarriage has also been reported. A single dose of candida glycoprotein given to mice on the eighth day of pregnancy caused an increased number of resorptions and a decreased number of fetuses.[296]

We have now seen hundreds and hundreds of women with various hormonal problems including menstrual irregularities, dysmenorrhea, and PMS who have improved dramatically with simple control measures to treat Candida. Our experience certainly reflects that reported in the medical literature.

SYMPTOMS ASSOCIATED WITH CHRONIC CANDIDIASIS

Now that the various mechanisms by which Candida can cause illness have been outlined, we would next like to describe some of the clinical features we see in patients with CC. We will only mention those symptoms that routinely clear with Candida treatment. **For each of the symptoms described below, we have seen hundreds of cases improve with simple Candida treatment measures. With some symptoms, we have seen thousands of cases improve with treatment.** An attempt will be made to explain the observed phenomena.

GASTROINTESTINAL TRACT: Sores in the mouth and a sore tongue are very commonly seen. Candida may, in some cases, directly invade these tissues, causing the discomfort. **Canker sores** may represent a host hypersensitivity response to food chemicals, Candida, or some other pathogen. Candida may play a permissive role in allowing other microorganisms to infect the mouth tissues. **Heartburn** is often described, and patients have often had a radiological or gastroscopic diagnosis of hiatus hernia with reflux esophagitis. Although Candida are well known to cause thrush-like lesions in the esophagus,[297,298] it is also likely that yeast-induced prostaglandins released by various tissues of the GI tract may produce gastroesophageal sphincter relaxation and increased intragastric pressure which could contribute to esophageal reflux.[299] This increased intragastric pressure along with the inflamed mucosal surfaces may also contribute to the **nausea, indigestion and epigastric distress** so often reported. Candida may also contribute more indirectly to these problems by interfering with the normal mucosal protection provided by a healthy prostaglandin balance. Candida-induced immune suppression may also facilitate other infective agents (such as Campylobacter and Giardia) to invade the upper gut. Abnormal levels of stress hormones associated with CC may also be a contributing factor.

Gas and bloating may be caused by the large amounts of CO_2 gas released by Candida as a metabolic by-product.[300] Other gas-producing organisms may also be present due to the general gut dysbiosis secondary to Candida-induced immune suppression. Gas, bloating, and lower abdominal discomfort may also be caused by impaired digestive processes and Candida-induced food allergy or intolerance.

Diarrhea is a frequent symptom, and may be caused by a direct infestation of the colon by Candida.[301,302] Both acute and chronic diarrhea have been reported.[303] We have now seen hundreds of cases of chronic diarrhea, of previously unknown etiology, cured by a few weeks of Candida treatment. One lady suffered for 42 years prior to being cured. Diarrhea may be caused by a Candida infection or by an allergic response to Candida present in the gut.

Adverse reactions to foods appears to be commonly associated with diarrhea, in some cases through IgE mediated responses,[304] but possibly through a variety of other immune and non-immune mediators.[305,306,307] Prostaglandins are now well recognized for their role in mediating a diarrheal response to foods. CC is often associated with food allergy/intolerance, probably secondary to the influence of Candida on the immune system.

Lactose intolerance can cause diarrhea that may be helped by ingesting acidophilus bacteria,[308] suggesting that the balance of gut flora may play an important role in lactose metabolism. Abnormal sympathetic nervous system response or elevated levels of stress-related neuro-chemicals may also be a factor in Candida-associated diarrhea. Histamine release associated with Candida may also contribute to diarrhea.

Constipation or alternating constipation and diarrhea is also frequently associated with chronic candidiasis. The frequent improvement in constipation and diarrhea reported from supplementing acidophilus bacteria to dietary products (like yogurt or acidophilus milk) or from direct ingestion of acidophilus again suggests the role of healthy intestinal flora for proper bowel function.[309] Constipation may also be an adverse reaction to certain foods, as it is often observed, along with other clinical manifestations, after ingesting wheat or other foods to which the patient is known to react. The mechanism by which constipation occurs is not clear.

Ano-rectal itching may be caused by the same local and host factors causing vaginitis, or may be a sensitivity to various contacts like colored or scented toilet paper or fabric softeners.

RESPIRATORY SYSTEM: Nasal congestion on a year-round basis is very common. This may represent an allergic or adverse reaction to foods, chemical odors, Candida or related fungal organisms and their metabolic by-products. This chronic nasal congestion, as well as **chronic sinusitis,** may also be a direct result of chronic Staphylococcus infection in these areas secondary to the pervasive action of Candida on the immune system.[310] **Sinus pressure and headaches** often result. Histamine release simulated by Candida may also account for chronic congestion.

It is very common for patients with seasonal rhinitis to have no candidiasis-related symptoms at all, but many of those with food allergies and almost all of those with symptoms related to exposure to chemical odors appear to have typical CC histories.

Asthma is common, and appears to be allergic in nature.[311,312,313,314,315] "Bronchial asthma associated with allergic candidiasis" was shown to improve with antimycotic drugs.[316] Although we have seen several patients with chronic asthma of many years' duration clear completely within a few hours to days of beginning a Candida antigen treatment program,[317,318,319,320,321] most asthmatic patients seem to react to a wide range of inhalants, foods, and chemical odors. Histamine produced in response to Candida may account for the asthma. Candida-induced immune system pathology may account for responses to many other antigens.

Many patients complain of **shortness of breath or a smothering feeling. Hyperventilation seems common.** Air entry seems very satisfactory on physical examination, and even in patients with asthma, the apparent difficulty in getting air appears to be much greater than would be expected with the observed amount of bronchospasm. Several possible mechanisms may explain this phenomenon: high stress hormones may trigger a partial fight-or-flight response with an associated attempt to maximally oxygenate tissues; red blood cell membrane defects (diminished flexibility) may interfere with the flow of blood through the small capillaries,[322] and also interfere with the diffusion of oxygen into these cells, thus interfering with general oxygenation of the tissues; the hyperventilation-like response may also be part of the latent tetany[323] described recently in the French medical literature, and may represent, in part, inadequate levels of tissue magnesium.[324,325] This theory is further strengthened by the excellent clinical response to magnesium supplementation along with effective Candida management.

CARDIOVASCULAR SYSTEM: Pounding heart, palpitations, and paroxysmal atrial tachycardia are common complaints in patients with candidiasis. Inappropriate neurotransmitter or toxins interfering directly with the pacemaker tissues may account for these symptoms. Of interest is the number of patients with candidiasis symptoms who have been diagnosed as having **mitral valve prolapse (MVP).** Papillary muscles that control the mitral valve may be affected in a manner similar to other muscle tissue. MVP has often been associated with a number of symptoms quite characteristic of candidiasis, including spastic colon,[326] migraine headaches,[327] and a wide variety of anxiety-associated symptoms.[328,329]

Generalized edema is common, and often subsides in a week or two with treatment. Although this may involve Na-K transport, it is also likely that the various hormones controlling fluid balance are affected in an as-yet unknown manner. Toxins may also produce edema.

Cold sweaty hands and feet are also common, and may reflect altered sympathetic nervous system outflow and reduced peripheral circulation due to Candida glycoprotein toxins.[330] Raynaud's phenomena may occur as an autoimmune response, which could be Candida related.

GENITO-URINARY SYMPTOMS: Many writers have indicated that Candida albicans is a well-known cause of **vulvovaginitis and penile candidiasis.** An occasional bout of acute vaginitis may be only a minor annoyance, but for many women, Candida vaginitis may recur very often or even become chronic. Symptoms may be very mild from the direct invasion of tissues by the Candida hyphae, but may become so severe as to be debilitating. The severe vaginal symptoms result from a host hypersensitivity or allergic response to the Candida.[331,332,333,334,335] Even small numbers of Candida organisms can produce rather severe symptoms in this situation. A lack of protective Lactobacillus bacteria in the mucous membrane may render the victim particularly susceptible to candidiasis. An immune system breakdown may also contribute to this state and may even contribute to some non-Candida vaginal infestations.

Candida may live in the mucous membranes of the urinary tract, and may account for **dysuria, frequency, irritable bladder, and may contribute to urinary tract infections and prostatitis.** Bacteria usually cause these urinary tract infections, but the bacteria may be present partly because the protective mucosal lining of the urinary tract has been damaged by Candida -- or because Candida has lowered the general resistance to infection.

Dysmenorrhea is common with chronic candidiasis. Although the mechanism is unclear, the favorable response to prostaglandin inhibitors seems to implicate prostaglandins. The precise role Candida plays in this and other prostaglandin effects is uncertain, but the frequently observed improvement in dysmenorrhea with treatment of candidiasis suggests some relationship.

MUSCULO-SKELETAL SYMPTOMS: A wide range of muscle symptoms are often seen in patients suffering from CC. These symptoms include **muscle soreness, tenderness, aching, stiffness, weakness, cramping, and easy fatigability.** In particular, the muscles of the upper back, shoulders, and neck often become tight and painful. Patients often state that their muscles always feel like they have just gotten through exercising. The muscles may be in a heightened tonic state due to high levels of circulating stress-related hormones (for reasons discussed below). Dr. Orian Truss has theorized that acetaldehyde may interfere with the flexibility of red blood cell membranes. This considerably reduces their ability to make the change from the discoid shape to the fusiform shape necessary for their passage through small capillaries. He has demonstrated that patients with candidiasis have a greatly reduced red blood cell filtration rate through a micro-pore filter, which increases back to normal after treatment.[336] This may reduce the rate of blood flow to the muscle tissues, impair the delivery of oxygen and nutrients (like glucose and fatty acids) to the tissues, and slow the excretion of metabolic by-products.

Defects similar to those found in red blood cell membranes may also interfere mechanically with transport of materials through the muscle cell membranes. It is also possible that the various enzyme systems responsible for cell membrane transport are inhibited, making it difficult to keep an optimum intracellular balance of Na, K, Ca, and Mg.

Defects in the ability to provide enough glucose and fatty acids (for reasons to be discussed) and defects in the ability to use these nutrients to produce energy may also interfere with normal muscle function.

Arthritic pains and even formal diagnoses of rheumatoid arthritis are common in patients with candidiasis. Autoimmunity associated with Candida may produce or contribute to arthritis. We have often seen remarkable improvement with simple Candida treatment in many patients with various types of arthritis, including rheumatoid arthritis.

SKIN: Acne is very common, and frequently continues well into middle age, or may even begin then. It frequently worsens premenstrually. **Dry skin with hyperkeratosis follicularis** is very common. **Seborrheic dermatitis** has been blamed onto intestinal candidiasis, and "vigorous therapy with oral nystatin" has produced long-lasting regression.[337] **Eczema and psoriasis**[338,339,340] are very common, and may be secondary to an allergic response to the Candida organisms.[341,342] We have seen a number of cases in which eczema and other resistant skin rashes have cleared-up completely with Candida antigen therapy. **Hives** and chronic urticaria[343,344] are also common, and are part of the allergic pattern so often associated with candidiasis.

CENTRAL NERVOUS SYSTEM: A wide variety of emotional symptoms are usually manifested by patients with candidiasis. **Anxiety and insomnia** are very common. **Irritability, tendency to anger, fears, panic attacks, and an impending sense of doom** are common, as are **worry, depression, and loss of interest in normally enjoyable activities. Depression,** in particular has been reported to be associated with chronic candidiasis.[345,346] These symptoms are presumably due to the effect of toxins on various enzyme systems. Acetaldehyde may combine with the amine groups of various neurotransmitters to form substances which may act like false neurotransmitters. These substances may bind to neurotransmitter receptor sites and thus competitively inhibit the action of neurotransmitters.[347]

Acetaldehyde may also bind with the sulfhydryl group on various enzymes, including acetyl CoA, which will interfere with many metabolic processes, including the production of acetylcholine.[348] A changed ratio of NAD to NADH may also occur, which could affect the production of serotonin. Dopamine is converted into norepinephrine, which converts to epinephrine, which is then converted into inactive metabolites. This cascade is mediated by a number of enzymes requiring co-factors. Any interference with these enzymes and co-factors could lead to excessive amounts of some neurotransmitters and inadequate amounts of others. These altered neurotransmitter relationships could certainly account for some of the intriguing fight-or-flight-type neurological symptom complexes frequently observed. Some patients become very angry, aggressive, argumentative, and abusive with minor provocation. Others become anxious, fearful, timid, phobic, and startle easily.

Intellectual function appears to be frequently impaired. Patients often describe **trouble concentrating, trouble remembering things, indecisiveness, and being fuzzy or dull-headed.**[349] In children, similar problems with intellectual function may be described as attention deficit disorder or learning disability, and may often be combined with hyperactivity.[350]

Although no good explanation is known for these impairments in intellectual function, they may result from neurotransmitter problems previously described. Proper intellectual function presumably requires processing of data by different areas of the brain, and could conceivably be interfered with by anything which blocked neurotransmitter action.

Migraine headaches are frequently observed, which may be due to yeast-induced alteration in levels of vaso-active hormones. Much medical literatue now suggests a link between food or chemical allergy and migraines.[351,352] **Tension or muscular contraction headaches** are also very common, and may also, in some cases, be a reaction to food or chemical allergy. The pulse test has often been advocated for assessing reactivity to specific foods - an elevation in pulse rate after ingesting the food suggests allergy. This pulse rate elevation is presumably due to elevation in stress-related hormones, and these same hormones released in response to food allergy could also affect the muscles in the base of the skull, leading to classical muscular contraction headaches.

Dizziness is common, and although it may be described as **vertigo, loss of balance, or light-headedness,** in many cases patients have trouble describing exactly how they feel, and may use such terms as a sense of unreality or feeling distant. Patients sometimes describe bumping into doorways, **incoordination, and dropping things. Blurry vision and trouble focusing** are frequently described, although the visual disturbance may be more a problem of perception or comprehension of what is visualized. These vague neurological symptoms may represent a low-grade intoxication-like state due to ethanol or acetaldehyde by-products.

Fatigue, weakness, and lack of endurance are almost always reported. These symptoms could be related to the impaired metabolism of carbohydrates, fats, and proteins, leading to low levels of available fuel. Impaired transport of these nutrients across cell membranes could also be a factor. The very basis for energy production, the ATP/ADP cycle, may be impaired by interference with the various involved enzyme systems, or lack of substrate. Low thyroid at the cellular level could also contribute to fatigue.

METABOLIC AND ENDOCRINE PROBLEMS: Patients often describe extreme **hunger and sugar cravings,** which may be constant or periodic. **Hypoglycemic symptoms are very common, which may include weakness, fatigue, shaking, anxiety, headache, trouble staying awake, and extreme hunger a few hours after eating. Weight gain is extremely common.** Many patients get sick if they miss a meal, and report the need to eat often. A good share of the patients with candidiasis report having been diagnosed as hypoglycemic, or having been tested for it but with negative results.

Candida-induced metabolic defects in metabolism may account for these clinical observations. When it is necessary to oxidize relatively large quantities of ethanol or acetaldehyde Candida by-products, NAD is converted to NADH, which results in excessive amounts of NADH in relationship to NAD. This may interfere with glycolysis as well as interfering with the citric acid cycle, which in turn inhibits gluconeogenesis (amino acid conversion to glucose) and fatty acid oxidation. This limits the ability of the body to derive energy from the sugar stores (glycogen), from the amino acids, and from the fats. Major energy sources then seem to be from carbohydrate-derived glucose absorbed directly from the intestines, for which the patient must compete with Candida and other gut flora.

Entry of glucose into the various cells may be inhibited by cell membrane defects, leading to relative insulin resistance and the need for increased amounts of insulin in order to provide adequate intra-cellular glucose. High insulin levels are known to stimulate lipogenesis (conversion of sugar to fat), storage of this fat in the fat cells, and inhibition of lipolysis. This appears to be the mechanism by which insulin induces obesity. In experimental subjects it makes them fat and keeps them fat, even when they eat no more than the controls who remain lean.

The preceding events may explain hypoglycemic symptoms. As the blood sugar falls in response to excessive insulin production, inadequate fuel is available for brain and muscle function, leading to fatigue, weakness, sleepiness, dizziness, and trouble concentrating, remembering, and thinking clearly. The "normal" person would compensate for the falling blood sugar, before any symptoms would arise, by releasing various hormones (including epinephrine, norepinephrine, growth hormone, cortisol, and glucagon) to counteract the insulin effect and to produce glucose by stimulating glycogenolysis and gluconeogenesis. In the patient with candidiasis, high levels of these insulin counter-regulatory hormones may be necessary to overcome the tendency towards low glucose availability to the various cells, and these increased hormones may account for some of the stress-type symptoms including palpitations, sweaty hands, shaking, anxiety, restlessness, insomnia, irritability, and anger. Hunger and food cravings are probably the cerebral component of glucose regulation designed to encourage eating in order to provide the needed fuel to power the body and to prevent and relieve these symptoms.

In some cases, a glucose tolerance test will be completely normal even when hypoglycemic symptoms experienced during the test are so severe that the patient cannot even leave the lab under his own power. In these cases, it is assumed that the high levels of insulin counter-regulatory hormones are able to get the serum glucose levels to normal ranges, but these hormones cause the many unpleasant symptoms. In spite of normal circulating levels of glucose, it is probable that inadequate amounts get into the cells. Symptoms which occur 5 to 6 hours after sugar ingestion may be withdrawal symptoms associated with food addiction. Autoimmune antibodies have also been described which interfere with insulin receptor sites leading to insulin resistance.

Although low serum levels of thyroid hormones are seldom found, patients almost all seem clinically hypothyroid, with low energy, low body temperature, coldness, dry hair and skin, fatigue, slowness of thought, and frequent constipation. This group of symptoms could be due to impaired transport of thyroid hormones into the various cells preventing them from performing their usual functions. Resistance to thyroid hormone has been described in the medical literature.[353,354] Recent research has focused on antibodies to thyroid hormones or thyroid receptor sites as a cause of clinical hypothyroidism

Premenstrual Syndrome has been reported in patients with CC:[355] Many of the symptoms reported in the literature describing premenstrual syndrome are identical to those observed in patients with candidiasis. These symptoms are often intensified during the premenstrual phase of the cycle, or in some cases, appear only at that time.[356] Candida produce steroid hormones similar to human female hormones,[357,358] which could somehow compete for binding sites with or competitively inhibit female hormones, or could change the balance of estrogen to progesterone. Receptor sites on Candida cells may also bind steroid hormones.[359] Cell membrane defects could interfere with the uptake of progesterone by various cells. Candida-induced interferencewith the immune system could contribute to an "allergic" type response to progesterone. Allergy treatment for progesterone allergy has produced "startlingly rapid and effective clearing of symptoms."[360]

PMS appears to be, at least partially, a nutritionally deficient state. Various studies, some double-blind, have shown an improvement in PMS with various nutrients.[361,362,363,364] These nutrients could have been depleted by competition by Candida with the host for available nutrients. The no sugar, low carbohydrate diet found to be helpful for controlling PMS symptoms is very similar to the one advocated for Candida treatment.

DEFINING CHRONIC CANDIDIASIS

With the preceding background on the role of Candida in causing pathology, we would now like to talk about defining illness caused by Candida organisms. It would be very helpful to have a specific, well defined set of symptoms that were always found with Candida, and that were produced only by Candida and by no other disease state. We could then have a clearly defined Candidiasis Syndrome. There is, however, no specific symptom unique to Candida. Any symptom that can be caused by Candida can also be caused by something else. Even vaginitis, caused in the vast majority of cases by Candida, can be caused by other organisms. Likewise, there are no groups of symptoms unique to candidiasis. Any group of symptoms could also be caused by something else. A person afflicted with a Candida infection may have only mild, local problems, may have virtually all of the clinical features described in the literature, or may have only some of the clinical features in varying degrees of severity.

The clinical picture produced by Candida may vary depending on a number of factors including:

1. **Site of involvement** will determine which organ systems are involved.
2. **Form of Candida** that predominates may determine whether the Candida invade into the deeper tissues (hyphae form), or merely cause local, surface involvement.
3. **Toxin production** may vary, depending upon the form of Candida (yeast forms may produce more toxins), diet of the host, strain of Candida (some strains produce more ethanol, other produce other toxins), and the numbers of Candida present. The predominant site of action of the various toxins may affect various enzyme systems, and determine what kind of symptoms are produced.

4. **Nutritional status** of the host, and specific nutrient deficiencies which may develop can account for various symptoms.
5. **Host immune response** may account for a number of allergic, autoimmune, or endocrine dysfunction symptoms.
6. **Other organisms** that are present due to the Candida-induced immune suppression may cause symptoms.

As a result of all these variable host and pathogen factors, we can see many combinations and permutations of symptoms. Perhaps no two patients ever present with exactly the same constellation of symptoms.

Even naming this condition (or these conditions) is a problem. Candida hypersensitivity syndrome (chosen by the allergists) implies a hypersensitivity component (which may or may not be present), and also implies a specific syndrome (a number of symptoms occurring together and characterizing a specific disease). There is, at this writing, no such tight group of symptoms unique to Candida.

Candida-related complex has been used by some writers, and has some strengths. "Related" implies that the features may not necessarily be caused directly or indirectly by the Candida, but may be merely associated. The term "complex" (Webster dictionary definition: a more or less complicated collection or system of related things or parts. Also defined as involved, perplexing, difficult, complicated, and intricate) certainly seems to fit well with the clinical features of the disease.

The problem of defining chronic candidiasis is much like that faced by a committee appointed by the Center for Disease Control to define Chronic Fatigue Syndrome. They ultimately established very clear diagnostic criteria by which a person can be clearly classified as having or not having CFS. This was an attempt to establish a homogeneous group of people on whom to do research to find better treatment tools. This was a major step forward in gaining acceptance and credibility for this very distressing illness. The committee members and anyone working with this disorder know the limitations of the diagnostic criteria. There may be a variety of causative agents for the syndrome, and there may be many people with the same organisms and slightly different features who may fall out of the group because of the definition. Establishing similar criteria for illness caused by Candida would be very useful, and many of us have agonized over this issue for years. A definition too broad would include a lot of people that don't have Candida, and a definition too narrow would exclude a lot of people who do have problems caused by Candida. We would like to propose a definition that may have some advantages. **Chronic candidiasis is a chronic condition characterized by (a) infection with Candida species and/or (b) a variety of symptoms in various body systems caused by Candida or by host responses to Candida.** This definition is broad enough to cover all chronic illness caused by Candida, and specific enough to include only those things actually caused by Candida. Although this definition is not helpful in making a specific diagnosis, diagnosis can still be made adequately as follows.

DIAGNOSING CHRONIC CANDIDIASIS

Diseases caused by microorganisms are generally diagnosed by one or more of the following techniques:

1.   Direct identification of the organism under a microscope, in a culture, or by the reaction of a swab with antibodies.
2.   Host antibodies formed to the organism itself or some toxin produced by the organism, assessed either with a skin test or by direct measurement of antibodies in the serum.
3.   Clinical features characteristic of that organism.

Although various lab tests like WBC count and differential, WBC's in the urine, and ESR give information about the nature of the infection, they do not tell us about the specific causative organism.

Each of these tests have their limitations. A December 1990 New England Journal of Medicine article described "the recent remarkable discovery that the bulk of microbes in the environment are refractory to in vitro cultivation by current techniques....we are made painfully aware of the real possibility that we have only begun to determine the full spectrum of infectious diseases."[365] Some infection-causing organisms that can be cultured grow in places from which taking samples is difficult. Giardia, for example, is best diagnosed from a duodenal biopsy. Stool and other samples are notorious for being negative even with a very active infection. Some organisms grow only on specialized media, or may grow rather poorly, even with very active disease. A colleague reported a patient who was the only contact of several men who contracted gonorrhea. Over 20 cultures were taken over a period of time before a positive one was reported.

Candida infections pose several diagnostic challenges. Because they are a common (if not normal) part of our flora, a positive culture does not necessarily indicate disease. Candida often live in areas, such as the esophagus, stomach, and intestines, from which direct sampling for culture is difficult. Previous treatment may have reduced superficial Candida to the point that mouth or vaginal swabs are negative, and yet invasive candidiasis can still be raging. Unless there are very high numbers of Candida on a swab, culture media usually used for bacteria will often produce negative results - special Candida culture media produce more accurate results. Allergic responses to Candida organisms may account for most of the clinical features, even when the organisms are present in relatively small numbers, a situation likely to produce negative cultures. Cultures and direct visualization are not very reliable indicators of CC. A recent study showed that "surveillance cultures from the oropharynx or stool were not helpful in identifying those patients who would develop an invasive fungi infection."[366] A recent report in the New England Journal of Medicine showed only 14 percent of women with suspected vaginal candidiasis had positive cultures, and extensive treatment did not significantly alter culture results.[367] The incidence of false positive and false negative cultures are unacceptably high.

Many attempts have been made to diagnose candidiasis using skin tests or measuring serum antibodies. Positive skin tests only indicate an immune response to Candida, and point out that the patient has been exposed to Candida. Although a strongly positive skin test may suggest a cause for someone's classical allergies, it does not give much help in knowing whether that patient has a significant infection with Candida, or is having features typical of CC. Many patients with the most severe invasive candidiasis have immune suppression (from the Candida organisms or for some other reason) and often have negative skin tests.

Literally hundreds of scientific articles have been written describing various blood tests for identifying candidiasis. Some workers have expressed their belief that high levels of various Candida-specific antibodies correlate well with CC, and have some experimental evidence to support that belief. Antibodies against up to 79 Candida antigens have been reported in the literature, but only a few of these have been used clinically, including antibodies to mannan[368,369,370] and cytoplasmic antigens[371,372,373,374]. Although these tests do have statistically significant correlations, there is still a high level of false positives and false negatives. More recent tests have been developed that identify, in patient's serum, Candida components (including mannan, cytoplasmic antigen, and uncharacterized antigens), Candida antigen/antibody immune complexes, and metabolic products (mannose and arabinitol). Assay techniques used include agargel diffusion, whole-cell agglutination, passive hemagglutination, latex agglutination,[375,376] counterimmunoelectro-phoresis,[377] indirect immunofluorescence, radioimmunoassay,[378] enzyme immunoassay,[379,380,381,382] two-dimensional crossed rocket immunoelectrophoresis,[383] and hemagglutination inhibition.[384,385] These tests, which reportedly indicate the presence of disseminating or invasive Candida, probably have few false positives, but seem to have significant levels of false negatives. One researcher reported four patients with proven systemic candidiasis on post-mortem exam in whom "serum antigen was undetectable despite examining multiple serum samples up until the time of death."[386] We ran a panel of these tests on approximately 50 patients with classical features of CC. We started all the patients on a trial of therapy. About 6 patients with negative tests responded very favorably to therapy, indicating a strong probability of CC. Other clinicians have also reported similar problems with false negative tests.

These antibody tests all suffer from a major problem. Severe cases of CC and invasive candidiasis often have immune suppression, and just don't respond "normally" to Candida. One test, devised for such people, holds some promise. Normal lymphocytes are incubated with serum from patients suspected of having candidiasis, then exposed to Candida antigenic material. If the serum suppresses the lymphoblastic response which would normally occur to such exposure, the test is positive for Candida-induced immune suppression. This test, however, may be negative in cases with immune suppression for reasons other than the Candida infection itself, in cases where immune suppression is minimal, or in other milder cases of CC.

In spite of their limitations, these various tests for candidiasis are proven, valid tests, used by many doctors clinically. They are just as valid and reliable as many of the other tests used for identifying infections with other microbes. No test for microbes available in clinical medicine is completely foolproof, and as more is discovered, more and more limitations are becoming known about laboratory tests. A December 1990 article in JAMA, for example, pointed out 4 cases of sub-acute bacterial endocarditis erroneously diagnosed as Lyme's disease because of positive serology tests for B burgdorferi.[387] Studies have shown many patients with AIDS having Tuberculosis, and yet have negative skin tests due to the immune suppression that limits their response to the TB antigen.

Antibody tests for virus infections are even more unreliable as a diagnostic test than for bacteria and fungi. Beginning in 1985, there was a flurry of activity using various antibody titers to diagnose Chronic Epstein-Barr Virus Syndrome or Chronic Fatigue Syndrome. Over 80% of people reportedly have IgG antibodies, but having high levels of the other antibodies (IgM, early antigen, and nuclear antigen) was supposedly proof of ongoing, chronic infection with the Epstein-Barr virus. Later studies showed this testing to be a very poor indicator of Chronic Fatigue Syndrome.

In a 1989 review article from Harvard entitled Diagnosis of Candida Infections,[388] the author concludes that "At present the laboratory tools available to clinicians for the diagnosis of invasive candidiasis are limited.... Blood cultures, even when they are tailored for optimal growth of fungi, are slow, insensitive, and nonspecific. Measurement of antibodies to Candida is not helpful in immuno-suppressed patients, who comprise the very group that is most vulnerable to invasive infections. Detection of circulating fungal products, particularly mannan, provides the desired level of specificity, but the clinical sensitivity of current assays is disappointing, and the technology for performing them is not readily portable to clinical laboratories. Commercially available latex agglutination kits detect uncharacterized antigen(s) and lack sensitivity and specificity... The clinician, who often is left to his or her own resources, must maintain a high index of suspicion and must be willing to treat empirically in high-risk situations."

HISTORY: The diagnosis of candidiasis is mainly made from the medical history. Sometimes there is a clear-cut history of the full-blown illness starting after a resistant infection for which a number of different antibiotics were used for a prolonged time. More often, the onset is gradual, with symptoms increasing in number and severity over a period of time. A careful history from a typical patient will often reveal that each new symptom was developed under conditions that favored yeast overgrowth. Symptoms (like yeast vaginitis, heartburn, fatigue, hypoglycemic symptoms with sugar craving, and weight gain) that develop during a pregnancy, along with the depression which may develop immediately afterwards, may remain for many years, although they may be reduced in severity as a relative degree of recovery occurs from the delivery. Most doctors have heard women complain of depression, weight gain, headaches, irritability, decreased sex drive, and many other symptoms following a hysterectomy. These symptoms have usually been blamed on emotional factors or on hormone replacement (which, of course, can enhance Candida growth). Gastrointestinal symptoms like gas, bloating, cramps, and frequent episodes of diarrhea may follow treatment for a respiratory infection, and worsened depression with anxiety, irritability, trouble concentrating, and muscle aches may begin after a flu-like illness treated with an antibiotic. Most doctors have heard patients describe just not feeling well and never quite recovering following a surgical procedure (especially when there were complications treated by antibiotics).

PHYSICAL EXAMINATION: There are no physical findings that are diagnostic of candidiasis. Clear cut evidence of infection by Candida may be found in the vagina, mouth, or on the skin, and most doctors are very comfortable with a diagnosis of localized candidiasis strictly on the basis of the very characteristic lesion produced on these surfaces. People with these local infections don't necessarily have the full-blown picture of CC. There are some fairly typical findings, depending on the nature of the symptoms. In those with year-round nasal congestion and chronic sinusitis, the nasal mucosa is often swollen, inflamed, and full of mucopurulent discharge. The tongue is often white-coated, and may have a geographic appearance. In those with intestinal symptoms, there may be generalized tenderness, worse over the colon, which may be in spasm. In those with muscle symptoms, neck muscles may be tense and tender, and muscles, in general, may be sensitive to pressure. The skin is often dry with hyperkeratosis follicularis, and may display dermographia. Adult acne, eczema, contact dermatitis, and athlete's foot are common. Again, none of these features are diagnostic of CC, but may help along with the history.

Many other medical conditions also have no definitive lab tests and no clear physical findings, yet we become comfortable in making diagnoses such as migraine headaches, muscular contraction headaches, depression, anxiety, insomnia, and dysmenorrhea based strictly on history. Perhaps we are more confident in diagnoses such as spastic colon, bursitis, and sprains in which physical findings are present, even when no confirmatory lab tests are available.

Symptom scoring systems have been developed for a number of medical conditions for which confirmatory laboratory tests are lacking. Based on answers to various questions, a person scores a certain number of points, and based on that score, they are diagnosed as not having, or having mild, moderate, or severe anxiety or depression. Scoring systems for stress have also been developed. Scoring systems don't help to diagnose cancer, but do help to predict probability of survival.

Scoring systems have been used in infectious diseases. Rheumatic fever is diagnosed based on having so many major and/or so many minor manifestations. The Center For Disease Control has developed a scoring system for diagnosing Chronic Fatigue Syndrome, based strictly on symptoms. If the patient has severe fatigue for more than six months, if other conditions that could cause that degree of fatigue are ruled out, and if they have at least 8 out of 11 of the common clinical symptoms associated with the disease, then they have, by definition, Chronic Fatigue Syndrome.

For primary-care physicians "in the trenches," diagnosing patients with infective agents is not always as easy and straight-forward as sometimes suggested in medical texts. Two of the more difficult infection syndromes to diagnose are chronic candidiasis and Chronic Fatigue Syndrome. There are many similarities in these two conditions, including the following:

1. They are both associated with a chronic infection.
2. Symptoms in both conditions are associated with or caused by inappropriate host immune responses.
3. Both conditions have multi-system symptoms, including emotional and cognitive difficulties.
4. Neither condition has any consistent, diagnostic physical signs on examination.

5. Antibody testing is of limited usefulness in making diagnosis.
6. Immune system changes are reported in each condition, but none are clearly diagnostic of the conditions.
7. Diagnosis is mainly based on clinical features.
8. Both conditions have been greatly popularized by the lay press.

There are also some important differences between these two conditions:

1. CC is caused by a specific microbe (Candida). CFS can be associated with a variety of viruses, and in some cases, all the clinical features can be caused by bacteria or non-infective processes.
2. CC responds beautifully and often dramatically to treatment. In fact, a clear response is necessary to confirm the diagnosis. No specific treatment has been developed for CFS, and it may or may not respond to a variety of treatment measures under investigation.
3. Specific diagnostic criteria have been established for CFS by an official government/medical agency (Center For Disease Control), giving CFS a certain "legitimacy." Specific diagnostic criteria for CC have not been officially sanctioned by any "official" agency.

Dr. William Crook has developed a very useful scoring system for help in diagnosing CC.[389] A certain number of points are given for various symptoms which typically improve with Candida treatment. Points are also given for historical events which enhance Candida growth (such as repeated antibiotic use, corticosteroid use, oral contraceptives, etc.). Those with high scores may be given a **presumptive diagnosis** of CC. A reliable **confirmatory diagnosis** can only be made after a positive response to a trial of Candida therapy.

In a sense, much of traditional medicine is based on the same presumptive diagnosis basis. Chronic diarrhea is often presumed to be due to Giardia or amoeba because of clinical features, even when lab tests are negative. A trial of therapy with Flagyl or similar drugs may be given, and a clearing of the diarrhea is viewed as confirmation that the initial presumption was correct. An ill patient with a positive throat culture for Strep or Hemophilus is presumed to be ill as a consequence of infection with a bacteria. Positive response to an antibiotic would confirm the diagnosis. Little or no response to a trial of therapy with an antibiotic, and a later positive Mono test, would suggest that the patient actually had infectious mononucleosis as the predominant problem, and that the bacteria identified on culture may have only been a minor, secondary invader.

DIAGNOSIS SUMMARY: Like all other infectious diseases, diagnosis for chronic candidiasis is based on results of history, physical, and laboratory testing when indicated. Although various cultures and serodiagnostic tests have been shown to be valid and somewhat useful, the high incidence of false negative and false positive results make them somewhat undependable. A number of experts on diagnostic tests for Candida have suggested implementing anti-Candida therapy when you have a high index of suspicion, even when the tests are negative.[390,391,392,393,394] In the final analysis, the only confirmatory test for chronic candidiasis is a favorable response to a trial of therapy.

DIFFERENTIAL DIAGNOSES: Since candidiasis can account for so many different symptoms, a complete list of differential diagnoses would be almost endless. Included here are a few major considerations when a complex pattern of symptoms appear which is similar to those described for CC.

Chronic infections caused by other organisms may produce symptoms similar to those of CC, Giardia, Amoeba, and other intestinal parasites may produce similar intestinal problems as well as various systemic symptoms. Chronic viral infections such as those caused by Epstein-Barr virus[395] and Cytomegalovirus[396] may have a wide range of physical and emotional symptoms very similar to those found in candidiasis. From 65%[397] to 85%[398] of those studied with chronic Epstein-Barr virus have been shown to suffer with allergies. **Since candidiasis and chronic viral states are both associated with impaired immunity, they may co-exist.** Many patients with CC also meet the CDC-established criteria for Chronic Fatigue Syndrome. It appears that the immune suppression which facilitates chronic virus states may be a consequence of Candida-suppressed immunity. Many of the patients that we see with Chronic Fatigue Syndrome clear up completely with Candida treatment, presumably because the recovering immune system is able to control the virus. Dr. Jesop reported a very dramatic improvement in a group of patients with chronic virus symptoms after treatment with Nizoral,[399] which is only known to be effective against Candida. In other cases, the immune suppression that facilitates chronic viruses may be a consequence of other factors, and a trial of Candida therapy may be a total failure.

Starvation and malnourishment can cause a wide range of physical and emotional problems. Experimental subjects, concentration camp victims, and populations with forced food rationing have been extensively studied.[400] Prolonged reduced food intake of 1500 to 2000 calories daily for men, and 1000 to 1500 calories daily for women are known to cause symptoms like fatigue, weakness, coldness, low body temperature, apathy, depression, irritability, trouble concentrating, trouble thinking clearly, reclusiveness, decreased sex drive, intestinal disturbances, paresthesia, dysesthesia, joint pain, frequent urination, and fluid retention. Many people with a typical candidiasis picture have been trying to live on less calories than that known to produce starvation symptoms! Others have been getting inadequate nutrients due to nutritionally inadequate food, or have limited food intake because of food allergy, or have impaired digestion. Candida organisms in the intestines may utilize enough of the ingested nutrients to produce nutritional deficiency states. A species of fungus that infests cockroaches has been shown to consume so many of their ingested nutrients that the cockroaches literally die of starvation.[401] Although a healthy diet high in vitamins and minerals may very gradually help these symptoms, the essentially unhealthy, high protein diet advocated for Candida treatment would not be the ideal way to improve these people.

Various toxic substances including organic solvents, other organic poisons, pesticides, herbicides, and heavy metals may poison various enzyme systems and cause symptoms similar to CC. For example, pentaborane poisoning produces a variety of multi-system physical, emotional, and cognitive problems very much like those observed in CC.[402] Newer testing techniques are emerging which enables detection of a wide range of these substances at relatively small concentrations. There appears to be an important relationship between nutritional status and vulnerability to the toxic effects of these substances. Steven Levine has demonstrated that fasted rats will die from certain toxic chemical exposures at levels only one-twenty-fifth of the level required to kill well nourished rats.[403]

"Allergies" may account for many of the symptoms seen in the patient with candidiasis, or may be confused with that condition. A wide range of adverse reactions to foods, chemicals, hormones, and drugs often occur in some patients, whether or not they have CC. There appears to be a number of mechanisms which can account for these reactions, and much controversy exists as to whether or not they should be classified as allergy. Besides IgE, which appears to cause the classical allergic pattern of hay fever, asthma, urticaria, eczema, and anaphylaxis, there are other parts of the immune system which may cause problems.[404] Non-immune factors may also be involved.[405,406,407] Prostaglandins are probably a major factor, at least in some cases, with these adverse reactions.[408,409] A lack of antioxidant vitamins, minerals, and other nutrients may also account for some of these reactions.[410] Steven Levine has shown that antioxidant supplements will often reduce or even eliminate some of these "allergic" reactions.[411] Reactions to chemicals in the environment can cause fatigue, weakness, dizziness, anxiety, headaches, various pains, intestinal symptoms, and a wide range of other multi-system symptoms.[412,413,414]

There may be a close relationship between these adverse reactions and toxic effects from environmental substances and natural food chemicals. For example, a chemically sensitive person may develop nausea, headaches, dizziness, and weakness from exposure to a tiny amount of car exhaust. All of us will develop the same symptoms if the exposure is great enough. If the specific chemical within a food which caused a severe reaction in a food sensitive person could be isolated and given to a healthy person in much higher concentrations, that person might also experience exactly the same kind of reaction. The difference between the chemically sensitive person and the normal person may only be a matter of degree. It is possible that much of the "allergic reactivity" so common today could be partially caused by a nutritional deficiency state. An improved tolerance to chemical exposure is very commonly observed as a response to good nutrition as well as to effective Candida treatment.

Autoimmune states and Endocrinopathy may cause problems typical of candidiasis.[415,416] The relationship between Candida and autoimmune endocrinopathy has previously described in this paper. Although some cases are associated with Candida,[417,418,419] and some cases improve with Candida treatment, there are obviously other organisms or other causes of autoimmunity in addition to Candida. Phyllis Saifer[420] has reported that many of the patients she sees have antibodies to thyroid hormones, thyroid glandular tissue,[421] ovarian hormones, and ovarian tissue.[422] It is probable that antibodies to many other endocrine hormones and glands including the adrenal and thymus will be shown in the future to account for a wide range of medical symptoms.

Somatization disorder, anxiety, and depression have been frequently blamed for a myriad of symptoms.[423,424] It has been suggested that when patients present vague, multisystemic symptoms with no clear-cut physical cause, "these patients use symptoms as a way to communicate, express emotion, and to be taken care of."[425] When depression or anxiety is found in association with many other symptoms, the entire problem is often blamed onto these two conditions. Although there are clearly multi-system diseases induced mainly by psychological problems (such as sexual abuse), many emotional problems are merely the result of biochemical disturbances produced by a variety of causes.

Identifying and treating clinical depression or anxiety, in a patient with many systemic symptoms, in our opinion is incomplete and inadequate when so many known physical causes can account for these problems. Although the drugs used for treatment may be reasonably effective in controlling some symptoms, they are not curative, and may relegate the patient to a life of drug taking and to incomplete control of symptoms which might otherwise be cured completely by finding and correcting the initiating cause of the problem.

Viewing all symptoms which don't fit clearly into known disease states as being caused by emotional or psychological problems is a great disservice to the patient. Many of the patients we see who clear-up completely with very little effort have been badly treated in the traditional medical community. Perhaps the worst offenders are those doctors in University centers who proclaim with complete certainty after a very expensive medical work-up that there is absolutely nothing physically wrong, and that the problem is therefore purely emotional. Some of these same doctors when asked whether these problems could be caused by Candida have told our patients with equal certainty that there is absolutely no way in which Candida could produce the symptoms from which they are suffering.

It would seem rational and in these patients' best interest when no reasonable cause for multiple symptoms typical of candidiasis is found, that before putting a label of emotional disorder on them (which will frequently stay with them for a lifetime and influence the opinion and treatment of all doctors who deal with them in the future) to at least give them one last test--a trial of Candida treatment. We have now treated thousands of patients given emotional illness labels, who have responded beautifully to Candida therapy.

TREATMENT OF CHRONIC CANDIDIASIS

1. ANTI-CANDIDA MEDICATION: A number of medications kill Candida and help control overgrowth, but it is not possible to completely eradicate Candida. The best that can be done is to reduce their numbers to a low enough level to alleviate symptoms. Several pharmacological agents are available:

NYSTATIN (Nilstat, Mycostatin): Nystatin is not absorbed from the intestine. Treatment is thus topical, and distant infections like vaginitis or skin infections will have only an indirect response to oral treatment. Candida infestation of the mouth or any direct involvement in the esophagus and stomach will respond better to oral powder or liquid than to Nystatin pills, which don't break down until they are lower in the intestines. The dosage of Nystatin commonly used to treat CC is 1/2 teaspoon of Nystatin oral powder, or 4 pills, four times daily. Truss reports that some patients achieve better results by increasing the Nystatin to 1 teaspoon (8 pills) four times daily. It appears to be very safe at that level. Up to 70 pills daily (equivalent to about 9 teaspoons) have been well tolerated by children undergoing chemotherapy for leukemia.

KETOCONAZOL (Nizoral) is reported to be active against all strains of Candida, with no resistance reported.[426,427,428,429,430] It is systemic and is reportedly more effective for mycelial invasion into deeper tissue and in disseminated candidiasis. It should be taken with meals, as it is dissolved and absorbed best in an acid media. Antacids, anticholinergics, and H2 blockers, when indicated, should be taken at least two hours after Nizoral is taken. Usual dosage is 200 to 400 mg. daily.

FLUCONAZOLE (Diflucan) is a newer systemic anti-candida drug, reportedly absorbed better than Nizoral. Usual treatment dosage is a loading dose of 200 mg. the first day, then 100 mg. taken once daily thereafter.

AMPHOTERICIN B is reported in the PDR to be "substantially more active in vitro against Candida strains than Nystatin...is extremely well tolerated and is virtually nontoxic in prophylactic doses. Although poorly absorbed from the gut, amphotericin B has a high degree of activity against Candida species in the intestinal tract." Although available for IV administration, this drug is available in the U.S.A. and Canada orally only in combination with tetracycline (Mysteclin-F in the U.S.A. and Resteclin in Canada).

CLOTRIMAZOLE (Mycelex Troche) is a topically active antifungal agent which has been approved for oropharyngeal candidiasis.[431,432] It is apparently inactivated in the upper GI system, and thus is not effective for Candida living in the intestines. There is also a high level of liver toxicity and unpleasant side effects from the use of systemic clotrimazole,[433] making it useful only for topical application (the Troche form can be slowly dissolved to topically treat tissues of the mouth and throat).

OVER THE COUNTER ANTI-CANDIDA PRODUCTS: There are a number of over-the-counter products with proven antifungal activity that contain caprylic acid,[434,435,436,437] tannic acid,[438] Pau D'Arco (Taheebo).[439] and garlic.[440,441,442,443,444,445] Deodorized garlic does not have the active ingredient allicin,[446,447,448,449] and has been shown to be ineffective against Candida. Although these products are reported as effective by some people, they do not have the extensive experimental evidence of efficacy as do the prescription drugs.

2. **LACTOBACILLUS:** Lactobacilli appear to have a number of interesting properties that make them useful in the treatment of candidiasis. **They manufacture antimicrobial substances that may be effective against a wide range of microorganisms, including Candida species.**[450,451,452] Even strains of Lactobacilli that do not survive in the human intestine or dead Lactobacilli that are given as supplements may have anti-microbial activity. A few of these antibiotic substances have been purified, named, and studied. Lactocidin and acidophilin are two such products.

Although much conflicting data exists, **some strains of Lactobacillus do apparently establish themselves in the intestinal tract and continue to grow in the ecological niche left by the killed Candida species.**[453,454,455] In addition to the role of controlling candidiasis, Lactobacilli may provide a number of other health benefits, including production of vitamins and digestive enzymes.

It has been shown that a good carbohydrate food supply needs to be provided in order for supplemented Lactobacilli to survive and become established in the intestines.[456,457] The low-carbohydrate diets, advocated by some for treatment of candidiasis, may not allow the optimal balance of intestinal flora conducive to good health.[458] Some evidence exists that a high-meat diet will produce a different balance of intestinal organisms than a high-complex carbohydrate diet,[459] and that putrefactive-type bacteria involved in high animal protein diets may produce toxic substances.[460]

For infants and children in the first few years of life, bifidus appear to be the predominant, natural strain of Lactobacillus.[461,462] Bifidus strains are generally recommended for patients under five years of age.

Bulgaricus species, used in yogurt and contained in many Lactobacillus products, are easy to grow in culture media, but do not appear to survive in the hostile environment of the human intestine.[463,464]

3.   **DIETARY MANAGEMENT:** A high-protein diet has been advocated by several authorities for Candida management. Although this diet seems to be very effective, we are concerned about the health aspects of a high-protein diet continued over the prolonged period necessary for effective Candida control. We suggest a two phase diet as follows:

There are three main categories of foods to avoid in the Phase 1 diet for the first month of treatment:

a.   **Avoid sugar, honey, and all refined carbohydrates.** These products have been stripped of their natural fungal inhibitors,[465] and seem to provide nutrients for rapid Candida growth.

b.   **Avoid foods which contain yeast or fungal products, including bread made with yeast, mushrooms, and aged products likely to contain fungus (like aged cheese, alcoholic beverages, vinegar, soy sauce, and brewer's yeast).** These fungal products may cause cross-reaction allergic responses in those sensitive to Candida and molds. Toxins produced by these fungal products (like cell wall mannans) may be additive to those produced by Candida.

c.   **Avoid fruit and fruit juice.** Fruit juice is rather refined, and the natural fungal inhibitors may be left behind in the pulp, allowing the yeast to grow rapidly in the fruit sugar. Even whole fruit may have enough readily digested sugar to be a problem for some people with CC. Many people are also allergic or intolerant to some fruits without being aware of it; avoiding fruit during the first month of therapy enables them to test themselves for fruit allergy as they gradually reintroduce fruits to their diet.

After continuing the Phase 1 diet for about one month, the patient can shift to the Phase 2 diet, which is more liberal. In this phase, the patient judiciously adds back whole fruit and some fungal products, watching closely for any adverse reactions. Any food causing symptoms should be avoided until a later time. If patients don't feel as well on the more liberal diet and can't pinpoint any specific food as the cause of problems, the Phase 1 diet should be followed for a few more weeks, and then foods added back more slowly, possibly only one new food a week until any problem foods are uncovered.

4.   **IMMUNOTHERAPY:** For many years Candida has been a well-known antigen for which the allergists have skin tested and treated with desensitization injections. Dermatologists have commonly used an allergy treatment approach for the itch associated with chronic yeast vaginitis,[466] giving injections of Candida antigen in increasingly larger concentrations.[467] Various workers have described successful treatment of vaginitis with desensitization that had failed to improve with conventional anti-Candida drugs.[468,469,470,471] A swiss researcher reported 87.9% favorable response in recurrent Candida vaginitis treated only with

immunotherapy. The results obtained may be the result of desensitization, which decreases the hypersensitivity reaction to Candida and may thus reduce itching and local irritation.[472] "Correction of secondary immunodeficiency due to the chronic antigen stimulus" was described in a case of chronic mucocutaneous candidiasis.[473]

There may also be an element of immunization which occurs as a result of continued introduction of killed Candida, producing a relative resistance to that organism in the same way that immunization to polio, tetanus, and measles produces resistance to those organisms.[474,475] There is great variability in the ease with which immunity to various organisms is produced, and while relative immunity to some pathogens can be established with only one vaccination, current recommendation for rabies immunization is for twenty to thirty vaccine injections.[476]

The medical literature describes various classical allergic problems (such as asthma, allergic rhinitis, chronic urticaria, and eczema) improving with desensitization using Candida antigen. We have also seen hundreds of these allergic patients cleared completely with Candida antigen as the only form of allergy management. The literature also reports that a variety of non-traditional allergic symptoms improve with Candida desensitization.[477] Drs. Truss, Crook and others also report these findings. We have seen many symptoms such as migraine headaches, sinus and muscular contraction headaches, fatigue, anxiety, aching, dizziness, and depression (symptoms not usually thought to be allergic in nature) also clear with Candida antigen treatment.

An improved allergy treatment technique called "neutralizing"[478,479,480,481,482] has been reported in the literature for many years. Although some allergists deny the existence of this phenomenon, and statements in the medical literature have suggested that "there is no good immunological explanation for the phenomenon,"[483] there has been much written about neutralizing, including a number of strongly supportive double-blind studies for both intradermal[484,485,486,487,488] and sublingual[489,490,491,492,493,494] routes of administration. Using allergy desensitization treatments at neutralization dilutions is safer, associated with less side effects, and often gives immediate relief of symptoms instead of the many months to years required by traditional treatment to work.

Instructional materials for neutralizing techniques are available from the following sources:

Injectable technique:
1. Food Allergy - Provocative Testing and Injection Therapy, Joseph B. Miller, M.D., Charles C. Thomas, Publisher, Springfield, Illinois, 1972.
2. Provocative Food Test Technique, James W. Willoughby, M.D., Annals of Allergy, Volume 23, November 1965.

Sublingual technique:
1. Clinical Ecology, L.D. Dickey, Charles C. Thomas, Publisher, Springfield, Illinois, 1976, pp. 544-557.
2. Testing and desensitization to food allergens by the use of oral antigens, L. Conway and J.C. Booren, Southwest Allergy Forum, El Paso, Texas, Jan. 16, 1973.

3. Sublingual procedures, G.O. Pfeiffer, Trans. American Society Ophthalmology Otolaryngology Allergy, Volume 104, 1970.
4. Sublingual therapy for food allergy, D.L. Morris, Annals of Allergy, Volume 27, 1969.

5. EXERCISE: Exercise does a great deal to improve many of the symptoms typically associated with candidiasis. Besides the help it provides in weight management, it seems to help in the following ways:
   a. Improves energy levels, strength, and endurance.
   b. Reduces insulin resistance, improves sugar metabolism, and reduces general hunger levels as well as specific food cravings.
   c. Reduces stress-related symptoms, including anxiety and depression, and elevates mood, possibly through endorphin production.
   d. Reduces allergy symptoms, and may improve immunity.
   e. Helps to normalize bowel function, and may help with miscellaneous symptoms, including those of premenstrual syndrome.

6. NUTRITIONAL SUPPLEMENTS: In some cases, nutritional supplements are helpful, and may be given depending upon the specific needs of the patient. A chronically debilitated patient may benefit from comprehensive vitamin and mineral coverage. Evidence for nutrient deficiency associated with gut candidiasis has been discussed, as has the immune impairment associated with nutrient defects. (Refer to Chapter 7.)

DURATION OF TREATMENT

The length of time for which treatment is indicted has become an important issue. A medical director of one major health insurance company indicated that they will only pay for three weeks of treatment, and that longer treatment constitutes preventative treatment, and that they don't pay for prevention.

Truss and others have advocated a trial of therapy period of at least 8 weeks before one decides whether or not the patient actually has CC. They then describe prolonged treatment courses of many months, and even several years in some cases. Treatment as suggested by these medical experts in the medical literature would not be covered by this insurance company. To resolve this issue, several important questions need to be answered.

1. Can a Candida infection be completely eliminated so that the patient is "cured"?
2. How long does it take to eradicate Candida or reduce the numbers below the symptom threshold?
3. How long does it take to reestablish immune competency so that symptoms are controlled without the need for continued anti-Candida medication.?
4. Does a flare-up of candidiasis represent a new infection in a previously cured patient, or does it represent a regrowth of the original Candida strain which had been incompletely treated?

A number of topical products for treating vaginal candidiasis suggest 1 week of therapy or 3 days in some cases, or even a 1 day treatment suppository is available. Although a simple, superficial Candida infection will be cured with this duration of treatment, more resistant infections will not. Good evidence of the chronicity of Candida vaginitis comes from the December 1990 study of women treated for extended periods with Nystatin orally, vaginally, or both, or with placebo. Eight weeks of treatment with either oral or vaginal Nystatin caused a proportional improvement of less than 50%, and 8 weeks of combined therapy caused proportional improvement of just slightly over 50%. There was no improvement in the number of positive cultures after the various blocks of treatment compared to before treatment began. The only group that did not worsen once active treatment was discontinued was the group who underwent 24 consecutive weeks of active treatment before the placebo. Other groups, even those with 16 weeks of active treatment, got worse again with the placebo. This study points out that even prolonged topical and/or oral therapy for Candida does not "cure" or eliminate the organisms even in those clinically improved, that even extended topical therapy is not enough to improve about half of cases, and that prolonged therapy of at least 24 weeks may be needed to adequately control the problem.

Although the standard therapy for most bacterial infections has been for a few days only, there are many infections which are well known to require prolonged therapy. Today's current policy by our local Public Health Department is that those with a positive skin test for Tuberculosis and negative chest X-rays are treated for 6 to 9 months with Isoniazid. (Note that these people are often treated with no firm diagnosis, and that some of them would obviously have not developed active disease, thus treatment in their case would be preventative). Those with positive X-rays are usually treated for at least 18 to 24 months with a combination of antibiotics. In immune compromised people, treatment for 3 years or so has been sometimes recommended.

Treatment for fungal infections of the toenails is suggested for **at least** 6 months, and longer if needed to produce clinical and laboratory evidence of a cure. The emphasis on treatment with fungal infections, including Candida, has been treatment until there is clinical and laboratory evidence of a cure. Maintenance therapy is even recommended. Various writers have suggested treating vaginal candidiasis for 6 months,[496] up to 14 months for the nails,[497] and for 3 years for chronic mucocutaneous candidiasis.[498]

Even after therapy for many months with systemic anti-Candida medication, vaginal and other forms of candidiasis return in a high incidence of cases.[499] An important new study points out that "we are dealing with recurrences in practically all cases and not with new infections."[500,501] These infections were not adequately treated, and thus returned. Extended treatment is therefore needed to control the infection, and in no way represents prevention of new infections (an important point for insurance considerations).

With effective treatment, nutritious diet, and other measures, most people will be able to control CC in 3 to 6 months, be able to stop medication, and seem to develop adequate immunocompetance to resist further infections. Some people, however, seem to be immunologically impaired, and require indefinite treatment. Improved treatment methods developed by Truss seem to permit immunocompetance to develop in people who might otherwise have never become well, and speed up the process in others.

OPPOSITION TO THE CONCEPT OF CHRONIC CANDIDIASIS

Although thousands of doctors from around the world have embraced the concept of CC and have treated millions of patients, many doctors have expressed strong opposition to the concept. A number of articles have appeared in various journals expressing opinions about this issue. There have even been several position papers dealing with CC. We would next like to describe this opposition literature, and critique it.

Negative Literature. All of the other criticisms of chronic candidiasis listed below contain no scientific references to discredit the concept–not one article!!

1. In all of the negative literature published about CC, not a single doctor has ever reported treating a single patient using Truss's full protocol! Not one doctor. Not one patient. After repeated, exhaustive, and recent world literature searches, there is really only one negative scientific study that even comes close to evaluating CC. Only nystatin was used, and none of the other components of Truss's treatment protocol was used. This could hardly be considered a fair or adequate evaluation of this condition.

Dismukes[501] selected a group of women with repeated vaginitis aggravated by antibiotics who had responded favorably in the past to topical antifungal agents, and who also exhibited various emotional and systemic features characteristic of CC. Four treatment groups were used: A - oral nystatin plus vaginal nystatin, B - oral nystatin plus vaginal placebo, C - oral placebo plus vaginal nystatin, and D - oral placebo plus vaginal placebo. Each patient received 8 weeks of treatment with each protocol. The authors concluded that "the three active-treatment regimens were more effective than placebo in relieving vaginal symptoms (P<.001)", and that "In women with presumed candidiasis hypersensitivity syndrome, nystatin does not reduce systemic or psychological symptoms significantly more than placebo. Consequently, the empirical recommendation of long-term nystatin therapy for such women appears to be unwarranted."

There are some major problems with this study, including the limitation admitted by the authors, that only the nystatin treatment was used, and none of the other treatments advocated by Truss were evaluated. Although the patients eventually got to the effective treatment dosage of nystatin recommended by Truss, only 4 weeks of treatment were given at this dosage. Truss recommends at least 8 weeks of treatment at this dosage along with diet, immunotherapy, and other treatment modalities before evaluating results of treatment. Many features of CC, particularly cerebral symptoms, may take considerably longer than that to show improvement.

The use of starch as a placebo has to be seriously questioned. Starch has been used by women for many years as a home remedy for intertriginous candidiasis, especially under the breasts. We have asked dozens of women how helpful this was for them, and a number of them have said that it was more effective than any creams their doctors had given to them. The favorable response of the so-called placebo group may well have been influenced by the starch.

Their conclusion that "nystatin does not reduce systemic or psychological symptoms more than placebo" is misleading, since there were a number of positive features in the study, including: overall improvement in group A; improvement in 4 systemic symptoms in group A; significant carry-over effects of nystatin on overall score; significant improved systemic score carry-over in sequence 1; "progressive beneficial effect on all three symptoms scores" from week 2 to week 6; "discernable difference between the effects of the double-drug group and those of the double-placebo group" from week 16 to weeks 20, 24, 28, and 32. (P=.06); significant improvement in oral-nystatin regimens versus oral placebo regimens on "somatization or distress arising from perceptions of bodily functions;" and a positive trend short of significance in a number of other reported results.

The effectiveness of nystatin treatment for vaginitis, reported as highly significant (P<.001), was not that impressive. According to Table 2, there was no improvement in vaginal pruritus, burning, or abnormal discharge in treatment groups AB versus CD, and no improvement in pruritus in groups ABC versus D. "No significant differences in the effects of treatment on the culture results [vaginal and rectal] were detected." Oral or vaginal nystatin alone only caused proportional improvement of less than 50%, only 10 percentage points better than placebo. Combined oral and vaginal nystatin treatment caused improvement of just over 50%, less than 20 percentage points better than placebo.

If this study had been done by someone with a bias towards proving the CC concept (instead of attempting to disprove it, as is the obvious intent of the authors), they could have easily reported it as positive, or at the least, could have mentioned the encouraging trends. Choosing to reject the results of those who failed to complete all four blocks of treatment instead of including their data (an arbitrary decision made by the researchers), may have made the difference in this study between positive and negative. (Of course no one experienced in using Truss's protocol would have used a study design like this one.)

Several important issues were pointed out in this study. The limitations of using vaginal and rectal cultures for diagnosing and evaluating treatment results were demonstrated very clearly. Only 14% of these women with strong presumptive evidence of vaginal candidiasis entering the study had positive vaginal cultures, and only 12% of them had positive rectal cultures. During the study, "the incidence of positive vaginal and rectal cultures at the end of each treatment block did not change significantly, ranging from 8 to 12.5 percent (vaginal cultures) and 7 to 10 percent (rectal cultures)." This study also demonstrates the pathetically poor results achieved by even prolonged treatment by traditional antifungal treatment regimens on this very distressing and very common health problem. This study also provides an example of diagnosing chronic or recurrent candidiasis strictly on the basis of history of a previous positive response to a trial of anti-fungal therapy. It also demonstrates the tremendous need for improved treatment modalities.

In a letter to us, Dr. Orian Truss described a re-analysis of the data showing a strongly positive treatment result. He has placed 25 of their original subjects on his full treatment protocol immediately after the study was completed; he has observed remarkable improvements.

Very few controlled scientific studies have been done to evaluate Truss's protocol on chronic vaginitis. One Swiss study, using women with at least 4 recurrent episodes of Candida vaginitis in the previous year, compared the effects of using nystatin along with a Truss-type diet, to treatment using only Candida-specific desensitization injections. At the end of 3 months, 90% of those treated with nystatin and diet had significant improvement, and 87.9% of those treated with immunotherapy alone were improved.[503] Other authors (reported earlier in this paper) have also reported improved results in Candida vaginitis with Candida immunotherapy compared to conventional antifungal treatment by itself.

2.   Renfro[504] evaluated a group of 100 patients with features suggestive of chronic fatigue syndrome. He compared those in the group who had heard of CC and suspected that they might have this problem, to those in the group who did not express such a concern. He states that 7 out of the 8 patients who expressed a concern that they might have chronic candidiasis were given a psychiatric diagnosis, as if to suggest that this ruled out any possibility that they could have candidiasis.

To compare a group of people based on what they had read and feared to another group who had not read the same things and did not share the same fears certainly doesn't seem very sound. To exclude any disease because a psychiatric diagnosis has been made is ridiculous. A great deal of psychiatric disturbances have been shown to have some organic basis.

3.   The **Executive Committee of the American Academy of Allergy and Immunology have published a position paper on Candidiasis hypersensitivity syndrome.**[505] They quote from Crook's Yeast Connection book to describe the syndrome. They do not reference a single piece of literature to support their conclusion that "the concept of the candidiasis hypersensitivity syndrome is unproven." The critique is as follows:

Critique

The Practice Standards Committee finds multiple problems with the candidiasis hypersensitivity syndrome.

1.   The concept is speculative and unproven.
   a.   The basic elements of the syndrome would apply to almost all sick patients at some time. The complaints are essentially universal; the broad treatment program (see Description of syndrome, particularly elements 1, 2, 3, and 7a) would produce remissions in most illnesses regardless of cause.
   b.   There is no published proof that Candida albicans is responsible for the syndrome.
   c.   There is no published proof that treatment of Candida albicans infection with specific antifungal agents (see Description 8) benefits the syndrome.
   d.   There is no proof that immunotherapy or provocation and/or neutralization with Candida albicans allergenic extract (see Description 9) benefit the syndrome.
   e.   There is no proof that the recommended special studies (see Description 6) are effective diagnostic tests for the purposes for which they are used.
2.   Elements of the proposed treatment program are potentially dangerous.
   a.   Resistant species of Candida albicans and of other pathogenic fungi may be produced by long-term oral use of the major antifungal agents (see Description 8).

b. Untoward effect from oral use of antifungal agents (see Description 8) are rare, but some inevitably will occur.

Their first complaint in 1a deals with the multi-system nature of CC. Their concern about the "universal" nature of the patient complaints in no way negates the observations of Truss and all the rest of us who see multi-system disease in the millions of patients that we have treated. Their assertion that the broad treatment program, especially the dietary part, would "produce remission in most illnesses regardless of cause" is absolute nonsense! If diets are such miracle workers in chronic health problems, why are diets not routinely used in medicine for treating all of these chronic problems? Healthy diets may help some chronic health problems, but responses are very slow and wouldn't account for the relatively short response time for Truss's treatment. The diet mentioned by Crook is, by his own admission, not a healthy diet for long term use, and wouldn't be expected to help other health conditions. In his introduction to the diet section of his Yeast Connection Book,[506] he describes his own belief system about healthy diets, and then states that "I had to re-orient my thinking and make a 180 degree turn-around before I could recommend diets high in protein and fat and low in carbohydrate." Our concern for the unhealthy nature of the diets recommended by Truss and Crook was the major motivation for us to write our own yeast control book.[507] Even our modified phase 1 diet, we believe, is unhealthy for long term use, and we strongly and repeatedly recommend that patients move to the healthier phase 2 diet after 4 weeks. Crook has also recently recommended similar improvements in diet after initial treatment with the stricter diet. For the committee to make this statement regarding diet and illness shows appalling ignorance of both Crook's diet and nutrition in general.

The committee's statement in 1b that "there is no published proof that Candida albicans is responsible for the syndrome" is absolutely untrue. The same proof exists in the medical literature relating Candida to various symptoms, as exists for other microbes and the symptoms associated with them. The medical literature is full of articles and letters to the editor written by doctors who have observed clinical features improve after treatment of a microbe that were not previously reported to be associated with that microbe. The same thing has happened with Candida. Even their own literature is full of accounts of Candida allergy treatment clearing up various allergic symptoms. Their own literature contains one of the earliest (1962) accounts of multi-system symptoms improving with Candida treatment.[508] Besides Truss' original article in the medical literature describing CC, a variety of other articles have also appeared describing the relationship of Candida to a host of symptoms.

The committee states in 1c that there is no proof that therapy with antifungal drugs benefit the syndrome. The literature widely quoted in this paper easily refutes that statement.

The statement in 1d that "there is no proof that immunotherapy or provocation and/or neutralization with Candida albicans allergenic extracts benefit the syndrome" again is completely untrue. There are numerous reports in the literature describing a wide range of symptoms improving with Candida desensitization; due to time and space, only a small number of them are reported in this paper.

The "special studies" pointed out in 1e were only mentioned as items of interest, work in progress, and special tests for some individuals to identify specific deficiencies. Crook specifically mentions that he does not use some of these tests in his practice, and certainly doesn't use them routinely, if at all, for making a diagnosis of CC.

4. The **Infectious Diseases Society of America** is also in the process of preparing a position paper.[509] Again, they don't offer any scientific evidence than Candida does not cause multi-system disease. Their strongest arguments that it does not exist are references to the position paper by the American Academy of Allergy and Immunology, other opinions expressed in the medical literature, and the findings of the Utah State Medical Association Unproven Health Practices Committee (to be discussed later). None of these references offer any scientific evidence of any kind that the syndrome does not exist.

The position statement is: "The existence of the yeast connection syndrome is scientifically unproven and the likelihood that the widely varied, systemic symptoms are related to Candida species in millions of individuals is improbable." This position is formulated on the following basis:

1. The results of any animal studies or clinical trials substantiating the disease have not been reported in the scientific literature cited in the Index Medicus.
2. The basis for the description of the syndrome is anecdotal.
3. The symptoms of the syndrome are widely heterogenous and non-specific.
4. It is highly probable that those patients who have benefitted from specific antifungal therapy have actually benefitted from a multifactorial placebo effect.
5. A large number of experts in the field of Candida infections and microbiology agree unanimously that the likelihood for the symptoms of the syndrome being related to Candida is very low. "They also express a concern that extensive treatment for candidiasis may result in substantial risk to public health care or inappropriate expenditures of patients' financial resources."

Their criticism, Point number 2, that "the description of the syndrome is anecdotal" can also be applied to every other infectious disease state. What we know about all infectious diseases is what doctors report seeing in the patients with the disorder, and in particular, what features they report clearing with effective treatment. Point number 3 is a valid complaint. But to suggest that these estimated millions of people who have benefitted from treatment were merely responding to a placebo effect, Point number 4, is a preposterous speculation on their part. Many of these patients have seen dozens of doctors, tried many unsuccessful treatment modalities, and then completely got well with anti-Candida therapy. To suggest that these long-lasting cures are merely placebo effects is a great insult to all these people and the physicians who have treated them. Point number 5 shows these authors to be incredibly arrogant and pompous. They claim to be experts in Candida and microbiology, and they may truly know a lot of old information published about aspects of Candida. Not a single one of these doctors, however, have ever reported treating a single person with chronic candidiasis using Truss' full protocol, and so they have no way of knowing whether his and thousands of other doctors' observations are true or not. They suggest that their own ponderings are more likely to be correct than the cumulative wisdom of all of those with extensive personal experience with this disorder.

5.   The **Utah State Medical Association Unproven Health Practices Committee** held a meeting to discuss the Candida controversy. Although the committee clearly knew several doctors in the state who were treating chronic candidiasis, they elected to hear from only 2 doctors who were known to be opposed to the concept. Those of us treating Candida had no invitation to attend, and were not even told the meeting was to be held. In a forty-five minute inquisition-like trial, the Unproven Health Practices Committee ruled that "treatment for chronic candidiasis must be considered an unproven health practice at this time." To compare this hearing to an inquisition is perhaps a little unfair - unfair to the memory of those long-departed Spaniards who at least had enough sense of fair play and justice to have the accused present at their own trial! Should not the committee have had a token representation from the other side so that it would look less like a witch hunt, and at least give the appearance of justice and fair play?

According to the minutes of this meeting, Dr. Charles Smith stated that "there is no known evidence which indicates that Candida normally growing in the gastrointestinal tract will create an immune-mediated illness," that Candida organisms invoke "an as yet undefined immune reaction." The research demonstrating specific immune system effects of Candida is extremely extensive, and the research described in this paper is only a small fraction of that available.
Dr. Smith also stated that "Koch's postulate has not been demonstrated in this disease." One would not expect Koch's postulate to be demonstrated in diseases that are caused by an organism that is a normal part of the flora and that cause immune-mediated illness in only part of those who are afflicted. Likewise, such criteria would not be very valid for evaluating the cause of Chronic Fatigue Syndrome, or to evaluate whether or not Proteus actually causes Rheumatoid Arthritis.

6.   A book review by **Constantine J. Falliers**, an allergist, is again very critical of the "yeast connection". He does not include a single shred of scientific evidence or discussion to discount Dr. Crook's extensive experience.[510] In this biting, sarcastic piece, he slams clinical ecologists, orthomolecular medicine, nutritionists, and anyone who believes in those concepts. Several patients who eventually came to us, asked one of the Salt Lake allergists about some scientific articles they might read to gain a better understanding of his side of the Candida controversy. This book review was the "scientific evidence" that he sent to them! It does not contain one scientific reference.

7.   In a letter to the editor of JAMA, Quinn and Venezio, expressed concern that the "Yeast Connection" book was responsible for iatrogenic disease, by convincing people with no organic disease that they were suffering from CC. They described Dr. Crook's heart-rending case histories as "an amusing collection of anecdotes and speculation." Again, they had absolutely no evidence to support their disbelief. They expressed concern regarding the "danger" and "expense" of therapy.[511]

Possible Reasons for Opposition to the Chronic Candidiasis Concept. Since there is absolutely no scientific evidence against the chronic candidiasis concept, there must be some reasons why the concept has met with such vocal opposition. If we knew what these reasons were, it might help us to understand the issues better. In our opinion, the following reasons are likely to be involved:

1. The expanded role of Candida in causing illness does not fit in well with the older concept that a specific microbe caused a single, discrete clinical illness. Understanding disease based on complex interrelationships between microbes and their hosts requires a major paradigm shift. Some doctors are threatened by having to give up their old body of knowledge with which they were comfortable, and learning a much more complex set of principles.

2. The American Academy of Allergy and Immunology has bitterly opposed new concepts of allergy and improved treatment techniques for 30 years or so, even though these ideas came from within their own ranks. Desensitization techniques using "endpoint titration" or sublingual routes of administration have been denounced in position statements[512] as unproven and unscientific, in spite of the fact that many double-blind studies have been done validating these procedures. Members of this organization have performed studies, often under the sponsorship of the organization, deceitfully designed and dishonestly reported, to discredit these techniques.[513] Several members have been convicted of illegal trade practices in their efforts to compete with allergists from other groups.

Members of the AAAI continue to write very derisive and sarcastic articles denouncing clinical ecology and those who believe in those concepts. Almost anything believed and practiced by those interested in environmental medicine is criticized and ridiculed. Because of their interest in food and chemical allergies, and their interest in both external as well as internal environmental factors (ecology of the gut), the doctors from the American Academy of Environmental Medicine have widely embraced Truss's concepts and treatment principles. Members of the AAAI would almost automatically reject this concept, just out of general principles.

3. Chronic candidiasis is basically an iatrogenic disease, often caused by repeated use of antibiotics and/or cortisone. To admit that this condition existed would be to accept some element of blame for having produced it. The allergists and infectious disease people probably use more broad-spectrum antibiotics and corticosteroids than any other group of doctors, and thus would be more at blame.

4. Allergists and infectious disease specialists consider themselves to be **the** experts in their respective areas. Since chronic candidiasis has both a strong allergic component and an infective component, this disease should fall within their realms. Since the disease was described and popularized by outsiders, their egos may not quite accept the idea that anyone else could develop valid concepts in their domains.

5. Most doctors have received very little training in the area of nutrition and nutrients, and feel uncomfortable using dietary treatments. There has long been a bias in traditional medicine against those doctors that do use dietary therapies and nutrients in their practices. Many of the doctors that have accepted the CC concept have been those that have prescribed diets, and have seen the dramatic changes in those who comply with Truss's diet.

There is even more of a bias against Chiropractors, Naturopaths, and Herbal therapists, many of whom have also embraced the CC concept and are treating it.

6. Doctors compete for the same patients, particularly conventional allergists and environmental allergists. Discrediting another specialty group's techniques and concepts may help to produce a larger flow of patients for your own group. There is also a tendency to judge techniques based on other doctor's failures. Most doctors will see some patients who have undergone a negative trial of therapy for CC.

Comments on Articles Critical of Chronic Candidiasis. Those critical of CC generally express similar concerns. Most are critical of the wide range of non-specific multi-system symptoms reported for this disorder. All of us that work with CC share this concern. It makes diagnosis and validation of the disease more difficult. Their disbelief in no way negates the observations of literally thousands of doctors who have verified the reports of Truss. Most of the clinical features of CC have been reported in the literature over the years, and their failure to accept this disease reflects their failure to search the literature adequately. The various facets of the disease fit in perfectly with a newer paradigm of pathogenesis of disease caused by microbes. There are many similar multi-system illness caused by other microbes reported in the recent literature such as typhus, Lyme's disease, chronic fatigue syndrome, and Rocky Mountain Spotted Fever.[514,515]

Several critics have reported that there is no published proof to support the concept, or to support the idea that antifungal or immunotherapy helped the disorder. These statements are obviously untrue, since many articles from the literature described in this chapter have provided proof for many facets of this disorder. Most of the proof we have described predates their article, was in their own journals, and in all probability was known to them. The "lack of proof" statements by the allergy committee are either flagrant, deliberate lies, or if they didn't really know about the reports in the literature, these committee members are guilty of being dishonest and irresponsible in claiming that there was no proof without an adequate literature search.

The authors' suggestion that proponents of the disease perform placebo-controlled trials, and the denunciation of the condition because double-blind studies have not been done, are both extremely hypocritical. They demand a kind of proof for chronic candidiasis that has never been expected of any other infectious disease state, while failing to provide a single shred of scientific evidence or other proof (except their own speculation) that it does not exist. Illness caused by infectious diseases are generally reported in the literature precisely how CC has been reported, and are usually accepted at face value.

Several writers describe seeing a few patients who were aware of CC, and thought that they might have this problem. These authors describe this concern as a form of iatrogenic disease. Compared to the millions of people suffering serious consequences from CC, this concern seems very trivial.

Several authors, in a seemingly noble concern for the safety of the patients, express concern about the dangers of therapy. The dangers involved in therapy for CC are likely to be considerably less than the dangers involved in widespread invasive testing and needless surgery imposed on many of these patients. Suicide, a common problem with depression, is likely to be a much greater risk in this population of people than any theoretical risk of anti-Candida treatment. The dangers of remaining immunocompromised due to Candida toxins is also likely to pose a greater threat to these patients than any theoretical production of resistant species of Candida with prolonged therapy.

Several writers were concerned about costs. Compared to the cost often incurred by these patients in countless investigative procedures and symptomatic treatment, the cost of nystatin or similar medication is very minimal. One patient described spending in excess of $8,000 over several years trying to find causes and cures for the group of symptoms that completely cleared with $100 worth of nystatin, along with diet. One young lady calculated that she and her insurance company spent more than $100,000 dollars in investigation costs, hospitalizations, and drug therapy over the previous 8 years for a multi-system disease which came on suddenly after a complicated delivery, and disappeared completely with a few short months of anti-Candida therapy.

Summary of Chronic Candidiasis Conflict. On one side of the conflict, Dr. Orian Truss published 3 important articles in the medical literature in 1978 describing an improved treatment protocol for chronic, resistance Candida albicans infections. Treatment involved high dose, long term oral (and where indicated, vaginal) nystatin, along with a low carbohydrate, yeast-free diet, and specific Candida desensitization injections using the end-point titration technique. He reported a series of patients treated with this protocol that experienced dramatic improvement in a wide variety of symptoms, including: depression, anxiety, irrational irritability, bloating, diarrhea, constipation, heartburn, indigestion, loss of self-confidence, inability to cope, lethargy, symptoms from contact with foods and chemical odors, acne, migraine headaches; and in women: urethritis, cystitis, repeated vaginal yeast infections, premenstrual tension and menstrual problems; and in children: hyperactivity, irritability, learning problems, recurrent ear infections, diaper rash, abdominal discomfort, diarrhea, constipation, poor appetite, and erratic sleep patterns. He also described a theory that would explain how Candida could produce all these problems, and in 1983 expanded these ideas into a referenced, full-sized book, written for both doctors and patients.

Many other doctors began using Truss' treatment protocol, and reports by these other doctors began to appear in the medical literature, confirming the original reports by Truss. At least 11 other full-sized books are written by doctors and other health professionals describing their experiences with the disorder, and outlining their own ideas about treatment. A number of texts and other books about health conditions, like endometriosis and PMS, included chapters about chronic candidiasis. At least 5 national conferences were held, taught by various doctors and university based researchers. Several medical societies, including the American Academy of Environmental Medicine, embraced the concept and regularly include presentations in their scientific meetings about chronic candidiasis. Thousands of doctors from around the world have tried Truss' treatment protocol, have observed the same results that he reported, and have collectively treated millions of people.

Although Truss is credited with developing the concept of chronic candidiasis and the treatment protocol, the medical literature pre-dating his reports also contains many references of Candida being associated with the various symptoms described by Truss. Specific immunotherapy and dietary interventions have also been described as being useful to control Candida-related problems.

A huge body of world literature supports the various theories that Truss has postulated to account for his observations. Hundreds of articles describe the identification of several toxins produced by Candida and describe their effects on various aspects of animal and human physiology. Candida-induced immune system damage is extensively described, and various autoimmune and endocrine disorders are linked to Candida in the literature. Improvement of these autoimmune and endocrine problems has been described after anti-Candida therapy, suggesting that Candida produced those specific problems. Allergies to Candida are extensively described in the literature. These allergic disorders, along with various conditions not previously identified as allergic, have been shown to improve with Candida-specific immunotherapy.

The proof that chronic candidiasis is a real condition is the same as the proof for any other illness caused by an infectious agent. Doctors report in the literature and at conferences the results they observe from treating the disorder. Those features which disappear with effective treatment are thought to be caused by the illness.

On the other side of the conflict, several doctors have written articles expressing their opposition to the concept of chronic candidiasis. Not one of these doctors have ever reported treating a single patient using Truss's protocol. They do not offer one shred of scientific evidence to support their opposition to the concept, while demanding more proof from those of us who do support the concept. Their criticisms seem to be economically and politically motivated.

CHRONIC CANDIDIASIS - PROVEN OR UNPROVEN?

Importance of the chronic candidiasis issue. Not only is the concept of chronic candidiasis being challenged, but in addition, the methods by which the medical community learns new ideas and teaches them to each other are being challenged. The concept of chronic candidiasis has evolved over the years, improved treatment techniques have been developed, medical literature reports have appeared, conferences have been held, and extensive use of the improved techniques has occurred, just like with every other disease concept that has been developed. If the concept of chronic candidiasis is considered unproven, and if the same criteria are used for other concepts and treatment techniques, then it is likely that no further progress will be made in medicine, and we will be forever stuck using existing technology.

Patient rights to receive the best possible care known to their doctors is in jeopardy. The ability of those doctors to practice in the way they best know how is being threatened.

Let us quote one case history to illustrate. A woman in her late twenties suffered for years with severe vaginal itching, discomfort, and discharge completely unresponsive to repeated, topical antifungal therapy. She also suffered from a wide range of severe physical and emotional symptoms. Treatment with nystatin and the rest of Truss's protocol helped her entire clinical picture, but only partially controlled the vaginitis. Nizoral seemed to help even more, but she tolerated it poorly, and only was able to take a limited dose for a short time. Diflucan produced dramatic and rapid relief of her entire symptoms complex. After a few weeks, she was informed by her insurance company that they would not pay for Diflucan, so she stopped it, and quickly deteriorated. A vaginal culture showed heavy Candida overgrowth. The insurance company's medical director stated that they didn't pay for chronic candidiasis, since it was considered experimental, and that unless we could prove that she had invasive Candida with a biopsy, or provide proof that she was severely immunocompromised by AIDS or cancer treatment, they wouldn't pay for her treatment. He further stated that they would not pay at all for oral nystatin powder, and would only pay for three weeks of therapy no matter what other medication we used, since that should be enough to cure her condition. Treatment for a longer time, he stated, was unjustified, would constitute prevention, and they do not pay for prevention! When we attempted to discuss this issue with him, he stated that he wasn't the expert, that he relied on two medical experts, an allergist and an infectious disease specialist, to make his decision. Further attempts to discuss the issue brought a threat that if we didn't quit "gaming him," he would have every single charge on every patient we submitted reviewed by his company. When we told him that they were already doing that, he blustered that he would get in touch with us when he and his experts decided how their company was going to handle the Candida issue. This patient, and several others, were told by employees of this company that if they went to see us, they could expect to have all their claims automatically denied and their medical records reviewed each visit.

In effect, this insurance company is setting themselves up as the expert in this field and telling us how to practice medicine. We are told the specific criteria we must use to make our diagnosis, what medications we can use, and how long we can treat. Even claims that have nothing to do with Candida are routinely denied, and weekly we are asked for piles of medical records. The situation is much worse for some of these patients, many of them with huge medical bills from previous ineffective testing and treatment and inability to work due to their medical problems. The vocal opposition of the opponents has given this insurance company, they believe, the mandate to discriminate against certain patients, and dictate how medicine is practiced in this state.

If a few self-serving, turf-protecting doctors can get the concepts and treatment techniques of another specialty group classified as unproven (thus unethical to treat and not paid for by insurance companies), what is to prevent other groups from doing the same thing to other treatment techniques? There is a very real danger that this type of in-fighting among specialty groups can lead to serious rifts in the medical community, further loss of freedom to practice medicine in the best way we know how, and increased control by insurance companies.

CONCLUSION

The Candida issue is an extremely important health issue. We strongly believe, along with a lot of other doctors, that we are in the middle of a Candida-induced epidemic in this country. The schools are filled with learning disabled and hyperactive children. Teenage suicide is rampant, and psychiatric hospitals are springing up all over to handle the anxiety, depression, and drug dependencies which are characteristic of this disorder. Severe headaches and other types of pain are epidemic, and millions of Americans are suffering extreme discomfort from multisystem problems, for which the medical community has only been providing symptomatic relief. Candidiasis is also rapidly becoming more common.[515,516,517] The very vocal opposition to chronic candidiasis is having some serious consequences.

Scientific proof that Candida can cause problems like hyperactivity, learning disabilities, depression, anxiety, and various psychiatric disorders is somewhat limited at the present time. There is, however, overwhelming proof that Candida infections can become chronic, and that Candida can cause a variety of multisystem health problems. Only a small part of that proof has been presented here.

On the other hand, there is only one scientific study in the medical literature (at this writing) with negative conclusions about chronic candidiasis.[518] This study only utilized part of Truss's treatment protocol for a relatively short time. It did show positive features and trends, about all that could be expected from such a study. It also provided some of the strongest evidence yet contained in the medical literature that candida vaginitis is chronic, responds poorly to even prolonged therapy, and has a strong tendency to recur. It certainly pointed out the need for improved treatment methods.

Which is the most believable, science or opinions? Which is more likely to be true, the opinions of those doctors who have never even treated a single person for chronic candidiasis, or the collective observations of thousands of doctors after treating millions of patients? This is not just a simple academic debate. If chronic candidiasis exists, then every physician who has a medical license to prescribe antibiotics, corticosteroids, immunosuppressive drugs, and H2 blockers has the potential for creating serious illness.

When the concept is finally accepted that Candida and other organisms can cause a wide variety of health problems through a variety of host-pathogen mechanisms, an exciting new era of medicine should be ushered in. Expanding these concepts should provide explanations for many disease states and symptoms now poorly understood. Curative treatment modalities will then become standard for conditions now only partially controllable through continued drug therapy. As doctors and health care professionals, we will then be able to offer an extended range of help to a wider variety of people.

1. Baker S. An epidemic in disguise. Omni March 1985; pp.85-127.
2. Thomas DC. New hope for allergy patients. Inn America April 6, 1983; pp. 77-84.
3. Bredell F. The spores that attack you when your immune system can't protect you. Bestways January 1984; pp. 22-26.
4. Thomas DC. The newest mystery illness. Redbook April 1986.

5. Baker N. We wouldn't give up on our son. Good Housekeeping Feb 1985.

6. Truss CO. The Missing Diagnosis. Birmingham, AL: Missing Diagnosis, Inc., 1982.

7. Crook WG. The Yeast Connection. Jackson, TN: Professional Books, 1983.

8. Connolly P. The Candida Albicans Yeast-Free Cookbook. New Canaan, CT: Keats Publishing Inc., 1985.

9. Wunderlich RC, Kalita DK. Candida Albicans: How to Fight an Exploding Epidemic of Yeast-Related Diseases. New Canaan, CT: Keats Publishing Inc., 1984.

10. Rose E. Lady of gray. An inspiring story of healing from environmental illness with systemic candidiasis. Butterfly Pub Co, 2210 Wilshire Blvd. Suite 845, Santa Monica, CA 1985.

11. Trowbridge JP, Walker M. The Yeast Syndrome. Bantam Books, NY 1986.

12. Hagglund HE. Why do I feel so bad (when the doctor says I'm okay)? IED Press, Oklahoma City, OK 1984.

13. LaPorte, RE. Insulin-dependent diabetes mellitus called "epidemiologist's dream". JAMA 1988;259:1614-1615.

14. Boubneres PF, Carel JC, et al. Factors associated with early remission of type 1 diabetes in children treated with cyclosporine. NEJM 1988;318:663-70.

15. Geffner ME, Lippe BM. The role of immunotherapy in type 1 diabetes mellitus. West J Med 1987;146:337-343.

16. Stahlheber PA, Peter JB. Multiple sclerosis: a clearer path to a complex diagnosis. Diagnostic Medicine. Jan 1984:1-5.

17. Nathanson N, Miller A. Epidemiology of multiple sclerosis: critique of the evidence for a viral etiology. Am J Epidemiol 1978;107:451.

18. Singh B, Milton JD, Woodrow JC. Anklyosing spondylitis, HLA-B27 and Klebsiella: a study of lymphocyte reactivity of anti-Klebsiella sera. Ann Rheum Dis 1986;45:190-7.

19. Ebringer A, Khalafpour S, Wilson C. Rheumatoid arthritis and Proteus: a possible etiological association. Rheumatol Int 1989;9:223-228.

20. Ebringer A, Corbett M, Macafee Y, et al. Antibodies to Proteus in rheumatoid arthritis. The Lancet August 10, 1985:305-307.

21. Bech K, Larsen JH, Hansen JM, Nerup J. Yersinia enterocolitica infection and thyroid disorders. Lancet 1974;2:951-2.

22. Granfors K, Jalkanen S, et al. Yersinia antigens in synovial-fluid cells from patients with reactive arthritis. NEJM 1989;320:216-21.

23. Cashman NR, Maselli R, Wollmann RL, Roos R, Simon R, Antel JP. Late denervation in patients with antecedent paralytic poliomyelitis. NEJM 1987;317:7-12.

24. Logigian EL, Kaplan RF, Steere AC. Chronic neurologic manifestations of Lyme disease. NEJM 1990;323:1438-44.

25. Hardebo JE. An association between cluster headache and herpes simplex. NEJM Jan 30, 1986:316.

26. Yeast/Human Interaction Symposium. Birmingham, Alabama. December, 1983.

27. Yeast/Human Interaction Symposium. San Francisco, California. March, 1985.

28. Yeast/Human Interaction Symposium. Dallas, TX 1982.

29. Yeast/Human Interaction Update Conference. Dallas, Tx 1987.

30. Yeast/Human Interaction International Symposium. Birmingham, AL 1988.

31. Goff JS. Infectious causes of esophagitis. Ann Rev Med 1988;39:163-9.

32. Kirillov VA, Preobrazhenski VN, Kasatkin NN, Seroshtanova AF. Comparative evaluation of various methods of treating patients with esophageal candidiasis. Klin Med (Mosk) 1989;67(4):58-60.

33. Debongnie JC, Beyaert C, Legros G. Touch cytology, a useful diagnostic method for diagnosis of upper gastrointestinal tract infections. Dig Dis Sci 1989;34(7):1025-7.

34. Morris AB, Sands ML, Shiraki M, Brown RB, Ryczak M. Gallbladder and biliary tract candidiasis: nine cases and review. Rev Infect Dis 1990;12(3):484-9.

35. Gordon SC, Watts JC, Veneri RJ, Chandler FW. Focal hepatic candidiasis with perihepatic adhesions: laparoscopic and immunohistologic diagnosis. Gastroenterology 1990;98(1):214-7.

36. Eisenberg ES. Intraperitoneal flucytosine in the management of fungal peritonitis in patients on continuous ambulatory peritoneal dialysis. Am J Kidney Dis 1988;11(6):465-7.

37. Cheng IK, Fang GX, Chan TM, Chan PC, Chan MK. Fungal peritonitis complicating peritoneal dialysis: report of 27 cases and review of treatment. Q J Med 1989;71(265):407-16.

38. Baetz-Greenwalt B, Debaz B, Kumar ML. Bladder fungus ball: a reversible cause of neonatal obstructive uropathy. Pediatrics 1988;81(6):826-9.

39. Bartkowski DP, Lanesky JR. Emphysematous prostatitis and cystitis secondary to Candida albicans. J Urol 1988;139(5):1063-5.

40. Swartz DA, Harrington P, Wilcox R. Candidal epididymitis treated with ketoconazole. NEJM 1988;319:1485.

41. Dupont B, Drouhet E. Fluconazole in the management of oropharyngeal candidosis in the predominantly HIV antibody-positive group of patients. J Med Vet Mycol 1988;26(1):67-71.

42. Arrieta Blanco FJ, et al. Efficacy of ketoconazole in the treatment of systemic candidiasis with pulmonary involvement. Rev Clin Esp 1988;182(2):114.

43. Cohen SR, Thompson JW. Otitic candidiasis in children: an evaluation of the problem and effectiveness of ketoconazole in 10 patients. Ann Otol Rhinol Laryngol 1990;99(6):427-31.

44. Colmenero C, Monux A, Valencia E, Castro A. Successfully treated candida sinusitis in an AIDS patient. J Craniomaxillofac Surg 1990 18(4):175-8.

45. Bach MC, Blattner S. Occult Candida thyroid abscess diagnosed by gallium-67 scanning. Clin Nucl Med 1990;15(6):395-9.

46. Isalska BJ, Stanbridge TN. Fluconazole in the treatment of candidal prosthetic valve endocarditis. BMJ 1988;6642:178-9.

47. Freischlag JA, Asbun HA, Sedwitz MM, Hye RJ, Sise M, Stabile BE. Septic peripheral embolization from bacterial and fungal endocarditis. Ann Vas Surg 1989;3(4):318-23.

48. Tanaka M, Abe T, Hosokawa S, Suenaga Y, Hikosaka H. Tricuspid valve Candida endocarditis cured by valve-sparing debridement. Ann Thorac Surg 1989;48(6):857-8.

49. Faix RG, Feick HJ, Frommelt P, Snider AR. Successful medical treatment of Candida parapsilosis endocarditis in a premature infant. Am J Perinatol 1990;7(3):272-5.

50. Kraus WE, Valenstein :N, Corey GR. Purulent pericarditis caused by Candida: report of three cases and identification of high-risk populations as an aid to early diagnosis. Rev Infect Dis 1989;10(1):34-41.

51. Corbett A. Candidiasis-endocrinopathy syndrome with progressive myopathy. Q J Med 1989;70(262):139-44.

52. Baley JE, Silverman RA. Systemic candidiasis: cutaneous manifestations in low birth weight infants. Pediatrics 1988;82(2):211-5.

53. Lindblad R, al-Obaidy A, Mobacken H, Rodjer S. Diagnostically usable skin lesions in Candida septicaemia. Mycoses 1989;32(8):416-20.

54. Bannatyne RM, Clarke HM. Ketoconazole in the treatment of osteomyelitis due to Candida albicans. Can J Surg 1989;32(3):201-2.

55. Piek JJ, Knot EA, Schooneveld MJ, Rietra PJ. Candidemia, look at the eye. Intensive Care Med 1988;14(2):173-5.

56. Despres E, Weber M, Jouart D, Sahel J, Flament J. Candida albicans uveopapillitis. Diagnostic and therapeutic discussion apropos of a case. Bull Soc Ophtalmol Fr 1990;90(1):105-8.

57. Coker SB, Beltran RS. Candida meningitis: clinical and radiographic diagnosis. Ped Neurol 1988;4(5):317-9.

58. Tonami N, Matsuda H, Oba H, Yokoyama K, Hisada K, Ikeda K, Yamashita J. Thallium-201 accumulation in cerebral candidiasis: unexpected finding on SPECT. Clin Nucl Med 1990;15(6):397-400.

59. Martinez GA, Bustillo JM, Garcia Martin C, Marti Cabanes J. Meningitis caused by Candida in a patient with acquired immunodeficiency syndrome. Neurologia 1987;2(5):256-7.

60. Ikeda K, Yamashita J, Fujisawa H, Fujita S. Cerebral granuloma and meningitis caused by Candida albicans: useful monitoring of mannan antigen in cerebrospinal fluid. Neurosurgery 1990;26(5):860-3.

61. Hernandez YL, Daniels TE. Oral candidiasis in Sjogren's syndrome: prevalence, clinical correlations, and treatment. Oral Surg Oral Med Oral Pathol 1989;68(3):324029.

62. Riestra Menendez S, Sleiman Halabi H, Suarez Gonzalez A, Rodrigo Saez L. Esophagitis caused by Candida albican. Rev Esp Enferm Apar Dig 1989;76(2):188-93.

63. Pope LM, Cole GT. Scanning Electron Microscopic Studies of Adherence of Candida-Albicans to the Gastrointestinal Tract of Infant Mice. Scanning Electron Microsc 1981; 3:73-80.

64. Minoli G, Terruzzi V, Ferrara A, et al. A Prospective Study of Relationships between Benign Gastric Ulcer, Candida, and Medical Treatment. Am J Gastroenterol 1984; 79/2:95-97.

65. Boero M, Pera A, Andriulli A, et al. Candida Overgrowth in Gastric Juice of Peptic Ulcer Subjects on Short and Long Term Treatment with Hsub 2-Receptor Antagonists. Digestion (Switzerland) 1983; 28/3:158-63.

66. Gotlieb JK, Andersen J. Occurrence of Candida in Gastric Ulcers. Significance for the Healing Process. Gastroenterology (USA) 1983; 85/3:535-37.

67. Triger DR, Goepel JR, Slater DN, Underwood JCE. Systemic Candidiasis Complicating Acute Hepatic Failure in Patients Treated with Cimetidine. Lancet 1981; 2/8251:837-38.

68. Dismukes WE, Wade JS, Lee JY, Dockery BK, Hain JD. A randomized, double-blind trial of nystatin therapy for the candidiasis hypersensitivity syndrome. NEJM 1990;323:1717-23.

69. Yasumoto R, Asakawa M, Umeda M, Tanaka S, Tsurusaki K, Mori K, Kakinoki K, Kawashima H. Clinical efficacy of flucytosine on urinary candidiasis. Hinyokika Kiyo 1988;34(9):1679-82.

70. Bagnolesi P, Camerini E, Romagnoli C, Vignali C, Medi F. Candidiasis of the kidney pelvis: importance of the urography/echography correlation. Radiol Med 1988;76(6):649-52.

71. Cohen HL, Haller JO. Unknown case 2: neonatal candidal pyonephrosis with an associated iatrogenic perirenal collection. J Ultrasound Med 1988;7(11):747-8.

72. Nielsen NS, Nepper-Rasmussen HJ, Hojhus J. Renal candida infections. Diagnosis by ultrasonography. ROFO 1988;149(4):417-9.

73. Bartone FF, Hurwitz RS, Rojas EL, Steinberg E, Franceschini R. The role of percutaneous nephrostomy in the management of obstructing candidiasis of the urinary tract in infants. J Urol 1988;140(2):338-41.

74. Gooding GA. Sonography of Candida albicans cystitis. J Ultrasound Med 1989;8(3):121-4.

75. Nito H. Clinical efficacy of fluconazole in urinary tract fungal infections. Jpn J Antibiot 1989;42(1):171-8.

76. Rajasingham KC, Challacombe SJ, Tovey S. Ultrastructure and possible processes involved in the invasion of host epithelial cells by Candida albicans in vaginal candidosis. Cytobios 1989;60(240):11-20.

77. Bennett JE. Candidiasis. In: Isselbacher KJ, Adams RD, Braunwald E, Petersdorf RG, Wison JD, eds. Harrison's Principles of Internal Medicine. New York: McGraw Hill, 1980:741-2.

78. Simonetti N, Strippoli V. Pathogenicity of the Y form as compared to M form in experimentally induced Candida albicans infections. Mycopathology and Mycology 1975;51(1):19-28.

79. Barlow AJE, Aldersley T, Chattaway FW. Factors present in serum and seminal plasma which promote germ-tube formation and mycelial growth of Candida albicans. J Gen Microbiology 1974;82:261-72.

80. Donaldson RM. Normal bacterial populations of the intestine and their relation to intestinal function. NEJM 1964; 270:938-45.

81. Vincent JG, Veomett RC, Riley RF. Antibacterial activity associated with Lactobacillus acidophilus. J Bact 1959; 78:477-84.

82. Kennedy MJ, Volz PA. Ecology of Candida albicans gut colonization: inhibition of Candida adhesion, colonization, and dissemination from the gastrointestinal tract by bacterial antagonism. Infect Immun Sep 1985; 49:654-63.

83. Haenel H. Human normal and abnormal gastrointestinal Flora. Am J Clin Nutr 1970; 23:1433-39.

84. Geertinger P, Bodenhoff J, Helweg-Larsen H, Lund A. Endogenous alcohol production by intestinal fermentation in sudden infant death. Z Rechtsmed 1982; 89:167-72.

85. Van Niel CB, Cohen AL. On the metabolism of Candida albicans. J Cell Comp Physiol 1942; 20:95-112.

86. Purohit BC, Joshi KR, Ramdeo IN, Bharadwaj TP. The formation of germtubes by Candida albicans, when grown with Staphylococcus pyogene, Escherichia coli, Klebsiella pneumonia, Lactobacillus acidophilus, and Proteus vulgaris. Mycopathologia 1977; 62:188.

87. Miller JA. Oral ecology: a matter of attachment. Science News June 21, 1986; 129:397.

88. Danley DL, Hilger AE, Winkel CA. Generation of hydrogen peroxide by Candida-albicans and influence on murine polymorphonuclear leukocyte activity. Infect Immun 1983; 40:97-102.

89. Friend BA, Shahani KM, Mathur BN. Newer Advances in Human Milk Substitutes for Infant Feeding. J Applied Nutr 1983; 35:88-115.

90. Haenel H. Human Normal and Abnormal Gastrointestinal Flora. Am J Clin Nutr 1970; 23:1433-39.

91. Wong J. Cancer and chemicals...and vegetables. Chemtech Feb. 1986; pp.100-107.

92. Bilsing L. Use nature's methods to control pests. Environ Fall 1985; 2:8-9.

93. Schmidt GL. Garlic: more than just a taste. Food Tech in New Zealand March, 1973; pp.13-15.

94. Raghunandana RS, Srinivasa R, Venkataraman PR. Investigations on plant antibiotics. J Sci Indus Res, August 1946; 1B:31-35.

95. Cavallito CJ, Bailey JH. Allicin, the antibacterial principle of Allium Sativum. 1. Isolation, physical properties, and antibacterial action. J Chem Soc 1944; 66:1950-51.

96. Bruggeman IM, Temmink JHM, Van Bladeren PJ. Glutathione- and Cysteine-mediated cytotoxicity of allyl and benzyl isothiocyanate. Toxicology & Applied Pharmacology 1986; 83:349-59.

97. Appleton JA, Tansey MR. Inhibition of growth of zoopathogenic fungi by garlic extract. Mycologia 1975; 67:882-85.

98. Barone FE, Tansey MR. Isolation, purification, identification, synthesis, and kinetics or activity of the anticandidal component of Allium sativum, and a hypothesis for its mode of action. Mycologia 1977; 69:793-825.

99. Yamada Y, Azuma K. Evaluation of the in vitro antifungal activity of allicin. Antimicrob Agents & Chemother Apr 1977; pp. 743-49.

100. Hasilik A. Perturbation of growth and metabolism in Candida albicans by 4-bromobenzyl isothiocyanate and iodoacetate. Naturforsch Jan-Feb 1973; 28:21-31.

101. Hrmova M, Sturdik E, Kosik M, Gemeiner P, Petrus L. Growth of Candida albicans on artificial D-glucose derivatives. Z Allg Mikrobiol 1983;23(5):303-12.

102. Li Y, Wei M, Tong S, Tian G. Optimum glucose content in culture media used for the detection of bacteria and molds. Yaowu Fenxi Zazhi 1983;3(3):141-6.

103. Samaranayake LP, Mac Farlane RW. The effect of dietary carbohydrates on the in vitro adhesion of Candida albicans to epithelial cells. J Med Microbiol 1982;1594):511-17.

104. Samaranayake LP, Geddes DAM, Weetman DA, MacFarlane RW. Growth and acid production of Candida albicans in carbohydrate supplemented media. Microbios 1983;37(148):105-15.

105. McClary DO. Factors affecting the morphology of Candida albicans. Ann Missouri Botan Garden 1952;39:137-64.

106. Barlow AJE, Aldersley T, Chattaway FW. Factors present in serum and seminal plasma which promote germ-tube formation and mycelial growth of Candida albican. J Gen Microbiology 1974;82:271.

107. Spellacy WN, Carlson KL. Plasma insulin and blood glucose levels in patients taking oral contraceptives. American Journal of Obstetrics and Gynecology 1965;95:474-8.

108. Walsh H, Hildebrandt RJ, Prystowsky H. Oral progestational agents as a cause of Candida vaginitis. American Journal of Obstetrics and Gynecology 1968;101:991-3.

109. Hesseltine HC. Nature of moniliasis (vulvar and vaginal). Rept Proc 3rd Intern Congr Microbiol 1939;518-9(1940)

110. Douglas LJ, Houston JG, McCourtie J. Adherence of Candida albicans to human buccal epithelial cells after growth on different carbon sources. FEMS Microbiol Lett 1981;12(3):241-3.

111. McCourtie J, Douglas LJ. Relationship between cell surface composition, adherence, and virulence of Candida albicans. Infect Immun 1984;45(1):6-12.

112. Pereira HA, Hoskins CS. The role of complement and antibody in opsonization and intracellular killing of Candida albicans. Clin Exp Immun Aug 1984; 57:307-14.

113. Nielsen H, Rorth M. Phagocytosis and killing of Candida albicans by blood monocytes from patients with non-seminomatous testicular carcinoma: effect of chemotherapy. Acta Pathol Microbiol Immun Scand Apr 1985; 93:85-89.

114. Baccarini M, Bistoni F, Lohmann-Matthes ML. In vitro natural cell-mediated cytotoxicity against Candida albicans: macrophage precursors as effector cells. J Immun Apr 1985; 134:2658-65.

115. Baccarini M, Vecchiarelli A, et al. Killing of yeast, germ-tube and mycelial forms of Candida albicans by murine effectors as measured by a radiolabel release microassay. J Gen Microbiol Mar 1985; 131:505-13.

116. Stiehm ER, Neumann CG, Swendseid ME, Lawlor GJ, Ferguson AC. Humoral and cellular aspects of immunity in malnutrition. Food and Immunology, Proceedings of a Symposium of the Swedish Medical Research Council, edited by Hambraeus L. Hanson LA. and McFarlane H, Almqvist and Wiksell International, Stockholm, 1977; pp. 69-85.

117. Neumann CG, Stiehm ER, Swendseid M. Immunoglobulin levels in Ghanaian children with protein-calorie malnutrition. Malnutrition and the Immune Response, edited by Suskind RM. New York, NY: Raven Press, 1977; pp.191-94.

118. Stiehm ER. Humoral immunity in malnutrition. Federation Proc. 1980; 39:3093-97.

119. Robbins SL. Infectious diseases. Textbook of Pathology with Clinical Application. Philadelphia, PA: W.B. Saunders Co., 1962; pp. 318.

120. Das M, Stiehm ER, Borut R, Feig SA. Metabolic correlates of immune dysfunction in malnourished children. Am J Clin Nutr 1977; 61:1949-52.

121. Zaikina NA. Trials of the new antifungal antibiotic 26/1 in the Candida carrier state in white mice. Inst Antibiotikov 1960;2:296-9.

122. Rogers TJ, Adams-Burton K, Mallon M, Hafdahl B, Rivas V, Donnelly R, O'Day K. Dietary ascorbic acid and resistance to experimental renal candidiasis. J Nutr 1983;113(1);178-83.

123. Kokushina TM. Effect of antibiotics and vitamin and hormone balance disorders on development of candidosis immunity. Leningr Inst Usoversh Vrachei 1964;41:102-6.

124. Paine Jr. TF. In vitro experiments with Monilia and Escherichia coli to explain moniliasis in patients receiving antibiotics. Antibiotics and Chemotherapy 1952;2:653-8.

125. Guentzel NG, Herrera C. Effects of compromising agents on candidosis in mice with persistent infections initiated in infancy. Infect & Immunity Jan 1982; pp. 222-28.

126. Kligman AM. Are fungus infections increasing as a result of antibiotic therapy? JAMA July 12, 1952; 149:979-83.

127. Huppert M, MacPherson DA, Cazin J. Pathogenesis of Candida albicans infection following antibiotic therapy. J of Bacteriology Feb 1953; pp. 171-76.

128. Martin E. Once-daily administration of ceftriaxone in the treatment of meningitis and other serious infections in children. Eur J Clin Microbiol Oct 1983; 2:509-15

129. Muth L, Eden T. High-dose tobramycin combined with clindamycin or lincomycin in the treatment of septic peritonitis and intraabdominal sepsis. Acta Chir Scand 1981; 147:339-46.

130. Brajtburg J, Elberg S, et al. Increase in colony-forming units of Candida albicans after treatment with polyene antibiotics. Antimicrob Agents Chemother Jan 1981; 19:199-200.

131. Gram HG. Antibiotics as a source of nitrogen for Candida albicans. Zentr Bakteriol Parasitenk, Abt I, Orig 1956;166:199-205.

132. Kesten S, Hyland RH, Pruzanski WR, Kortan PP. Esophageal candidiasis associated with beclomethasone dipropionate aerosol therapy. Drug Intell Clin Pharm 1988;22(7-8):568-9.

133. Nishikawa F. Effects of cortisone acetate on oral inoculation with Candida albicans in germ-free mice. Keio J Med 1969;18(1):47056.

134. Lourin DB, Fallon N, Browne HG. The influence of cortisone on experimental fungus infections in mice. J Clin Invest 1960;39:1435-49.

135. DeMaria A, Buckley H, Von Lichtenberg F. Gastrointestinal candidiasis in rats treated with antibiotics, cortisone, and azathioprine. Infect Immun 1976;13(6):1761-70.

136. Seligmann E. Virulence enhancement of Candida albicans by antibiotics and cortisone. Proc Soc Exp Biol Med 1953;83:778-81.

137. Henry B, Fahlberg WJ. The potentiating effect of hydrocortisone acetate and tetracycline on monilial infection in mice. Antibiotics and Chemotherapy 1960;10:114-20.

138. Samonis G, Anaissie EJ, Rosenbaum B, Bodey GP. A model of sustained gastrointestinal colonization by Candida albicans in healthy adult mice. Infect Immun 1990;58(6):1514-7.

139. Samonis G, Anaissie EJ, Rosenbaum B, Bodney GP. A model of sustained gastrointestinal colonization by Candida albicans in healthy adult mice. Infect Immun 1990;58(6):1514-7.

140. Figus IA, Papp I, Vitez A, Bajtai A. Esophageal and gastric candidiasis. Orv Hetil 1990;131(6):279-81.

141. Singh S, Kochhar R, Dutta U. Severe duodenal candidiasis in a patient with IgA deficiency and T cell defects. Indian J Gastroenterol 1990;Jan 15 (1):95-6.

142. Kochhar R, Talwar P, Singh S, Metha SK. Invasive candidiasis following cimetidine therapy. Am J Gastroenterol 1988;83(1)102-3.

143. McGroarty JA, Soboh F, Bruce AW, Reid G. The spermicidal compound nonoxynol-9 increases adhesion of Candida species to human epithelial cells in vitro. Infect Immun 1990:58(6):2005-7.

144. Eastman NJ. Hellman LM. Williams Obstetrics, 13th edition, New York, NY: Appleton-Century-Crofts, 1966; pp. 334.

145. Moors MA, Jones SM, Klyczek KK, Rogers TJ, Buckley HR, Blank KJ. Effect of Friend leukemia virus infection on susceptibility to Candida albicans. Infect Immun 1990:58(6):1796-801.

146. Douglas LJ. Adhesion of Candida species to epithelial cells. In: CRC Critical Rev in Microb. M.O. Leavy Leary, ED., CRC Press, Inc;, Boca Raton, Fl.1987;15:27-43.

147. Rotrosen D, Calderone R, Edwards Jr. JE. Adherence of Candida sp. to host tissues and plastic surfaces. Rev Infect Dis. 1986;8:73.

148. Lee JD, King RD. Characterization of Candida albicans adherence to human vaginal epithelial cells in vitro. Infect Immun 1983;41:1024.

149. McCourtie J, Douglas LJ. Relationship between cell surface composition, adherence and virulence of Candida albicans. Infect Immun 1984;45:6.

150. Calderone RA, Cihlar R, Lee D, Hoberg K, Scheld WM. Yeast adherence in the pathogenesis of Candida albicans endocarditis: studies with adherence-negative mutants. J Infect Dis;1985;710.

151. Kwon-Chung KJ, Lehman D, Good C, Magee PT. Genetic evidence for role of extracellular proteinase in virulence of Candida albican. Infect Immun 1985;49:571.

152. Borg M, Ruchel R. Expression of extracellular acid proteinase by proteolytic Candida sp. during experimental infection of oral mucosa. Infect Immun 1988;56:626.

153. Slutsky B, Buffo J, Soll DR. High-frequency switching of colony morphology in Candida albican. Science 1985;230:666.

154. Soll DR, Langtimm CJ, McDowell J, Hicks J, Galask R. High-frequency switching in Candida strains isolated from vaginitis patients. J Clin Microbiol 1987;25:1611.

155. Soll DR, Staebell M, Langtimm C, Pfaller M, Hicks J, Gopala Rao TV. Multiple Candida strains in the course of a single systemic infection. J Clin Microbiol 1988;26:1448.

156. Edwards Jr. JE, Gaither T, Shea JO, Rotrosen JD, Lawley T, Wright S, Frank MM, Green I. Expression of specific binding sites on Candida with functional and antigenic characteristics of human complement receptors. J Immun 1986;137:3577.

157. Gilmore BJ, Retsinas E, Lorenz J, Hostetter M. An iC3b receptor on Candida albicans: structure, function and correlates for pathogenicity. J Infect Dis 1988;157:38.

158. Eigentler A, Schulz TF, Larcher C, Breitwieser E, Myones BL, Petzer A, Dierich M. C3bi binding protein in Candida albicans: temperature-dependent expression and relationship to human complement receptor Type 3. Infect Immun 1989;57:616.

159. Yamabayashi H. Zymosanlike substance extracted from Candida albicans. Med J Osake Univ 1958;9:11-21.

160. Lingappa BT, Prasad M, et al. Phenethyl alcohol and tryptophol: autoantibiotics produced by the fungus, Candida albicans. Science 1969; 163:192-94.

161. Nosal R, Menyhardtova Z, Nosalova V. Pharmacological effect of glycoprotein from Candida albicans. Zb Pr Ustavu Exp Farmakol SAV 1978; 1:207-15.

162. Jeffries GH. Diseases of the hepatic system. Cecil-Loeb Textbook of Med 13th edition. Philadelphia, PA: W.B. Saunders Company, 1971; pp. 1404.

163. Weber D. Personal communication. 1985.

164. Burge H. Bioaerosols: prevalence and health effects in the indoor environment. J Allergy Clin Immun 1990;86:687-701.

165. Iwata K. A review of the literature on drunken symptoms due to yeasts in the gastrointestinal tract. Proceedings of the Second International Specialized Symposium on Yeasts. Univ. Tokyo Press 1972; pp.. 260-68.

166. Zwerling MH, Owens KN, Ruth NH. "Think yeast" - the expanding spectrum of candidiasis. J So Carolina Med Assoc Sept 1984; pp.454-56.

167. Van Niel CB, Cohen AL. On the metabolism of Candida albicans. J Cell Bio 1942; 20:95-112.

168. Truss OC. Metabolic abnormalities in patients with chronic candidiasis. J Orthomolecular Psychiatry 1984; 13:70.

169. Chattaway FW, Odds FC, Barlow AJE. Production of hydrolytic enzymes and toxins by pathogenic strains of Candida albicans. J Gen Microbiol 1971; 67:255-63.

170. Cutler JE, Friedman L, Milner KC. Biological and chemical characterization of toxic substances from Candida albicans. Infec Immunity 1972; 6:616-27.

171. Iwata K, Uchida K. Canditoxin, a new toxic substance isolated from Candida albicans. III. Repurification of the toxic substance and physicochemical properties of the purified fraction. Igaku To Seibitsugaku 1967; 75:192-95.

172. Iwata K. Toxins produced by Candida albicans. Contrib Microbiol Immun 1976 (Pub 1977); pp. 77-85.

173. Yamamoto, Y, Iwata K. Studies of glycoprotein toxins produced by a Candida albicans strain. 1. Purification procedures and physicochemical properties. Shinkin to Shinkinsho 1980; 21:264-73.

174. Balonova T, Vrbovsky L, et al. Embryotoxic effects of orally administered glycoprotein isolated from Candida albicans in rats. Eval Embryotoxic Mutagen Carcinog Risks New Drugs, Proc Symp Toxicol Test Saf New Drugs, 3rd 1976 (Pub 1979); pp. 91-4.

175. Yamamoto Y, Iwata K. Studies of glycoprotein toxins produced by a Candida albicans strain. 2. Limulus amebocyte lysate-gelling activity of one of the toxins and the cellular mannan isolated from the same strain. Shinkin to Shinkinsho 1980; 21:274-85.

176. Iwata K, Yamamoto Y. Glycoprotein toxins produced by Candida albicans. Sci Pub - Pan Am Health Organ 1977 (Pub 1978) 356 (Proc Int Conf Mycoses, 4th); pp. 246-57.

177. Balanova T, Vrbovsky L, Ujhazy E, Sikl D. Embryotoxic effects of orally administered glycoprotein isolated from Candida albicans in rats. Eval Embryotoxic Mutagen Carcinog Risks New Drugs, Proc Symp Toxicol Test Saf New Drugs, 3rd. 1976 (Pub 1979):91-4.

178. Trnovec T, Gajdosikova A, Greguskova M. Induction of pentylenetetrazol convulsions by polysaccharide-protein complex isolated from Candida albicans. Exp Mol Pathol 1980;33(3):251-8.
179. Ito K, Tanaka T. Formation of amine by pathogenic fungi. Formation of tyramine from N-acetyltyramine by pathogenic fungi. Bull Pharm Res Inst, Osaka 1973; 100:1-11.
180. Iwata K, Uchida K. Canditoxin, a new toxic substance isolated from a strain of Candida albicans. V. Enzymic activity, with special reference to phosphatase. Igaku To Seibutsugaku 1968; 77:159-64.
181. Uchida K, Iwata K. Canditoxin, a new toxic substance isolated from a strain of Candida albicans. VII. Properties of the intracellular alkaline phosphatase. Igaku To Seibutsugaku 1968; 77:171-74
182. Vrbovsky L, Ujhazy E, et al. Embryotoxic effects of intravenously administered glycoprotein isolated from Candida albicans in mice. Eval Embryotoxic Mutagen Carcinog Risks New Drugs, Proc Symp Toxicol Test Saf New Drugs, 3rd 1976 (Pub 1979); pp. 83-9.
183. Iwata K, Uchida K, et al. Studies on the toxins produced by Candida albicans with special reference to their etiopathological role. Yeasts Yeast-like Microorg Med Sci Proc Int Spec Symp Yeasts, 2nd 1972 (Pub 1976); p. 184-90.
184. Cutler JE. Toxic substances in Candida albicans. New Orleans, LA: Tulane Univ, 1972; pp. 1-87.
185. Masler L, Sikl D, et al. Extracellular polysaccharide-protein complexes produced by Candida albicans. Folia Microbiol 1966; 11:373-78.
186. Kobayashi I, Kondoh Y, Shimizu K, Takana K. A role of secreted proteinase of Candida albicans for the invasion of chick chorio-allantoic membrane. Microbiol Immun 1989;33(9):709-17.
187. de Bernardis F, Morelli L, Ceddia T, Lorenzini R, Cassone A. Experimental pathogenicity and acid proteinase secretion of vaginal isolates of Candida parapsilosis. J Med Vet Mycol 1990;28(2):-125-37.
188. Calderone RA. Host-parasite relationships in candidosis. Mycoses 1989;32 Suppl 2:12-7.
189. Chia JK, Clark JB, Ryan CA, Pollack, M. Botulism in an adult associated with food-borne intestinal infection with Clostridium botulinum. NEJM 1986; 315:239-41.
190. Bartlett JC. Infant botulism in adults. NEJM 1986; 315:254-55.
191. Kemp DR, Gin D. Bowel-associated dermatosis-arthritis syndrome. Med J Aust 1990;152(1-):43-5.
192. Haggerty RJ. Diseases due to chemical factors: common accidental poisoning. Cecil - Loeb Textbook of Medicine. 13th edition. Philadelphia, PA: W.B. Saunders Co., 1971; pp 66.
193. Silverman JJ, Hart RP, et al. Posttraumatic stress disorder from pentaborane intoxication. JAMA 1985; 254:2603-08.
194. Yarborough BE, Garrettson LK, et al. Severe central nervous system damage and profound acidosis in persons exposed to pentaborane. Clin Toxicol 1985; 7:23.
195. Carlson E. Synergistic Effect of Candida Albicans and Staphylococcus Aureus on Mouse Mortality. Infect Immun 1982; 38:921-24.
196. Carlson E. Enhancement by Candida Albicans of Staphylococcus Aureus, Serratia Marcescens, and Streptococcus Faecalis in the Establishment of Infection in the Mouse. Infect Immun 1983; 39:193-97.
197. Carlson E. Effect of Strain of Staphylococcus Aureus on Synergism with Candida Albicans Resulting in Mouse Mortality and Morbidity. Infect Immun 1983; 42:285-92.
198. Yamamoto Y, Iwata K. Studies on glycoprotein toxins produced by a Candida albicans strain. IV. The effects on peripheral blood lymphocytes. Shinkin to Shinkinsho 1981; 22:304-13.
199. Yamamoto Y, Iwata K. Biological activities of glycoproteins produced by Candida albicans. Shinkin to Shinkinsho 1983; 24:76-82.
200. Cutler JE, Friedman L, Milner, KC. Biological and chemical characterization of toxic substances from Candida albicans. Infec Immunity 1972; 6:616-27.

201. Witkin SS. Defective Immune Responses in Patients with Recurrent Candidiasis. Infections in Med May/June 1985; 129-32.

202. Lee KW, Balish E. Effect of T-Cells and Intestinal Bacteria on Resistance of Mice to Candidosis. J Reticuloendothelial Soc 1982; 31:233-40.

203. Bartizal KF, Salkowski C, Balish E. The Influence of a Gastrointestinal Microflora on Natural Killer Cell Activity. J Reticuloendothelial Soc 1983; 33:381-90.

204. Hilger AE, Danley DL. Alteration of polymorphonuclear leukocyte activity by viable Candida-albicans yeast cells. Abstr Ann Meet Am Soc Microbiol 1979; 79:368.

205. Danley DL, Polakoff J. Rapid killing of monocytes in vitro by Candida albicans yeast cells. Infect Immun Jan 1986; 51:307-13.

206. Barnaba V, Zaccari C, et al. Suppressor T cells role in the unresponsiveness to Candida albicans in chronic mucocutaneous candidiasis. Boll Ist Sieroter Milan 1985; 64:126-30.

207. Mikhno IL, Barshtein YA. Experimental mixed infection with Candida and staphylococcal cultures. Mikrobiol 1976; 38:188-96.

208. Yamamoto Y, Iwata K. Studies on glycoprotein toxins produced by a Candida albicans strain. 111. Their effects on complement and peripheral leukocytes. Shinkin to Shinkinsho 1981;22(3):223-33.

209. Iwata K, Uchida K. Cellular immunity in experimental fungus infections in mice: the influence of infections and treatment with a candida toxin on spleen lymphoid cells. Mykosen Sullp 1978;1:72-81.

210. Lombardi G, Di Massimo AM, Del Gallo F, Vismara D, Piccolella E, Pugliese O, Colizzi V. Mechanism of action of an antigen nonspecific inhibitory factor produced by human T cells stimulated by MPPS and PPD. Cell Immun 1986;98(2):434-43.

211. Budtz-Joergensen E. Inhibition of leukocyte migration by the agarose plate technique. Application to antigen from Candida albicans and Fusobacterium nucleatum. Acta Allergol 1977;32(1):15-26.

212. Kototila MP, Rogers AL, Beneke ES, Smith CW. The effects of soluble Saccharomyces cerevisiae mannan on the phagocytosis of Candida albicans by mouse peritoneal macrophages in vitro. J Med Vet Mycol 1987;25:85.

213. Sung S-S, Nelson RS, Silverstein SC. Yeast mannans inhibit binding and phagocytosis of zymosan by mouse peritoneal macrophages. J Cell Biol 1983;96:160.

214. Speert DP, Silverstein SC. Phagocytosis of unopsonized zymosan by human monocyte-derived macrophages: maturation and inhibition by mannan. J Leuk Biol. 1985;38:655.

215. Salvin SB, Cheng S-L. Lymphoid cells in delayed hypersensitivity. II. In vitro phagocytosis and cellular immunity. Infec Immunity 1971;3(4):548-52.

216. Diamond RD, Oppenheim F, Nakagawa Y, Krzesicki R, Haudenschild CC. Properties of a product of Candida albicans hyphae and pseudohyphae that inhibits contact between the fungi and human neutrophils in vitro. J Immun 1980;125(6):2797-804.

217. Diamond RD, Krzesicki R, Nakagawa Y, Oppenheim F. Characterization of a product of Candida albicans hyphae which inhibits contact between hyphae and neutrophils. Excerpta Med 1980;480:233-6.

218. Rogers TJ, Balish E. Effect of a systemic candidiasis on blastogenesis of lymphocytes from germfree and conventional rats. Infect Immun 1978;20(1):142-50.

219. Yamamoto Y, Iwata K. Studies on glycoprotein toxins produced by a Candida albicans strain. IV. The effects on peripheral blood lymphocytes. Shinkin to Shinkinsho 1981;22(4):304-13.

220. LaForce FM, Mills DM, Iverson K, Cousins R, Everett ED. Inhibition of leukocyte candidacidal activity by serum from patients with disseminated candidiasis. J Lab Clin Med 1975;86:657.

221. Verhaegen H, DeCock W, DeCree J. In vitro phagocytosis of Candida albicans by peripheral polymorphonuclear neutrophils of patients with recurrent infections. Case reports of serum-dependent abnormalities. Biomedicine 1976;24:164.

222. Cates KL, Grady PG, Shapira E, Davis AT. Cell-directed inhibition of polymorphonuclear leukocyte chemotaxis in a patient with mucocutaneous candidiasis. J Allergy Clin Immun 1980;65:431.
223. Walker SM, Urbaniak SJ. A serum-dependent defect of neutrophil function in chronic mucocutaneous candidiasis. J Clin Pathol 1980;33:370.
224. Kennedy CRC, Valdlmarsson H, Hay RJ. Chronic mucocutaneous candidiasis with a serum-dependent neutrophil defect: response to ketoconazole. J R Soc Med 1981;74:158.
225. Wright CD, Herron, MJ, Gray GR, Holmes B, Nelson RD. Influence of yeast mannan on human neutrophil functions: inhibition of release of myeloperoxidase related to carbohydrate-binding property of the enzyme. Infect Immun 1981;32:731.
226. Wright CD, Bowie JU, Nelson RD. Influence of yeast mannan in release of myeloperoxidase by human neutrophils: determination of structural features of mannan required for formation of myeloperoxidase-mannan-neutrophil complexes. Infect Immun 1984;43:467.
227. Rest RF, Farrell CF, Naids FL. Mannose inhibits the human neutrophil oxidative burst. J Leuk Biol 1988;43:158.
228. Hajime Y. Zymosanlike substance extracted from Candida albicans. J Osaka Univ 1958;9:11-21.
229. Durandy A, Fischer A, LeDeist F, Drouhet E, Griscelli C. Mannan-specific and mannan-induced T-cell suppressive activity in patients with chronic mucocutaneous candidiasis. J Clin Immun 1987;7:400.
230. Lombardi B, Di Massimo AM, Del Gallo F, Vismara D, Piccolella E, Pugliese O, Colizzi V. Mechanism of action of an antigen stimulated by MPPS and PPD. Cell Immunol 1986;98(2):434-43.
231. Witkin SS, Yu I-R, Ledger WJ. Inhibition of Candida albicans-induced lymphocyte proliferation by lymphocytes and sera from women with recurrent vaginitis. Am J Obstet Gynecol 1968;147:809.
232. Fischer A, Ballet J-J, Griscelli C. Specific inhibition of in vitro Candida-induced lymphocyte proliferation by polysaccharide antigens present in the serum of patients with chronic mucocutaneous candidiasis. J Clin Invest 1978;62:1005-13.
233. Nelson RD, Herron MF, McCormack JR, et al. Two mechanisms of inhibition of human lymphocyte proliferation by soluble yeast mannan polysaccharide. Infect Immun 1984;43:1041-6.
234. Podzorski RP, Herron MJ, Fast DJ, Nelson RD. Pathogenesis of Candidiasis. Arch Surg 1989;124:1290-4.
235. Wright CD, Bowie JU, Gray GR, Nelson RD. Candidacidal activity of myeloperoxidase: mechanisms of inhibitory influence of soluble cell mannan. Infections and Immunity 1983;42(1):76-80.
236. Hobbs JR, Brigden D, Davidson R, et al. Immunological aspects of candidal vaginitis. Proc Roy Soc Med 1977;70:11-14.
237. Theofilopoulos AN, Dixon FJ. The biology and detection of immune complexes. Adv Immun 1979;28:89-220.
238. Canales L, Middleman RO 111, Louro JM, South MA. Immunological observations in chronic mucocutaneous candidiasis. Lancet 1969;2:567.
239. Twomey J, Waddell CC, Krantz S, O'Reilly R, L'Esperance P, Good RA. Chronic mucocutaneous candidiasis with macrophage dysfunction, a plasm inhibitor, and co-existent aplastic anemia. J Lab Clin Med 1975;85:968.
240. Witkin SS. Defective immune responses in patients with recurrent candidiasis. Infections in Medicine May/June 1985:129-32.
241. Rogers TJ, Balish E. Immunity to Candida albicans. Microb Rev 1980;44:660-82.
242. Kirkpatrick CH, Rich RR, Bennett MD. Chronic mucocutaneous candidiasis: Model-building in cellular immunity. Ann Intern Med 1971;74:955-78.
243. Kirkpatrick CH, Soble PG. Chronic mucocutaneous candidiasis. in Nahmias AJ, O'Reilly RJ. eds: Immunology of Human Infection. Part 1. New York, Plenum. 1981:495-514.

244. Ahonen P, Myllarniemi S, Sipila I, Perheentupa J. Clinical variation of autoimmune polyendocrinopathy-candidiasis-ectodermal dystrophy (APECED). NEJM 1990;322:829-36.
245. Saifer PL, Becker N. Allergy and autoimmune endocrinopathy: APICH syndrome. In: Brostoff J, Challacombe SJ, eds. Food Allergy and Intolerance. Philadelphia, W.B. Saunders. 1987:781-93.
246. Dolen J, Varma SK, South MA. Conversations on allergy and immunology: Chronic mucocutaneous candidiasis-endocrinopathies. CUTIS 1981;28(6):592-64.
247. Appelboom TM, Flowers FP. Ketoconazole in the treatment of chronic mucocutaneous candidiasis secondary to autoimmune polyendocrinopathy-candidiasis syndrome. CUTIS 1982;30:71-2.
248. Peterson PY, Semo R, Blumenschein G, et al. Mucocutaneous candidiasis, anergy and a plasma inhibitor of cellular immunity: reversal after amphotericin B therapy. Clin Exp Immun 1971;9:595-602.
249. Kirkpatrick CH. Mitogen and antigen-induced lymphocyte responses in patients with infections diseases. In: Oppenheim JJ, Rosenstreich, eds. Mitogens in Immunobiology. New York, Academic Press. 1976:639-65.
250. Fischer A, Ballet J-J, Griscelli C. Specific inhibition of in vitro Candida-induced lymphocyte proliferation by polysaccharide antigens present in the serum of patients with mucocutaneous candidiasis. J Clin Invest 1978;62:1005-13.
251. Mathur S, Melchers 111 JT, Ades EW, Williamson HO, Fudenberg HH. Anti-ovarian and anti-lymphocyte antibodies in patients with chronic vaginal candidiasis. J Reproductive Immun 1980;2:247-62.
252. Kirkpatrick Ch, Rich RR, Smith TK. Effect of transfer factor on lymphocyte function in anergic patients. J Clin Invest. 1972;51:2948-58.
253. Schulkind ML, Adler WH, Altemeier WE, et al. Transfer factor in the treatment of a case of chronic mucocutaneous candidiasis. Cell Immun 1972;3:606-15.
254. Sokolova GA, Karaev ZO, Silnitskii PA, Sardyuko NV, Ivanova LA. Functional characteristics of the endocrine and immune systems in patients with visceral candidiasis. Ter Arkh 1989;61(11):81-5.
255. Miller C. Chemical Susceptibility and "Candida Albicans." Human Ecologist 1980; 3-11.
256. Candida Albicans - Yeast Growth and Chemical Sensitivity. Human Ecology Found Quarterly Fall 1980; 3:6-7.
257. Cheung G, Heuser B, Raxien B, Wojdani A. Concomitant increase of delayed onset food sensitivity with acute candidiasis. 1985 Annual Meeting of AAOA Atlanta.
258. Svec P. Mechanism of action of glycoprotein from Candida albicans. J Hyg Epidemiol Microbiol Immun 1974; 18:373-76.
259. Yamamoto Y, Iwata K. Biological activities of glycoproteins produced by Candida albicans. Shinkin to Shinkinsho 1983; 24:76-82.
260. Nosal R. Release of histamine from isolated rat adipose cells as a result of their treatment with a glycoprotein from Candida albicans in vitro. Zh Gig Epidemiol Mikrobiol Immun 1974; 18:372-73.
261. Nosal R. Histamine release from isolated rat mast cells due to glycoprotein from Candida albicans in vitro. J Hyg Epidemiol Microbiol Immun 1974; 18:377-78.
262. Rea WJ. Presentation to the Third Annual International Symposium on Man and His Environment in Health and Disease. Dallas, Texas, 1985.
263. Buisseret PD, Heinzelmann DI, Youlten LJF, Lessor MH. Prostaglandin-synthesis inhibitors in prophylaxis of food intolerance. Lancet Apr 29, 1978; 1:906.
264. Jones VA, Shorthouse M, McLaughlan P, Workman E. Food intolerance: a major factor in the pathogenesis of irritable bowel syndrome. Lancet Nov. 22, 1982; pp. 1115-17.
265. Witkik SS, Hirsch J, Ledger WJ. A macrophage defect in women with recurrent Candida vaginitis and its reversal in vitro by prostaglandin inhibitors. Am J Obstet Gynecol 1986;155:790-5.
266. Liebeskind A. Candida albicans as an allergenic factor. Annals of Allergy. 1962;20:394-6.

267. Antipov EV, Mironova EP. Microflora in the sputum of persons engaged in the production of penicillin and streptomycin. Kazan Med Zh 1976;57(4):396-7.

268. Young G, Krasner RI, Yudkofsky PL. Interactions of oral strains of Candida albicans and lactobacilli. J Bacteriol 1956;72:525-9.

269. Kovak EK. Provocation of systemic mycoses by therapeutic agents. Int Congr Chemother Proc 5th 1967;4:85-8.

270. Raloff J. Roaches: the battle continues. Science News, June 14, 1986;129:379.

271. Antipov EV, Mironova EP. Microflora in the sputum of persons engaged in the production of penicillin and streptomycin. Kazan Med Zh 1976;57(4):396-7.

272. Wilkins TJ. Receptor autoimmunity in endocrine disorders. NEJM 1990;323:1318-24.

273. Johnson JH, Crider BP, McCorkie K, Alford M, Unger RH. Inhibition of glucose transport into rat islet cells by immunoglobulins from patients with new-onset insulin-dependent diabetes. NEJM 1990;322:653-9.

274. Bech K, Larsen JH, Hansen JM, Nerup J. Yersinia enterocolitica infection and thyroid disorders. Lancet 1974;2:951-2.

275. Weiss M, Ingbar S, Winblad S, Kasper DL. Demonstration of a saturable binding site for thyrotropin in Yersinia enterocolitica. Science 1983;219:1331-3.

276. Ingbar SH, Weiss M, Cushing GW, Kasper DL. A possible role for bacterial antigens in the pathogenesis of autoimmune thyroid disease. In: Pinchera A, Ingbar SH, McKenzie JM, Fenzi GR, eds. Thyroid autoimmunity. New York: Plenum Press, 1987:35-44.

277. Neufeld AI, MacLaren NK, Blizzard RM. Autoimmune polyglandular syndromes. Ped Ann 1980;9:154-62.

278. Arulanantham K, Dwyer JM, Genel M. Evidence for defective immunoregulation in the syndrome of familial candidiasis. NEJM 1979;300:164-8.

279. Kendell-Taylor P, Lambert A, Mitchell R, Robertson WR. Antibody that blocks stimulation of cortisol secretion by adrenocorticotrophic hormone in Addison's disease. BMJ 1988;296:1489-91.

280. Whitaker J, Landing BH, Esselborn VM, Williams RR. Syndrome of familial juvenile hypoadrenocorticism, hypoparathyroidism and superficial moniliasis. J Clin Endocrinol 1956;16:1374-87.

281. Wuepper, KD, Fudenberg HH. Moniliasis, 'autoimmune' polyendocrinopathy, and immunologic family study. Clin Exp Immun 1967;2:71.

282. Tomar RH, Lawrence A, Moses AM. Moniliasis and anergy in hypoparathyroidism: treatment with transfer factor. Ann Allergy 1979;42:241.

283. Valdimarsson H, Higgs JM, Wells RS, Yamamura M, Hobbs JR, Holt FJL. Immune abnormalities associated with chronic mucocutaneous candidiasis. Cell Immun 1973;6:348.

284. Irvine WJ, Barnes EW. Addison's diseases, ovarian failure and hypoparathyroidism. Clin Endocrinol Metab 1976;4:379.

285. Horowitz SD, Hong R. Chronic mucocutaneous candidiasis. In the pathogenesis and treatment of immunodeficiency. Monographs in Allergy 1977, vol. 10. Farber, New York.

286. Block MB, Pachman LM, Windhorst D, Goldfine ID. Immunological findings in familial juvenile endocrine deficiency syndrome associated with chronic mucocutaneous candidiasis. Am J Med Sci 1977;261:213.

287. Blizzard RM, Gibbs JH. Candidiasis: studies pertaining to its association with endocrinopathies and pernicious anemia. Ped 1968;42:231.

288. Mathur S, Virella G, Koistinen J, Horger EO.III, Mahvi RA, Fudenberg HH. Humoral immunity in vaginal candidiasis. Infect Immun 1977;15:287.

289. Mathur S, Goust JM, Horger EO.III, Fudenberg HH. Immunoglobulin E anti-Candida antibodies and candidiasis. Infect Immun 1977;18:257.

290. Mathur S, Goust JM, Horger EO.III, Fudenberg HH. Cell-mediated immune deficiency and heightened humoral immune response in vaginal candidiasis. J Clin Lab Immun 1978;1:129.

291. Edwards JE Jr, Gaither T, Shea JO, Rotrosen D, Lawley T, Wright S, Frank MM, Green I. Expression of specific binding sites on Candida with functional and antigenic characteristics of human complement receptors. J Immun 1986;137:3577.

292. Gilmore BJ, Retsinas E, Lorenz J, Hostetter M. An iC3b receptor on Candida albicans: structure, function and correlates for pathogenicity. J Infect Dis 1988;157:38.

293. Mathur S, Melchers JT.III, Ades EW, Williamson HO, Fudenberg HH. Anti-ovarian and anti-lymphocyte antibodies in patients with chronic vaginal candidiasis. Journal of Reproductive Immunology 1980;2:247-62.

294. Stevens LJ, Ballweg ML. The endometriosis-candidiasis link. In: Overcoming Endometriosis: New help from the Endometriosis Association. Congdon and Weed, Inc., New York 1987:198-219.

295. Nagy B, Sutka P, Ziwe-el-Abidine M, Kovacs I, Forgacs V, et al. Candida guilliermondii var. guilliermondii infection in infertile women. Mycoses 1989;32(9):463-8.

296. Vrbovsky L, Ujhazy E, Balonova T, Siki D. Embryotoxic effects of intravenously administered glycoprotein isolated from Candida albicans in mice. Eval Embryotoxic Mutagen Carcinog Risks New Drugs, Proc Symp Toxicol Test Safe New Drugs, 3rd 1976 (Pub 1979):83-9.

297. Kobayashi RH, Rosenblatt HM, et al. Candida esophagitis and laryngitis in chronic mucocutaneous candidiasis. Pediatrics 1980; 66:380-84.

298. Dudley JP, Rosenblatt HM, et al. Candida laryngitis in chronic mucocutaneous candidiasis: its association with Candida esophagitis. Ann Otol Rhinol and Laryngol 1980; 89:574-75.

299. Sanders KM. Role of prostaglandins in regulating gastric motility. Am J Physiol 1984; 247:G117-G126.

300. Levitt MD. Intestinal Gas. Proceedings of the Nutrition Society 1985; 44:145-46.

301. Svec P. Mechanism of action of glycoprotein from Candida albicans. J Hyg Epidemiol Microbiol Immun 1974; 18:373-76.

302. Bensaude RJ. Contribution of proctosigmoidoscopy in colonopathies caused by Candida albicans. Ann Gastroenterol Hepatol Oct-Nov 1984; 20:275-78.

303. Talwar P, Chakrabarte A, Chawla A, Mehta S, Walia BN, Kumar L, Chugh KS. Fungal diarrhoea: association of different fungi and seasonal variation in their incidence. Mycopathologia 1990;110(2):101-5.

304. Atkins FM. The multiple etiology of food hypersensitivity. Nutrition Reviews Aug 1983; 41/8:245-47.

305. Anderson JA. Non-immunologically-mediated food sensitivity. Nutrition Reviews Mar 1984; 42:109-16.

306. Breneman JC. Overview of food allergy: historical perspective. Ann Allergy Aug 1983; 51:220.

307. Kjell AAS. The critical approach to food allergy. Ann Allergy 51:257-59.

308. Friend BA, Shahani KM. Nutritional and therapeutic aspects of Lactobacilli. J of Applied Nutr 1984; 36/2:127-28.

309. Smith RP. The implantation or enrichment of Bacillus acidophilus and other organisms in the intestine. British Med J Nov. 22, 1924; pp. 950.

310. Rutgeerts L, Verhaegen H. Intravenous miconazole in the treatment of chronic esophageal candidiasis. Gastroenterology Feb 1977; 72:316-18

311. Obtulowicz K, Pawlik B, Gluszko P. Myco flora in bronchial asthma. Allergy Immun 1981; 27:28-34.

312. Tsukioka K. Studies on the mechanism developing bronchial asthma due to Candida-albicans. A comparative study of clinical features among Candida induced asthma and house dust induced asthma. Jpn J Allergol 1981; 30:519-530.

313. Okudaira H, Hongo O, Ogita T, et al. Serum immuno globulin E and immuno globulin E antibody levels in patients with bronchial asthma atopic dermatitis eosinophilic granulomas of the soft tissue Kimuras disease and other disease. Ann Allergy 1983; 50:51-54.

314. Tsukioka K. The mechanism developing bronchial asthma due to Candida-albicans in atopic patients with bronchial asthma. Jpn J Allergol 1982; 31:1029-34.

315. Nakazawa T, Toyoda T, et al. Antibodies in asthmatics showing late asthmatic responses to Candida-albicans. Jpn J Allergol 1977; 26:640-44.

316. Pronina EV, Karaev ZO, Alferov VP. Increased sensitivity to Candida in patients with bronchial asthma. Pediatriia 1990;5:14-18.

317. El-Hefny AM. The arthus reaction to Candida albicans in asthma patients. Acta Allergologica 1968; 23:303-311.

318. Itkin IH, Dennis M. Bronchial hypersensitivity to extract of Candida albicans. J of Allergy 1966; 37:187-194.

319. Kabe J, Aoke Y. et al. Relationship of dermal and pulmonary sensitivity to extracts of Candida albicans. Am Rev Resp Dis 1971; 104:348-357.

320. Kurimoto Y. Relationship among skin tests, bronchial challenge, and serology in house dust and Candida albicans allergic asthma. Ann Allergy 1975; 35:131-41.

321. Tsukioka K, Hirono S. A clinical evaluation of the effectiveness of hyposensitization in bronchial asthma induced by Candida albicans. Arerugi Oct 1985; 34:922-30.

322. Palmer AA, Betts WH. The axial drift of fresh and acetaldehyde hardened erythrocytes in 25 mm capillary slits of various lengths. Biorheology 1975; 12:283-92.

323. Durlach J. Deficit magnesique, tetanie et dystonie neuro vegetative: Donnees nouvelles sur les formes neuromusculaires du deficit magnesique chronique. Mag Bull 1981; 3:121-36.

324. Durlach J. Clinical aspects of chronic magnesium deficiency. Magnesium in Health and Disease. New York, NY: Spectrum Pub., 1980; pp. 885-909.

325. Seelig MS, Berger AR, Speilholz N. Latent tetany and anxiety, marginal magnesium deficit, and normocalcemia. Dis of the Nerv Sys 1975; 36:461-65.

326. Galland LD, Baker SM, McLellan RK. Irritable bowel, mitral valve prolapse, and associated condition. Letter to the editor. JAMA July 19, 1985; 254/3:357-58.

327. Spence JD, et al. Increases prevalence of mitral valve prolapse in patients with migraine. Can Med Assoc J 1984; 131:1457-60.

328. Jeresaty RM. Mitral valve prolapse: an update. JAMA Aug 9, 1985; 254/6:793-95.

329. Truss CO. Metabolic abnormalities in patients with chronic candidiasis: the acetaldehyde hypothesis. J Orthomolecular Psychiatry 1984; 13/2:24-25.

330. Nosalova V, Trnovec T, et al. The effect of polysaccharide-protein complex isolated from Candida albicans on regional blood flow in rats. Experientia 1979; 35:341-42.

331. Ferguson AC, Kershnar HE, Collin WK, Stiehm ER. Correlation of cutaneous hypersensitivity with lymphocytic response to Candida albicans. Am J Clin Path 1977; 68:499-504.

332. Stiehm ER. Chronic cumocutaneous candidiasis; clinical aspects, pp. 96-99, in Edwards JE. Jr. (moderator): Severe Candida infections: clinical perspectives, immune defense mechanisms and current concepts of therapy. Ann Int Med 1978; 89:91-106.

333. Tomsikova A, et al. An immunologic study of vaginal candidiasis. Int J Gynaecol Obstet 1980; 18:398-403.

334. Kudelko NM. Allergy in chronic monilial vaginitis. Ann Allergy May 1971; 29:266-67.

335. Palacios, HJ. Hypersensitivity as a cause of dermatologic and vaginal moniliasis resistant to topical therapy. Ann Allergy Aug 1976; 37:110-13.

336. Truss CO. Metabolic abnormalities in patients with chronic candidiasis: the acetaldehyde hypothesis. J Orthomolecular Psychiatry 1984; 13/2:16-24.

337. Buslau M, Hanel H, Holzmann H. The significance of yeasts in seborrheic eczema. Hautarzt 1989;40(10);611-13.

338. Rosenberg EW, Belew PW. Improvement of psoriasis of the scalp with ketoconazole. Arch Dermatol 1982; 118:370-71.

339. Wachowiak W, Stryker GV, Marr J, et al. The occurrence of monilia in relation to psoriasis. Arch Derm Syph 1929; 19:713-31.

340. Crutcher N, Rosenberg EW, et al. Oral Nystatin in the treatment of psoriasis. Arch Dermatol (in press).

341. Liebeskind A. Candida albicans as an allergenic factor. Ann Allergy 1962; 20:394-96.

342. Leyden JL, McGinley KJ, Kligman AM. Role of micro-organisms in dandruff. Arch Dermatol 1976; 112:333-38.

343. Numata T, Yamamoto S, Yamura T. The role of mite dermatophagoides-farinae house dust and Candida-albicans allergens in chronic urticaria. J Dermatol 1980; 7:197-202.

344. Nijo S, Inouye T. Candida-albicans allergy may be 1 of the causes of chronic urticaria. Symposium on Urticaria, Osaka, Jpn, July 17, 1982.

345. Crook WG. Depression associated with Candida albicans infections. JAMA 1984;252(22):2928-9.

346. Edwards DA. Depression and Candida. JAMA 1985;253(23):3400.

347. Truss CO. Metabolic abnormalities in patients with chronic candidiasis: the acetaldehyde hypothesis. J Orthomolecular Psychiatry 1984; 13/2:26.

348. Truss CO. Metabolic abnormalities in patients with chronic candidiasis: the acetaldehyde hypothesis. J Orthomolecular Psychiatry 1984; 13/2:6,24,26.

349. Da Prato RA. Chronic endotoxemia in atypical candidiasis: a hypothesis. Research Perspectives in Allergy and Immunology: A Continuing Nutritional Education Series by Ecological Formulas, 1984.

350. Crook WG. Case histories. The Yeast Connection. Jackson, TN: Professional Books 1983; pp.195-207.

351. Grant ECG. Food allergies and migraine. Lancet May 5, 1979; pp. 966-68.

352. Mansfield LE. Food allergy and adult migraine: double-blind and mediator confirmation of an allergy etiology. Ann Allergy 1985; 55:126-29.

353. Lamberg BA, Liewendahl K. Thyroid hormone resistance. Annals of Clinical Research 1980;12:243-53.

354. Refetoff S, Syndromes of thyroid hormone resistance. Am J Physiology 1982;243:E88-98.

355. Schinfeld JS. PMS and candidiasis: study explores possible link. The Female Patient 1987;12:67-73.

356. Nazzani A, Lumbard D, Horrobin D. The PMT Solution. Montreal: Eden Press, 1985.

357. Kolata G. Steroid Hormone Systems Found in Yeast. Science August 31, 1984; pp. 913-14.

358. Candida Fungal Metabolites.

359. Loose DS, Schurman DJ, Feldman D. A corticosteroid binding protein and endogenous ligand in Candida albicans indicating a possible steroid-receptor system. Nature October 8, 1981; 293: 477-79.

360. Mabray CR, Burditt ML, et al. Treatment of common gynecologic-endocrinologic symptoms by allergy management procedures. Obstet & Gyn 1982;59:560-4.

361. Abraham GE, Hargrove JT. Effect of vitamin B6 on premenstrual symptomatology in women with premenstrual tension syndromes: a double blind crossover study. Infertility 1980;3:155-65.

362. Kerr GD. The management of the premenstrual syndrome. Curr Med Research & Opinion. 1977;4:29-34.

363. Barr W. Pyridoxine supplements in the premenstrual syndrome. The Practitioner 1984;228:425-7.

364. Abraham GE, Lubran MM. Serum and red cell magnesium levels in patients with premenstrual tension. Am J Clin Nutr 1981;34:2364-6.

365. Eisenstein BI. New opportunistic infections-more opportunities. NEJM 1990;323:1625-6.

366. Escuro RS, Jacobs M, Gerson SL, Machicao AR, Lazarus HM. Prospective evaluation of a Candida antigen detection test for invasive candidiasis in immunocompromised adult patients with cancer. Am J Med 1989;87(6):621-7.

367. Dismukes WE, Wade JS, Lee JY, Dockery BK, Hain JD. A randomized, double-blind trial of nystatin therapy for the candidiasis hypersensitivity syndrome. NEJM 1990;323:1721.

368. de Repentigny L, Reiss E. Current trends in immunodiagnosis of candidiasis and aspergillosis. Rev Infect Dis 1984;6:301-12.
369. Hasenclever HF, Mitchell WO. Antigenic studies of Candida III Comparative pathogenicity of Candida albicans group A, group B, and Candida stellatoidea. J Bacteriol 1961;82:578-81.
370. Summers DF, Grollman AP, Hasenclever HF. Polysaccharide antigens of the Candida cell wall. J Immunol 1964;92:491-9.
371. Ellsworth JH, Reiss E, Bradley RL, Chmel J, Armstrong D. Comparative serological and cutaneous reactivity of candidial cytoplasmic proteins and mannan separated by affinity for concanavalin. A J Clin Microbiol 1977;5:91-9.
372. Syverson RE, Buckley HR, Gibian JR. Increasing the positive predictive value of the precipitin test for the diagnosis of deep-seated candidiasis. Am J Clin Pathol 1978;70:826-31.
373. Macdonald R, Odds FC. Inducible proteinase of Candida albicans in diagnostic serology and in the pathogenesis of systemic candidosis. J Med Microbiol 1980;13:423-35.
374. Syverson RE, Buckley HR, Campbell CC. Cytoplasmic antigens unique to the mycelial or yeast phase of Candida albicans. Infect Immun 1975;12:1184-8.
375. Bailey JW, Sada E, Brass C, Bennett JE. Diagnosis of systemic candidiasis by latex agglutination for serum antigen. J Clin Microbiol 1985;21:749-52.
376. Kahn FW, Jones JM. Latex agglutination tests for detection of Candida antigens in sera of patients with invasive candidiasis. J Infect Dis 1986;153:579-85.
377. Kerkering TM, Espinel-Ingroff A, Shadomy S. Detection of Candida antigenemia by counterimmunoelectrophoresis in patients with invasive candidiasis. J Infect Dis 1979;140:659-64.
378. Weiner MH, Coats-Stephen M. Immunodiagnosis of systemic candidiasis: mannan antigenemia detected by radioimmunoassay in experimental and human infections. J Infect Dis 1979;140:989-93.
379. Felice G, Yu B, Armstrong D. Immunodiffusion and agglutination tests for Candida in patients with neoplastic disease: inconsistent correlation of results with invasive infections. J Infect Dis 1977;135:348057.
380. Warren RC, Bartlett A, Bidwell DE, Richardson MD, Voller A, et al. Diagnosis of invasive candidosis by enzyme immunoassay of serum antigen. Br Med J 1977;1:1183-5.
381. Lew MA, Siber GR, Donahue DM, Maiorca F. Enhanced detection with an enzyme-linked immunosorbent assay of Candida mannan in antibody-containing serum after heat extraction. J Infect Dis 1982;145:45-56.
382. Segal E, Berg RA, Pizzo PA, Bennett JE. Detection of Candida-antigen in sera of patients with candidiasis by an enzyme-linked immunosorbent assay-inhibition technique. J Clin Microbiol 1979;10:116-8.
383. Axelsen NH, Kirkpatrick CH. Simultaneous characterization of free Candida antigens and Candida precipitins in a patient's serum by means of crossed immunoelectrophoresis with intermediate gel. J Immunol Methods 1973;2:245-9.
384. Weiner MH, Yount WJ. Mannan antigenemia in the diagnosis of invasive Candida infections. J Clin Invest 1976;58:1045-53.
385. Meunier-Carpentier F, Armstrong K. Candida antigenemia as detected by passive hemagglutination inhibition in patients with disseminated candidiasis or Candida colonization. J Clin Microbiol 1981;13:10-4.
386. Burnie JP. Latex tests in the early diagnosis of systemic candidosis. Serodiangn and Immunother 1987;1:3-5.
387. Kaell AT, Volkman DJ, Gorevic PD, Dattwyler RJ. Positive lyme serology in subacute bacterial endocarditis. JAMA 1990;264:2916-8.
388. Lew MA, Diagnosis of systemic candida infections. Ann Rev Med 1989;40:87-97.
389. Crook WG. The Yeast Connection. Jackson, TN: Professional Books, 1983; pp. 30-33.
390. Platenkamp GJ. Application of serological tests in the diagnosis of invasive candidiasis. Mycoses 1988;31:27-33.

391. Pizzo PA, Robischaud KJ, Gill FA, Witebsky FG. Empiric antibiotic and antifungal therapy for cancer patients with prolonged fever and granulocytopenia. Am J Med 1982;72:101-12.

392. Lew MA. Diagnosis of systemic Candida infections. Ann Rev Med 1989;40:87-97.

393. Gupta TP, Ehrinpreis MN. Candida-associated diarrhea in hospitalized patients. Gastroent 1990;98(3):780-5.

394. Escuro RS, Jacobs M, Gerson SL, Machicao AR, Lazarus HM. Prospective evaluation of a Candida antigen detection test for invasive candidiasis in immunocompromised adult patients with cancer. Am J Med 1989;87(6):621-7.

395. Jones JF, Ray CG, et. al. Evidence for active Epstein-Barr virus infection in patients with persistent, unexplained illnesses: elevated anti-early antigen antibodies. Ann of Internal Med 1985; 102:1-7.

396. Collaborative DHPG Treatment Study Group. Treatment of serious cytomegalovirus infections with 9-(1,3-Dihydroxy-2-propoxymethyl)Guanine in patients with AIDS and other immunodeficiencies. NEJM 1986; 314:801-805.

397. Straus SE, Tosato G, Armstrong G, et. al. Persisting illness and fatigue in adults with evidence of Epstein-Barr virus infection. Ann of Internal Med 1985; 102:7-16.

398. Jones JF. Epstein-Barr Virus. Med Facts from National Jewish Center For Immunology And Respiratory Medicine 1984; pp. 1-4.

399. Jessop C. Presentation at the Chronic Fatigue Syndrome Symposium, sponsored by the University of California and San Francisco Department of Public Health (and others), April 15, 1989. Reported in American Medical News, May 26, 1989.

400. Keyes A. Biology of Human Starvation. Minneapolis, MN: University of Minnesota Press, 1950.

401. Raloff J. Roaches: the battle continues. Science News, June 14, 1986; 129:379.

402. Silverman JJ, Hart RP, Garrettson K, Stockman SJ, Hamer RM, Schulz C, Narasimhachari N. Posttraumatic stress disorder from pentaborane intoxication: Neuropsychiatric evaluation and short-term follow-up. JAMA 1985;254:2603-8.

403. Levine S. Unified stress theory of diseases. Allergy Research Review Spring 1984; 3/1:4.

404. Saavedra-Delgado AM, Metcalf DD. The gastrointestinal mast cell in food allergy. Annals of Allergy Aug 1983; 51/2:185-89.

405. Lessof MH. Food intolerance. Proceedings of the Nutrition Society 1985; 44:121-25.

406. Atkins FM. The multiple etiology of food hypersensitivity. Nutrition Reviews Aug 1983; 41/8:245-48.

407. Taylor SL. Food Allergies. Food Technology Feb 1985; pp. 98-105.

408. Manku MS, Horrobin DF, Morse N, et al. Reduced levels of prostaglandin precursors in the blood of atopic patients: defective delta-6-desaturase function as a biochemical basis for atopy. Prostaglandins, Leukotrienes and Med 1982; 9:615-28.

409. McCormick JN, Neill WA, Simm AK. Immuno-suppressive effect of linoleic acid. Lancet 1977; 2:508.

410. Epstein FH. Oxygen-derived free radicals in postischemic tissue injury. NEJM 1985; 312/3:159-63.

411. Levine SA, Reinhardt JH. Biochemical-pathology initiated by free radicals, oxidant chemicals, and therapeutic drugs in the etiology of chemical hypersensitivity disease. J Orthomolecular Psychiatry 1983; 12/3:166-83.

412. Strickland BR. Implications of food and chemical susceptibilities for clinical psychology. Int J Biosocial Res 1982; 3/1:39-43.

413. Pearson DJ, Rix KJB, Bentley SJ. Food allergy: how much in the mind? A clinical and psychiatric study of suspected food hypersensitivity. Lancet June 4, 1983; pp.1259-61.

414. Crook WG, Harrison WW, Crawford SE, Emerson BS. Systemic manifestations due to allergy: report of fifty patients and a review of the literature on the subject (sometimes referred to as allergic toxemia and the allergic tension-fatigue syndrome). Pediatrics 1961; 27:790-99.

415. Doniach D, Bottazzo GG, Drexhage HA. The autoimmune endocrinopathies. Chapter 31, Clinical Immunology, editor Peter Lackman. London: Blackwell Publishers, 1982.

416. Volpe R. Autoimmunity in the endocrine system. Monographs on Endocrinology, Springer-Verlag, N.Y., 1981; Vol. 20.

417. Dolen J, Varma S, South MA. Chronic mucocutaneous candidiasis-endocrinopathies. Cutis 1981; Vol. 29.

418. Appelboom T, Flowers F. Ketoconazole in the treatment of chronic mucocutaneous candidiasis secondary to autoimmune polyendocrinopathy-candidiasis syndrome. Cutis July 1982; Vol. 30.

419. Wuepper K, Fudenberg H. Moniliasis, autoimmune polyendocrinopathy and immunologic family study. Clin Exp Immunol 1967; 2:71-82.

420. Saifer PL. Presentation at the Yeast-Human Interaction Symposium. San Francisco, March 1985.

421. Thielemans C, et al. Autoimmune thyroiditis: a condition related to a decrease in T-Suppressor cells. Clin Endocrinology 1981; 15:259-63.

422. Dempsey A, DeSwiet M. Premature ovarian failure associated with the Candida endocrinopathy syndrome. British J of Obstet & Gyn May 1981; 88:563-65

423. Smith GR, Monson RA, Ray DC. Psychiatric consultation in somatization disorder. NEJM 1986; 314:1407-13.

424. Smith GR, Monson RA, Ray DC. Patients with multiple unexplained symptoms: their characteristics, functional health, and health care utilization. Arch Intern Med 1986; 146:69-72.

425. Quill TE. Somatization disorder: one of medicine's blind spots. JAMA 1985; 254:3075-79.

426. Hanifin JM. Ketoconazole - an oral antifungal with activity against superficial and deep mycoses. J Am Acad Dermatol 1980; 2/6:537-39.

427. Graybill JR, Herndon JH, Kniker WT, Levine HB. Ketoconazole treatment of chronic mucocutaneous candidiasis. Arch Dermatol 1980; 116/10:1137-41.

428. Hanifin JM. Ketoconazole - an oral antifungal with activity against superficial and deep mycoses. J Am Acad Dermatol 1980; 2:537-39.

429. Graybill JR, Herndon JH, et al. Ketoconazole treatment of chronic mucocutaneous candidiasis. Arch Dermatol 1980; 116:1137-41.

430. Hay RJ, Wells RS, et al. Treatment of chronic mucocutaneous candidosis with ketoconazole: a study of 12 cases. Rev Infect Dis Jul-Aug 1980; 2:600-05.

431. Kirkpatrick CH, Alling DW. Treatment of chronic oral candidiasis with Clotrimazole Troches. NEJM 1978; 299:1201-03.

432. Yap BS, Bodey GP. Oropharyngeal candidiasis treated with a troche form of Clotrimazole. Arch Intern Med June 1979; 139:656-57.

433. Personal communication with the Medical Director of Miles Laboratories, Inc.

434. Tsukahara T. Fungicidal action of caprylic acid for Candida albicans. 1. Quantitative observations of the action. Jpn J Microb 1961; 5/4:383-94.

435. Tsukahara T. Fungicidal action of caprylic acid for Candida albicans II. Possible mechanisms of the action. Jpn J Microb 1962; 6/1:1-14.

436. Neuhauser I. Successful treatment of intestinal moniliasis with fatty acid-resin complex. Arch Int Med 1954; 93:56-60.

437. Hoffman C, Schweitzer TR, Dalby G. Fungistatic properties of the fatty acids and possible biochemical significance. Food Res Nov-Dec 1939; 4:539-45.

438. Lotter L. Evaluation of antifungal properties of Tanalbit. Test results from Valley Microbiology Services, 3118 Depot Road, Hayward, Ca. 94545.

439. Austin FG. Schistosoma mansoni chemoprophylaxis with dietary lapachol. Am J of Tropical Med and Hygiene 1974; 23/3:412.

440. Moore GS, Atkins RD. The fungicidal and fungistatic effects of an aqueous garlic extract on medically important yeast-like fungi. Mycologia 1977; 69:341-48.

441. Prasad G, Sharma VD. Efficacy of garlic (Allium sativum) treatment against experimental candidiasis in chicks. Br Vet J 1980; 136:448-51.
442. Moore GS, Atkins RD. The fungicidal and fungistatic effects of an aqueous garlic extract on medically important yeast-like fungi. Mycologia 1977; 69:341.
443. Tynecka Z, Gos Z. The inhibitory action of garlic (Allium sativum L.) on growth and respiration of some microorganisms. Acta Microbiol Polonica 1973; 5:51-62
444. Sandhu DK, Warraich MK, Singh S. Sensitivity of yeasts isolated from cases of vaginitis to aqueous extracts of garlic. Mykosen 1980; 23:691-98.
445. Adetumbi MA, Lau BHS. Allium sativum (garlic) - a natural antibiotic. Med Hyp 1983; 12:227-37.
446. Yamada Y, Azuma K. Evaluation of the in vitro antifungal activity of allicin. Antimicrob Agents Chemotherapy Apr 1977; 11:743-49.
447. Block E. The chemistry of garlic and onions. Sci Am 1985; 252:114-19.
448. Folk remedies point to new drugs. C&EN January 7, 1985; pp. 34.
449. Garlic - not to be sniffed at. The Economist Feb 15, 1986; pp. 82
450. Vincent JG, Veomett RC, Riley RF. Antibacterial Activity Associated with Lactobacillus Acidophilus. J Bact 1959; 78:477-84.
451. Shahani KM. Nutritional and Healthful Aspects of Cultured and Culture-Containing Dairy Foods. J Dairy Sci 1979; 62:1685-94.
452. Collins EB, Hardt P. Inhibition of Candida albicans by Lactobacillus Acidophilus. J Dairy Sci. 1980; 63:830-32.
453. Hensgens C, Klastersky J. Intestinal colonization with Lactobacilli strains in neutropenic patients. Biomedicine 1976; 25:11-15.
454. Pettersson L. Survival of Lactobacillus acidophilus NCDO 1748 in the human gastro-intestinal tract. Proc XXI Int Dairy Congr ICU, 1982; pp. 301.
455. Robins-Browne RM, Levine MM. The fate of ingested Lactobacilli in the proximal small intestine. Am J Clin Nutr April 1981; 34:514-19.
456. Laxatives and Anti-Diarrheal. Food and Drug Adm; March 21, 1975.
457. Rettger LF, Cheplin HA. Bacillus acidophilus and its therapeutic application. Arch Inter Med 1922; 29:357-67.
458. Goldin BR, et al. Effect of diet and Lactobacillus acidophilus supplements on human fecal bacterial enzymes. J Nat Can Inst 1980; 64:255-61.
459. Thompson GE. Control of intestinal flora in animals and humans: implications for toxicology and health. J of Envir Path & Toxic 1977; 1:113-23.
460. Goldin B, Gorbach SL. Alterations in fecal microflora enzymes related to diet, age, Lactobacillus supplements, and dimethylhydrazine. Cancer 1977; 40:2421-26.
461. Barbero GJ, et al. Investigations on the bacterial flora, pH, and sugar content in the intestinal tract of infants. J of Ped 1952; 40:152-63.
462. Shahani KM, Ayebo AD. Role of Dietary Lactobacilli in Gastrointestinal Microecology. Am J Clin Nutr 1980; 33:2448-57.
463. Browne RM, Levine MM. The Fate of Ingested Lactobacilli in the Proximal Small Intestine. Am J. Clin Nutr 1981; 34:514-19.
464. Smith RP. The Implantation or Enrichment of Bacillus Acidophilus and Other Organisms in the Intestine. British Med J 1924; 11:948-50.
465. Sturdik E, Heriban V, et al. Mechanism of anti yeast activity of juglone a naturally occurring 1 4 naphtho quinone. Biologia 1983; 38:343-52.
466. Personal communication B. Kent Remington, M.D., Dermatologist, Calgary, Alberta, Canada.
467. Palacios, HJ. Hyper sensitivity as a cause of dermatologic and vaginal moniliasis resistant to topical therapy. Ann Allergy 1976; 37:110-13.
468. Palacios HJ. Hypersensitivity as a cause of dermatologic and vaginal moniliasis resistant to topical therapy. Ann of Allergy 1976;37:110-13.

469. Tomsikova A, Tomaierova V, Kotal L, Novackova D. An immunologic study of vaginal candidiasis. Int J Gynaecol Obstet 1980;18)6):398-403.

470. Kudelko NM. Allergy in chronic monilial vaginitis. Ann of Allergy 1971;29:266-7.

471. Holti G. Candida Allergy. Symposium on Candida Infections Eds: Winner HI, Hurley R, E & S Livingstone Ltd., Edinburgh and London 1966:73-81.

472. Rosedale N, Browne K. Hyposensitization in the management of recurring vaginal candidiasis. Ann Allergy Oct 1979; 43:250-53.

473. Montero MP, Dominguez CF, Vigna GA. Chronic mucocutaneous candidiasis. A case report. Rev Alerg Mex 1990;37(1):29-31.

474. Segal E, Sandovsky-Losica H, Nussbaum S. Immune responses elicited by vaccinations with Candida albicans ribosomes in cyclophosphamide treated animals. Mycopathologia Feb 1985; 89:113-18.

475. Levy R, Segal E, Barr-Nea L. Systemic candidiasis in mice immunized with Candida albicans ribosomes. Mycopathologia Jul 1985; 91:17-22.

476. Kilbourne ED. Viral Disease. Textbook of Medicine. Philadelphia, PA: W.B. Saunders Co, 1971; pp. 400.

477. Liebeskind A. Candida albicans as an allergenic factor. Annals of Allergy 1962;20:394-6.

478. Dickey LD. Editors Introduction. Clinical Ecology. Thomas 1976; pp. 6.

479. Lockey SD, Sr. Reactions to hidden agents in foods, beverages and drugs. Ann Allergy 1971; 29:461.

480. Drug reactions and sublingual testing with certified food colors. Ann Allergy 1973; 31:423.

481. Hosen H. Hydrocarbons and other gases, as related to the field of allergy and clinical ecology, pp. 262.

482. Rapp DJ. Food allergies: treatment for hyperkinesis. J Learn Disabilities 1979; 12:608.

483. Rapp DJ. Allergies and the hyperactive child. New York: S & S, 1979.

484. Reisman RE. American Academy of Allergy: Position statements - controversial technique. J Allergy Clin Immun 1981; 67:333.

485. Boris M, Schiff M, et al. Bronchoprovocation blocked by neutralization therapy. J Allergy Clin Immun 1983; 71:92.

486. Rea WJ, Podell RN, et al. Intracutaneous neutralization of food sensitivity: a double-blind evaluation. Arch Otolaryngology 1983.

487. McGovern JJ, Rapp DJ, Gardner RW, et al. Double-blind studies support reliability of provocative-neutralization test. Arch Otolaryngology 1983.

488. Miller JB. A double blind study of food extract injection therapy: a preliminary report. Ann Allergy 1977; 38:185-91.

489. Rapp DJ. Weeping eyes in wheat allergy. Trans Soc Opthal Otolaryngol Allergy 1982; 18:159-60.

490. Pfeiffer GO. Sublingual allergy therapy. Trans Am Soc Opthal Otolaryngol Allergy 1963; 4:82.

491. Pfeiffer GO, Dickey LD. Sublingual therapy in allergy (Instructional course number eight). Trans Am Soc Ophthal Otolaryngol Allergy 1964; 5:37.

492. O'Shea J, Porter S. Double-blind study of children with hyperkinetic syndrome treated with multi-allergen extract sublingually. J Learn Disabilities 1981; 14:189-91.

493. King D. Can allergic exposure provoke psychological symptoms? A double-blind test. Biological Psychiatry 1982; 16:3-7.

494. Rapp DJ. Double-blind confirmation and treatment with milk sensitivity. Med J Australia 1978; 1:571-72.

495. Rapp DJ. Food allergy treatment for hyperkinesis. J Learn Disabilities 1979; 12:42-50.

496. Sobel JD. Recurrent vulvovaginal candidiasis. A prospective study of the efficacy of maintenance ketoconazole therapy. NEJM 1986;315:1455-8.

497. Mobacken H, Moberg S. Ketoconazole treatment of 13 patients with chronic mucocutaneous candidiasis. A prospective 3-year trial. Dermatologica 1986;173:229-36.

498. Montero MP, Calderon F, Vigna Garcia A. Chronic mucocutaneous candidiasis. A case report. Rev Alerg Mex 1990;37(1):29-31.

499. Sobel JD. Recurrent vulvovaginal candidiasis. A prospective study of the efficacy of maintenance ketoconazole therapy. NEJM 1986;315:1455-8.

500. Gehring W, Spate W, Gehse M, Gloor M, Braun KJ. Results of a combination treatment with natamycin and butylscopolamine in cases of intestinal Candida colonization. Mycoses 1990;33(3):140-5.

501. Cole GT, Lynn KT, Seshan KR. Evaluation of a murine model of hepatic candidiasis. J Clin Microbiol 1990;8:1828-41.

502. Dismukes WE, Wade JS, Lee JY, Dockery BK, Hain JD. A randomized, double-blind trial of nystatin therapy for the candidiasis hypersensitivity syndrome. NEJM 1990;323:1717-23.

503. Corthay P, Terki N, Perez T, Lech B. Traitement des vaginites a Candida albicans: comparaisons de mesures dietetiques et de o'immunotherapie specifique. Med et Hygiene 1989;47:2009-13.

504. Renfro L, Feder HM Jr, Lane TJ, Manu P, Matthews DA. Yeast connection among 100 patients with chronic fatigue. Am J Med 1989;86:165-8.

505. Anderson JA, et al. Candidiasis hypersensitivity syndrome. J Allergy Clin Immunol 1986;78:271-3.

506. Crook WG. The yeast connection: a medical breakthrough. Jackson, Tenn.: Professional Books, 1983:67-74.

507. Remington DW, Higa BW. Back to health: a comprehensive medical and nutritional yeast control program. Provo, Utah: Vitality House International, 1986.

508. Liebeskind A. Candida albicans as an allergenic factor. Annals of Allergy 1962:20:394-6.

509. Edwards, J. Infectious Disease Society of America Position statement on the yeast connection. Unpublished

510. Falliers CJ. The yeast connection: a medical breakthrough. J of Asthma 1986;23(1):35-6.

511. Quinn JP, Venezio FR. Ketoconazole and the Yeast Connection. JAMA 1986;255(23):3250.

512. Reisman RE. American Academy of Allergy: Position statements - controversial technique. J Allergy Clin Immun 1981;67:333.

513. Remington DW. A critique on sublingual provocative neutralization therapy. Presentation to the Utah State Association Joint Committee Meeting. July, 1990.

514. Yecheskel S, Yechiel S, Maier, M. Delayed neurologic display in murine typhus. Arch Intern Med 1989;149:949-51.

515. Rosenblum MJ, Masland RL, Harrell GT. Residual effects of rickettsial disease on the central nervous system: results of neurologic examinations and electroencephalograms following Rocky Mountain spotted fever. Arch Intern Med 1952;90:444-55.

516. Kauffman CA, Jones PF. Candidiasis: a diagnostic and therapeutic challenge. Postgrad Med 1986;80(1):129-34.

517. Perfect JR. Fluconazole therapy for experimental cryptococcoses and candidiasis in the rabbit. Rev Infect Dis 1990;12(3):S299-302.

518. Cantani A, Mastrantoni F. Recent advances in Candida albicans mycoses in children. Riv Eur Sci Med Farmacol 1989;11(1):17-20.

519. Dismukes WE, Wade JS, Lee JY, Dockery BK, Hain JD. A randomized, double-blind trial of nystatin therapy for the candidiasis hypersensitivity syndrome. NEJM 1990;323:1717-23.

Index

Cytomegalovirus 209, 230
Depression 6, 12, 42, 49, 73, 79, 80-82, 91,
    100, 104, 202, 220, 227, 228, 230, 231, 232,
    235, 236, 245, 246, 249
Dermatitis 213, 220, 228
Desensitization 85, 234, 235, 240, 241, 246
Diabetes 42, 55, 93-95, 103-104, 202, 215
Diarrhea 6-8, 18, 29, 33, 63, 66-67, 73-74, 76,
    81-82, 204, 207, 209, 215, 217, 227, 229,
    246
Die-off symptoms 61-62, 68
Dieting 12, 15, 33, 64, 75, 77, 79, 92, 94, 97-
    100, 103-105, 108-109, 112, 214
Diflucan 24
Diphtheria 201, 210,
Dizziness 4, 6, 11, 62, 82, 91, 112, 209, 221,
    222, 231, 235
Dopamine 220
Dysbiosis 210, 217
Dysmenorrhea 216, 219, 228
Eczema 1, 4, 11, 73, 80, 82, 213, 214, 220,
    228, 231, 235,
Edema 219
Electrolytes 97
Endocrine 202, 204, 212, 215, 216, 221, 224,
    231, 247
Endorphin 236
Energy 5, 12, 49, 64, 68, 89, 97-98, 100-103,
    106, 108, 109, 220, 221, 222, 236
Enzymes 5-6, 12, 33, 49, 61, 63, 84, 89, 90,
    92, 97-98, 100-101, 103, 214, 215, 220, 233
Epstein-Barr virus 85, 227, 230
Ernsberger, Dr. Paul 103
Erythromycin 69, 75, 205
Esophagus 7
Estrogen 113, 117, 208, 215, 216, 223
Ethanol 4-5, 15, 80, 206, 210, 221, 223
Exercise 21, 36, 49-50, 63, 84, 95, 102-103,
    108-109, 116, 236
Exotoxin 210
Fat 16, 30, 36, 42-43, 46, 49, 64, 75, 85, 89,
    95, 97-107
Fat-burning enzymes 49, 101, 103
Fat-storage enzymes 97-98
Fat thermostat 49, 95-99,
    102-106, 109
Fatigue 4-5, 12, 16, 36, 42, 68, 73, 80, 82, 91,
    104, 202, 209, 221, 222, 224, 227, 228, 230,
    231, 235, 240, 243, 245

Fatty acids 17, 33, 46, 85, 101, 106, 112, 116,
    220
Fears 51, 73, 91, 106, 220, 240
Feet 1, 9, 82, 219
Fever 62
Fingernails 3, 23
Flagyl 66
Flu 12, 15, 61, 104, 227
Follicularis 220, 228
Food Addiction 61-2, 64, 68, 82-84, 94, 102,
    105, 222
Food deprivation 15, 45, 55, 77, 92, 98, 101
Formaldehyde 80
Framingham study 104
Fredericks, Dr. Carlton 95
Fungal 1, 2, 4, 25, 41-42, 44, 205, 206, 212,
    218, 227, 234, 237
Fuzzy thinking 11
Garlic 25, 233
Gastritis 7, 204
Gastrointestinal 3, 7-8, 73, 208, 214, 216, 227
Genitourinary 9
Giardia 8, 66, 217, 225, 229, 230
Glucagon 91, 222
Gluconeogenesis 100, 222
Glucose 89-93, 100, 206, 220, 222
Glutathione 36
Glycogen 89-90, 93-94, 100
Glycogenolysis 222
Glycolysis 222
Glycoprotein 210, 213, 216, 219
Hay fever 4, 79, 82, 213, 231
Headaches 1, 4, 6, 7, 9-12, 42, 53, 62, 79-82,
    91, 202, 209, 214, 218, 219, 221, 227, 228,
    231, 235, 246, 249
Heartburn 7-8, 16, 68, 76, 81-82, 217, 227,
    246
Herpes 202
Hiatus hernia 227
Histamine 213, 217, 218
Hives 1, 6, 11, 73, 80, 82, 220
Hormone 5-7, 9, 11, 16, 46, 50, 61, 63, 65,
    85, 89-94, 99, 102, 109, 111-114, 117, 208,
    212, 215, 216, 217, 218, 219, 221, 222, 223,
    227, 231
Hydrogen peroxide 206
Hyperactivity 73, 221, 246, 249
Hyperkeratosis 228
Hypersensitivity 203, 212, 213, 216, 219,
    224, 235, 240